Combating Teen Smoking

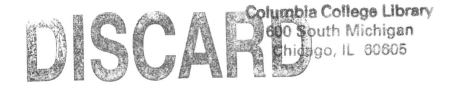

Combating Teen Smoking

Research and Policy Strategies

Peter D. Jacobson · Paula M. Lantz
Kenneth E. Warner · Jeffrey Wasserman
Harold A. Pollack · Alexis A. Ahlstrom

Ann Arbor
THE UNIVERSITY OF MICHIGAN PRESS

Copyright © by the University of Michigan 2001
All rights reserved
Published in the United States of America by
The University of Michigan Press
Manufactured in the United States of America
♾ Printed on acid-free paper

2004   2003   2002   2001   4   3   2   1

A CIP catalog record for this book is available from the British Library.

Library of Congress Cataloging-in-Publication Data

Combating teen smoking : research and policy strategies / Peter D.
    Jacobson . . . [et al.].
        p.   cm.
    Includes bibliographical references and index.
    ISBN 0-472-09771-7 (cloth : alk. paper) — ISBN 0-472-06771-0
(pbk. : alk. paper)
        1. Teenagers—Tobacco use—United States—Prevention. 2.
Youth—Tobacco use—United States—Prevention. 3. Smoking—United
States—Prevention. 4. Medical policy—United States. I. Jacobson,
Peter D.
HV5745 .C66   2000
362.29'67'08350973—dc21   00-12322

Dedication

We dedicate this book to Ted Klein, a friend and colleague who sponsored our work. In 1997, two of the authors (Jacobson and Warner) met with Ted to discuss ways to address teen smoking. At that time, Ted was in the process of selling his public relations business and asked for our input on how to allocate some of his money to achieve his tobacco control goals. After considerable discussion, he provided generous support for a study of teen smoking that resulted in this book. Ted died in June 2000, in time to review the final manuscript but before its publication.

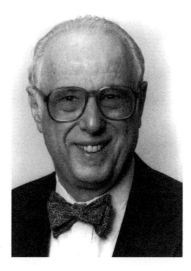

Ted was a wonderful colleague throughout this endeavor. He believed very strongly that both government and private citizens have a social responsibility to discourage kids from smoking, and gave actively of his time and resources to achieve that goal. Ted's vision was to engage scholars, tobacco control advocates, and public health practitioners in fighting tobacco use. To this effort, as to so much else in his life, Ted brought verve, commitment, ideas, intellectual vision, and a sense that the goal was worthy and achievable. He raised questions, pushed the team to think about how policymakers could use the research, and sought out the opinions of numerous scholars and advocates to make sure the project was going in the right direction.

Ted embodied the essence of humanity—the willingness to devote himself to causes in which he believed deeply. He brought insight, creativity, and dedication to everything he did. Nothing seemed to discourage his elemental optimism. Even though he was in constant pain during the last few years, he never complained or sought sympathy. With him, the next idea, the next goal was what he wanted to discuss—not his illness.

Above all, though, he was a warm and wonderful individual. We are deeply indebted to Ted for his support and for his model of how to live a caring and contributing life.

Preface

Smoking is "cool." Smoking is glamorous. Addicted to tobacco? Not me. I can quit anytime I want. Health hazards of smoking? Not a problem—I'll quit long before it harms me. And besides, I'll be so old by then that it won't matter anyway. For many adolescents, the future extends no further than the end of the school term. How can they be expected to be concerned with health hazards that may be decades away when they cannot even concern themselves with what to do next summer?

This reasoning seems to be the simplest explanation for why adolescents smoke. For policymakers and health educators, adolescents' thought processes present a rather amorphous and moving target. What constitutes cool? How can tobacco use be made "uncool"? For researchers, saying that smoking is cool expresses a range of different influences that must be described and studied in much finer detail.

By saying that smoking is cool, adolescents are, at a minimum, suggesting that tobacco use takes place in a social context. Both the decision to initiate smoking and the decision to continue smoking are made with reference to other influences, such as peers, parents, and other family members.

Our goal in this book is to explain what we know about adolescent tobacco use and to address ways of reducing it. The book is written for public officials, tobacco control advocates, and individuals in the community who are interested in reducing adolescent tobacco use. Discouraging youth tobacco use requires both public policy changes and community involvement. Government can take the lead by changing public policy to make it more difficult for adolescents to smoke and can provide financial support for community-based programs and interventions. But it is appropriate that groups and individuals from the community take the lead in defining the problems or issues that are most important in their neighborhoods and social environments and in designing and implementing the interventions that have the best chance for success. Governmental involvement is necessary, but it is important to stimulate a range of community-based responses that can complement and even inform governmental policies.

Acknowledgments

We would like to thank several individuals for making this book possible. First and foremost, we are indebted to Ted Klein for funding our work. Not only did Ted provide the financial backing, but his intellectual support and guidance were an integral part of writing the book.

Ted's vision was to involve a new generation of scholars, advocates, and public health practitioners in fighting tobacco use. As part of that vision, he provided additional funding so that students at the University of Michigan School of Public Health could participate in the research. To distinguish these students from other research assistants, we have called them Ted Klein scholars. So far, there have been two Ted Klein scholars, Alexis Ahlstrom, M.P.H., one of the authors, and Julie Berson, M.P.H. Fulfilling the idea for this funding, Julie has been working in tobacco prevention at the Karmanos Cancer Clinic in Detroit. We very much appreciate the work she did as a Ted Klein scholar.

We would also like to thank the many people who took time to participate in interviews about the future of tobacco control policy. We have benefited greatly from their insight, and many of their suggestions are incorporated into this book. We also thank Lori Pbert, Ph.D., who reviewed the manuscript and offered many useful suggestions; Unto Pallonen, Ph.D., for sharing his insights on computer systems; Deborah Kleinman, for excellent research assistance on chapter 5; Brenda Payne and Sue Corner, who painstakingly prepared the manuscript; and Stanley Siegelman, who provided expert editorial review.

As part of preparing this book, we convened an advisory panel consisting of Ted Klein, Thomas Houston, M.D., Judith Ockene, Ph.D., and Nancy Rigotti, M.D. We appreciate their involvement and their suggestions for how to think about the challenging issues herein.

Contents

Introduction

The use of tobacco products in the United States, especially among adolescents, has generated a major public debate over whether and how to control tobacco products. How extensively should the use of tobacco be regulated? Should we invest more to reduce adolescent smoking patterns? Should the nicotine content of cigarettes be regulated? Which level of government—local, state, or federal—should take the lead in tobacco control efforts? These are just a few of the questions animating a lively public policy debate.

For many years, the tobacco industry, through its ability to influence the political process at the state and federal levels, was able to shape the policy debate to its advantage. This is no longer true. Although the industry remains a formidable political force, it must now share how the policy debate is framed with its public health opponents. A few examples demonstrate how the political environment has shifted in the 1990s.

Within the past few years, we have witnessed events that were unimaginable 15 years ago, when the tobacco industry enjoyed enviable political dominance. That dominance is now being severely challenged on several fronts. Many people may remember the sight of chief executive officers from the tobacco industry testifying before a somewhat skeptical congressional committee that nicotine is not addictive. Then, when Senator Robert Dole, running in the 1996 presidential election, declared that cigarettes were not addictive, he was met by an outpouring of public derision and had to retreat hastily. At about the same time, the Food and Drug Administration (FDA), reversing previous policy that it lacked jurisdiction over tobacco products, attempted to regulate tobacco by adopting a youth-oriented set of policies.[1]

Meanwhile, states began suing the tobacco industry to recover their health care costs associated with smoking among Medicaid recipients.

Even though the tobacco industry had rarely lost in defending lawsuits brought by individuals to recover damages suffered by using tobacco, the states' litigation added a new and more threatening dimension. For a while, it seemed that rarely a day passed without another damaging disclosure of tobacco industry documents detailing how the industry had misled the public about the harms caused by its products.

The increasing public scrutiny of the tobacco industry and the accompanying litigation encouraged the industry and its public health critics to settle their differences. An initial settlement was reached in 1997, but it required congressional action to implement. Throughout much of 1997 and 1998, Congress debated the legislation (named the McCain Bill after being introduced by Republican senator John McCain of Arizona) but was unable to enact or agree on any compromise legislation. A massive and effective media campaign by the tobacco industry depicted the legislation as a "big government" solution and caused serious defections from earlier support. After the attempted legislative solution failed, the two sides continued negotiating and skirmishing in the courts. Finally, the states' litigation against the tobacco industry was settled in November 1998. As we discuss in chapter 1, the eventual settlement agreement was substantially less onerous to the tobacco industry than the proposed 1997 agreement would have been. Money from the settlement is now being distributed to the states.

At the same time as the political and policy debates have been unfolding, researchers have continued examining all facets of the use and health effects of tobacco. The research includes attempts to understand why adolescents begin smoking and whether genetic predispositions are related to nicotine addiction, as well as studies concerned with which tobacco control strategies are most effective in reducing tobacco use and how to help regular smokers quit. By now, the research is so voluminous that it is difficult even for specialists, let alone interested nonexperts, to keep up to date on all developments. Given the debate over how to allocate the settlement funds and how to regulate the use of tobacco products, policymakers, tobacco control advocates, and interested citizens need accessible information on the latest research findings to help shape public policy.

About This Book

Objectives

In this book, we synthesize the vast amount of research and policy thinking on how to discourage teen smoking in the United States. Our primary objective is to provide a comprehensive report on the status of tobacco control with regard to children and adolescents (whom we define as children between 12 and 17 years old). (Our reasons for focusing on adolescents are discussed in chapter 1.) In providing a comprehensive synthesis and analysis of existing information, we hope to contribute to the development of an informed research agenda and to the design and adoption of reasonable and effective policy measures. Right now, a lot of information is available about tobacco control and adolescent use of tobacco products (especially cigarettes), but this information is fragmented and not easily accessible to the nonspecialist. One of our goals is to provide a compendium of what we know about adolescents and tobacco use—and to point out, as well, those areas in which we still require additional knowledge to deal with the problem effectively. We need to know, in brief, what research exists, what gaps remain, what programs have been developed, which programs have been evaluated, and how effective the programs have been. Another goal is to address why most children do not become regular smokers, even though most experiment with cigarette smoking. This book provides one convenient source of the available research and thinking on adolescent tobacco control for policymakers, tobacco control advocates, researchers, and interested lay persons to reflect on and use.

In this book, we focus our attention on the following areas:

- The literature on adolescent use of tobacco products, focusing on data trends and data availability, major themes and arguments, and existing reports
- Any studies evaluating the effectiveness of programs or laws dealing with adolescent tobacco use, including the effects of price and tax increases
- Smoking prevention and cessation programs aimed at adolescents
- Innovative programs that are underway but have not yet been evaluated.

For comparison purposes, we also consider the literature on the prevention of teenage alcohol and substance use, to assess the applicability of programs in those areas to tobacco control efforts.

We focus on synthesizing information updating the Institute of Medicine's (IOM) and Surgeon General's reports from 1994.[2] But since the entire tobacco policy environment has changed since then, we frame a research and policy agenda that reflects new circumstances and opportunities to discourage youths from consuming tobacco products.

Organization

This book is divided into two parts. In part 1, "Adolescent Smoking in Context," we discuss the nature of the adolescent smoking problem. Chapter 1 establishes the policy context regarding adolescent smoking. In chapter 2, we set forth basic trends in adolescent smoking behavior and identify the available data sources. Chapter 3 describes the social context in which adolescent tobacco use occurs, such as peer and parental influences. While there is a considerable amount of literature as to why adolescents smoke, there is less attention in the literature to understanding why most adolescents do not smoke, which we also consider.

Part 2, "Strategies for Adolescent Smoking Prevention and Control," is devoted to reviewing alternative strategies that policymakers can pursue to prevent and control adolescent tobacco use.[3] Most of part 2 reviews programs that have already been evaluated, but we also discuss innovative programs now emerging that have not yet been subject to formal evaluations. To organize the information, we have categorized the relevant tobacco control efforts into the following areas: (1) school-based educational interventions, (2) community interventions, (3) cessation programs, (4) youth access restrictions, (5) regulatory restrictions on tobacco products and use, (6) mass media/public education, (7) tobacco advertising restrictions, and (8) tobacco excise taxes.

In chapter 4, we describe the extensive literature evaluating adolescent smoking prevention interventions and youth smoking cessation programs. Understanding the content and efficacy of past prevention interventions is critical for assessing new efforts and deciding how to allocate tobacco control funds. In chapter 5, we consider the various media and advertising influences on adolescent smoking behavior. In particular, this chapter explores how industry insights into adolescent behavior can be used to redirect antismoking messages. We also consider the evidence on the effects of advertising and advertising bans on youth smoking behavior.

In chapter 6, we consider various influences on the price of tobacco products and how higher prices might influence teen smoking. Since most tobacco control advocates endorse strategies to raise cigarette prices, it is important to understand just how teens will react. Chapter 7 discusses various strategies for regulating youth smoking, such as laws restricting youth access to tobacco, the effects of clean indoor air laws, and alternatives for product regulation. The chapter also assesses changes over time in state and local restrictions on youth access to tobacco.

In our "Conclusion and Recommendations," we synthesize our findings and present recommendations that policymakers can consider in designing and implementing an effective tobacco control program. We also describe a preliminary research agenda that other researchers can build on to assist policymakers in developing smoking control programs. As part of the research agenda, we stress the need for policymakers, tobacco control researchers, and tobacco control advocates to evaluate programs initiated to reduce adolescent tobacco use. We do not offer a magic solution that will lead to dramatically reduced smoking initiation rates. Instead, we advocate a comprehensive, long-term strategy that will discourage adolescent tobacco use.

As this book will demonstrate, considerable uncertainties remain about which tobacco control strategies are likely to be successful. But here we show that there is sufficient positive information for policymakers to implement both short- and long-term policy prescriptions. Throughout this book, we intend to provide policymakers with information about what works and about how they can develop and implement a sound tobacco control strategy to discourage adolescent smoking.

Conceptual Approach

At the heart of our conceptual approach is the argument that a coherent strategy focusing on the use of tobacco products by youths can be developed and translated into effective public policy and interventions. Teenage smoking rates are of particular concern because considerable research has shown that few people initiate smoking behavior once past their teenage years.[4] By age 18, most people who will ever smoke routinely have already become or are in the process of becoming habitual smokers. As long as it remains difficult to quit smoking, tobacco will remain the major preventable cause of morbidity and mortality, although premature deaths can be avoided through effective smoking cessation programs. In the long term, strategies to avoid teenage smoking in the first place are likely to prove effective and consequential. As a result, a significant aspect of the policy and research agenda should be to develop cost-effective measures for reducing youth smoking initiation rates.

We believe that tobacco control advocates have yet to develop a comprehensive strategy to achieve these longer-term goals. Starting in 1994 with both the surgeon general's report, which focused on youth smoking, and the IOM's report, which focused on nicotine addiction in children, tobacco control advocates showed heightened emphasis on a comprehensive research and policy strategy. The IOM has released a report arguing in favor of the kind of comprehensive approach we are recommending.[5] The Centers for Disease Control (CDC) has completed a similar document outlining the best tobacco control practices.[6] Whether this represents an emerging consensus among tobacco control advocates on how best to proceed remains to be seen.

As we detail in chapter 1, tobacco control advocates disagree as to where tobacco control resources should be concentrated—on reducing adolescent smoking or on comprehensive approaches that would include adult cessation. Essential to dramatically reducing the public health burden of tobacco, along with teen smoking initiation rates, are the notions of complementarity and comprehensiveness in tobacco control. By this we mean that tobacco control resources should be devoted (in greater amounts) to both youth prevention and adult issues. An effective long-term strategy to reduce youth smoking initiation rates should be viewed as complementary to a more comprehensive approach that includes adults. For instance, there is reason to believe that a parallel strategy of encouraging addicted adults to quit smoking while simultaneously addressing youth smoking prevention efforts would be a cost-effective strategy for reducing morbidity and mortality costs. There is a large opportunity for targeting smoking cessation programs to adults and eventually migrating to cessation programs for nicotine-addicted adolescents. Of equal importance, getting adults not to smoke would be a good model for encouraging youths not to use tobacco products.

One of the defining characteristics of tobacco control—regardless of whether or not one adopts a youth-oriented focus—is recognition that a successful assault on the disease burden created by smoking necessarily must be multidimensional.[7] Individual interventions do work on their own. For example, smoking cessation treatments do help a subset of smokers to quit, tax increases clearly discourage children from smoking and reduce smoking by adults, and prohibitions on smoking in public places clean the air for nonsmokers and decrease smoking prevalence and daily consumption among ongoing smokers. Yet, alone, each of these interventions is only tinkering on the fringe. Collectively, these and other interventions may exhibit powerful synergism. The smoker committed to participating in a cessation treatment, for instance, stands a better chance of quitting if the external environment discourages smoking, as when smoking is prohibited in public places. That same smoker is more likely to succeed in quitting if the price of cigarettes rises due to a tax increase.

Developing appropriate public policy is integral to successfully achieving the goals of reduced tobacco use. While aspects of our approach will rely on tobacco control groups and community organizations for design and implementation, we want to help policymakers identify the most promising policy interventions to maximize the effectiveness of tobacco control resources devoted to preventing youth smoking.

Research Methods

We conducted an extensive literature review and synthesis of published research addressing interventions to reduce youth smoking. Through Medline, a database of health-related journals and reports, we identified articles reporting evaluations of smoking prevention and control initiatives involving youth. While we reviewed some pre-1994 literature, our focus was on what has been learned since 1994, when both the IOM's and surgeon general's reports were published.

In addition, we collected and reviewed information on emerging initiatives and interventions that have not yet been evaluated or received much attention in the peer-reviewed literature. We monitored reports of new strategies distributed through several different electronic mailing lists. We also conducted a series of informal interviews with tobacco control advocates in the United States to identify emerging trends and promising innovations to discourage youth smoking. For example, we discuss in this book the emergence of computer-based systems in tobacco control, peer-based interventions, and penalizing youth for tobacco possession and use. It should be noted that our discussion of innovations is neither comprehensive nor systematic in a scientific sense. Instead, we are trying to identify emerging trends and to provide information about some of the new and creative interventions that are being implemented and evaluated.

This project also builds on and expands work that the authors have been conducting in tobacco research for many years. In that sense, this report represents a synthesis of some of our prior research as applied to youth tobacco use. That research will be referred to at appropriate points in this book.

Background

In recent years, several outstanding books have been published that document the history of the tobacco industry and various attempts to control the health harms produced by tobacco use. For example, Richard Kluger's monumental history chronicles how the industry attained its prominence and how the public health community has responded to growing evidence associating tobacco use with myriad health hazards.[8] In the following sections, we provide a general overview of the tobacco story.

The Nature and Magnitude of the Health Consequences of Tobacco Consumption

A prominent article published in 1993[9] compared the leading disease causes of death with "the actual causes of death" (i.e., those health risk behaviors and environmental exposures that can lead to illness and ultimately death). Accounting for 1.1 million annual deaths among Americans, half of all mortality, these "actual causes" represent the principal challenge to public health in the twenty-first century. Topping the list was tobacco consumption, the source of nearly one-fifth of all deaths among Americans.

Almost single-handedly, smoking has transformed lung cancer from a virtually unknown disease at the turn of the twentieth century to the leading cause of cancer death at its conclusion. Including mortality associated with environmental tobacco smoke and with interactions with other exposures (especially radon), smoking is responsible for more than 90 percent of the lung cancer deaths that befall Americans each year. Smoking is also the leading cause of chronic obstructive pulmonary disease mortality, accounting for at least 85 percent of deaths attributable to emphysema and chronic bronchitis. Although smoking accounts for only 17 percent to 30 percent of cardiovascular disease deaths, the dominance of heart disease as the leading disease cause of death accords this illness its dubious status as a contender, with lung cancer, as the chief tobacco-produced source of mortality. In addition to the "big three," smoking contributes to a host of less common causes of death, and it creates an enormous burden of preventable morbidity and disability.[10]

The enormity of the toll of smoking stems from a combination of the widespread prevalence of the behavior (more than 45 million Americans smoke), its intensity (smokers take 10–12 puffs per cigarette on an average of more than 25 cigarettes per day), and the chemical composition of the smoke inhaled (over 4,000 chemicals, including tobacco-specific nitrosamines, ammonia, formaldehyde, napthalene, carbon monoxide, hydrogen cyanide, arsenic, benzo(a)pyrene, and polonium 210); 43 of the chemicals are known human carcinogens.[11] Over a typical smoking "career" of 50 years, a lifelong smoker inhales these 4,000 chemicals 4 to 5 million times. Given such exposure, it is perhaps nothing short of remarkable that an estimated one-half of lifelong smokers do not die as a consequence of the behavior. Indeed, there may be no more impressive testimony to the strength of the human organism.

However, considering its burden on the other half of the smoking population, this chemical onslaught has taken a toll unparalleled in the course of human history. In the United States, the toll will subside over time, a reflection of a gradual and continuing decline in smoking rates dating from the 1960s. The prevalence of smoking has dropped from approximately 45 percent in 1963, the year prior to publication of the first surgeon general's report on smoking and health,[12] to 25 percent in 1997.[13] Among men, smoking prevalence has been cut in half. Despite a rising population, total cigarette consumption in the United States has fallen from 633 billion cigarettes in 1981 to 479 billion in 1997. Adult per capita cigarette consumption—a common measure of consumption that adjusts for population growth—has fallen almost annually since 1973.[14] Based on projections of the demographics of smoking, even in the absence of stronger tobacco control education and policy than exist at present, and assuming no change in youth initiation of smoking, prevalence should continue to fall in the United States over the next two decades or so, "bottoming out" at around 18 percent of adults.[15] But even at these diminished prevalence levels, the toll of smoking will remain substantial throughout at least the first half of the new century.

Children, as well as adults, are at increased risk of tobacco-produced disease both from smoking and from exposure to environmental tobacco smoke (ETS). Each day, about 3,000 children begin smoking cigarettes. With regard to adolescent tobacco use, the harms are not immediately evident. Aside from shortness of breath and coughing spells, most diseases attributable to tobacco use are latent, that is, not obvious until two or three decades later. Because nicotine, one of the active ingredients in tobacco, is strongly addictive, adolescents who regularly smoke cigarettes find it hard to quit, thus significantly increasing their chances of suffering some type of tobacco-related disease.

ETS exposure in the home is an important predictor of increased morbidity in children. Children exposed to secondhand smoke had more annual days of restricted activity, bed confinement, and school absence than did children not exposed to ETS.[16] As many as 300,000 children under the age of three suffer from lower respiratory tract infections each year as a result of ETS exposure.[17] Other problems include an increased prevalence of chronic middle ear disease, up to 26,000 new cases of asthma annually, and increased prevalence of sudden infant death syndrome (SIDS).[18]

Still, the achievements of America's "antismoking campaign," dating from publication of the 1964 surgeon general's report, rank tobacco control among, and perhaps at the top of, the major public health success stories of the second half of the twentieth century.[19] The consumption declines previously described suggest the magnitude of the shift in smoking behavior since the early 1960s, but in fact they considerably understate the extent of the accomplishments. In the absence of the then new knowledge about the dangers of smoking, as well as the publicizing of it that constituted the heart of the early antismoking campaign, smoking prevalence almost certainly would have continued to climb, reflecting the rapid rise of smoking rates among women. It is certainly plausible, even probable, that total smoking prevalence would have exceeded 50 percent by the end of the 1960s or early 1970s. Adult per capita cigarette consumption would have exceeded 6,000 cigarettes per year, compared to 4,345 in 1963—the highest level ever attained in the United States—and 2,333, today's figure. According to one analysis, the first two decades of the antismoking campaign should be credited with avoiding nearly 3 million premature deaths through the year 2000.[20]

Reflecting on America's tobacco control victories when juxtaposed against the enormity of the continuing problem, one can consider America's situation as either a cup half full or a cup half empty. The picture for the rest of the world is far bleaker. The World Health Organization predicts that today's global smoking population of 1.1 billion will mushroom to 1.6 billion by the year 2030. By then, tobacco will have become the leading cause of death in developing countries as it is today in developed countries. Currently the cause of 4 million deaths per year worldwide, tobacco will kill 10 million of the globe's citizens annually beginning near the end of the third decade of the twenty-first century.[21] No other behavioral, environmental, or biological cause of death will come close.[22]

The magnitude of America's continuing tobacco-produced death toll, combined with the success of the nation's multifaceted smoking control endeavors, make tobacco control an excellent candidate for examining why a comprehensive approach to disease intervention is essential. Lessons from the tobacco story certainly have relevance to other health behavior dilemmas within the United States, and they generalize to other countries' efforts to come to grips with their own emerging and existing epidemics of tobacco-produced disease.

The Development of Smoking as a Normative Behavior

While American public health leaders like to fantasize about a "tobacco-free" country, the prospects for eliminating tobacco from the list of primary causes of morbidity and mortality verge on the nonexistent in the foreseeable future. The fascinating history of tobacco use, eloquently related by Goodman and others,[23] demonstrates the viselike grip that tobacco and nicotine, its principal dependency-forming constituent, have long held on the members of all societies exposed to "the golden leaf." The earliest recorded evidence of tobacco use in the Americas dates from the ninth century, and in the intervening 1,000-plus years, people have developed an extraordinary array of methods of consuming tobacco, including as a suppository for medicinal purposes. In India at present, tobacco is consumed in about a dozen distinct forms by millions of people.[24] Although the principal early purposes of tobacco use were medicinal and religious, history reveals evidence of social use, multiple times per day, in several North American tribes in the early years of the second millennium.

Tobacco use spread rapidly throughout Europe and Asia beginning in the sixteenth century, when explorers of the New World first brought tobacco back. So potent was the hold of nicotine that smokers defied official prohibitions of its use. Most notably, in the late sixteenth century, Sultan Murad IV of Turkey declared smoking punishable by beheading or being drawn and quartered, yet thousands of Turks persisted in inhaling the intoxicating fumes and, in many cases, suffering the consequences. This experience is more than an interesting historical footnote. It demonstrates that official tobacco control policies have existed for centuries and that tobacco smoking has persisted in the face of far more draconian penalties than any contemplated today. One might credit Murad IV not only as the first government official to develop tobacco control policy but also, through its enforcement, as the first person to prove that smoking was hazardous to health.

Thus, suspicions about the dangers of smoking have existed for at least four centuries. In 1604, writing in a document entitled *Counterblaste to Tobacco*, King James I of England called smoking " a custome lothsome to the eye, hatefull to the nose, harmefull to the braine, dangerous to the Lungs and in the blacke stinking fume thereof, nearest resembling the horrible Stigian smoke of the pit that is bottomelesse."[25]

Despite this early insight, true scientific understanding of the hazards is a strictly twentieth-century phenomenon, primarily dating from the second half of the century.[26] In large part, this reflects the fact that smoking became a widespread threat to health beginning only in the second decade of the twentieth century, with the refinement of the easy-to-inhale cigarette. Prior to 1913, the harsh tobaccos used in cigarettes made cigarette smoking a minor form of tobacco consumption. Cigars, pipes, snuff, and chewing tobacco dominated the tobacco market. Rarely inhaled deeply and frequently, these forms of tobacco consumption, although hazardous to health, posed only a minor risk compared to that which would become associated with cigarette smoking.

In 1913, Camel cigarettes introduced the "American blend" of tobaccos, a combination of flavorful tobaccos imported from Turkey and Egypt with milder American tobaccos that permitted deep inhalation for the first time. Camel also introduced what is widely regarded as the field's first modern advertising campaign. The pairing of flavor and ease of inhalation with creative advertising has been credited with inaugurating the modern era of the cigarette.[27] Other factors that contributed to the rapid emergence of cigarette smoking included the relatively low cost of the new cigarettes, the addictiveness of easily inhaled nicotine, and the convenience of packaged cigarettes: in an increasingly harried daily life, tobacco users appreciated the ease and brevity of the cigarette smoking experience. The latter constituted a principal reason why cigarettes were included in soldiers' rations in World War I and in every war thereafter until the Gulf War. Before the Gulf War, the military also made cigarettes available through the commissary at significantly reduced prices.

Previously considered effeminate, cigarette smoking was converted into a normative behavior among males by the return to America of tens of thousands of newly addicted soldiers. Through effective marketing, the cigarette manufacturers managed to associate smoking with athleticism and romance. A veritable Who's Who of baseball stars, such as Lou Gehrig and Joe DiMaggio, advertised cigarettes widely. Smoking became de rigueur in seduction scenes in the movies, epitomized by the cigarette dangling from Humphrey Bogart's lips whenever he was sweet-talking an attractive lady in one of his films. In the 1950s, America's most respected newsman, Edward R. Murrow, chain-smoked his way through his television news and commentary broadcasts.[28] When the cohort of men born in the decade 1911–20 reached their age of peak smoking prevalence—in their late twenties to middle thirties—fully 70 percent smoked cigarettes. As recently as the early 1960s, more than half of adult males smoked.[29]

In contrast, at no time did a majority of women smoke. Smoking by women was considered socially unacceptable during the first two to three decades of the century and "daring" thereafter until World War II opened the "man's world" to women (e.g., with so many men overseas fighting, women began working in factories in large numbers). The cigarette industry exploited the image of smoking as risqué in multiple ways. In early cigarette ads, women urged their male companions, who were smoking, to "blow some my way." In a precursor to the "liberated woman" advertising campaign for Virginia Slims in the late 1960s, ad agencies staged marches through downtown New York with defiant women smoking. Through such techniques, the agencies tried to link smoking by women to the suffragette movement.

By the 1940s, women were beginning to smoke in large numbers. Indeed, it is striking to note that in four 10-year birth cohorts of women, those born from 1901 to 1940, all reached their rates of peak smoking prevalence within the single five-year period of 1958–63. For the oldest of the four cohorts, born during the century's first decade, this meant that their tobacco use peaked at an average age of 52.5.[30] (By comparison, women born from 1951 to 1960 achieved their peak prevalence in 1976, at an average age of 20.5.) From the 1930s through the early 1960s, the diffusion of smoking among women was paralleling that experienced among men approximately three decades earlier. Unlike men, however, women's smoking prevalence peaked at about a third. The growth of smoking among women was interrupted by the advent of the national antismoking campaign, inaugurated in January 1964 with publication of the first surgeon general's report.[31]

The antismoking campaign has never been a single "campaign" in the conventional sense. Rather, it has consisted of an unorchestrated mix of varied private and public sector efforts, first, to educate the public about the hazards of smoking and, subsequently, to protect non-smokers from exposure to environmental tobacco smoke. As one indication of the overall impact of the campaign, consider the subtle shift in the norms surrounding the act of smoking. In the middle of the century, it was considered impolite to light a cigarette without offering one to companions. Beginning in the 1970s, however, the question asked by a smoker contemplating lighting up switched from "Would you like a cigarette?" to "Do you mind if I smoke?" By the 1990s, in many social circles, the latter question had been mooted by the expectation that the answer would be "Yes." Even before then, antismoking advocates had adapted the latter question into the colloquy "Do you mind if I smoke? Do you mind if I die?" Today, many smokers generally ask nothing and refrain from smoking in the presence of nonsmokers.

Who Smokes and Why?

Although our primary focus in this book is on children, it is useful to understand general adult smoking patterns for comparison purposes. In 1995, 24.7 percent of adult Americans were smokers, down from a high of 42.4 percent in 1965.[32] A larger percentage of men smoke than do women (27.6 percent and 22.1 percent, respectively), but the gap between the two genders has declined gradually over time. Racial and ethnic differences in smoking prevalence are substantial, ranging from 16.9 percent for Asians/Pacific Islanders to twice as much, 34.1 percent, for American Indians and Alaskan Natives. Race/ethnicity and gender differences in smoking prevalence are presented in table 1.

Race/ethnicity prevalence differences mask other differences in smoking behaviors that affect disease outcomes. More African American males smoke than do white males, but African Americans smoke fewer cigarettes per day. Possibly mitigating the potential health advantage of lower daily consumption is African Americans' preference for mentholated cigarettes, believed to have an anesthetizing effect on the throat, which may lead to deeper inhalation. Menthol may also contribute to a higher rate of addiction.[33]

Smoking rates vary substantially by age, with prevalence declining in the fourth and subsequent decades of life. In the older ages, differential death rates for smokers and nonsmokers account for a significant fraction of the prominent decrease in smoking prevalence.[34] Smoking cessation, the principal determinant of the decline in prevalence with age, rises significantly with age. Cessation rates appear to have leveled off during the 1980s and early 1990s, with concern that they may actually have fallen in the late 1990s.

A real challenge to students of the demographics of smoking is assessing smoking initiation, a phenomenon that occurs almost exclusively during childhood and adolescence. Much concern has been expressed about the documented increase in 30-day smoking prevalence among eighth, tenth, and twelfth graders during the first half of the 1990s, a trend that has, fortunately, reversed in the most recent years. In the 1999 Monitoring the Future survey, 34.6 percent of high school seniors had smoked within the past 30 days, down from nearly 37 percent in 1996. The comparable 1999 figures for tenth and eighth graders are 25.7 percent and 17.5 percent.[35] Troubling, however, is the question of how one should assess "smoking" by children; while 30-day prevalence rates were rising during the 1990s, measures of regular and heavy smoking (e.g., half a pack or more per day) were not.

Data on youth smoking also raise perplexing questions about racial and ethnic differences. Most notably, the rates of smoking by African American students were dramatically lower than those for whites, although the gap has narrowed in recent years. Yet smoking rates among young adult African Americans often exceed those of comparably aged whites. The difference is explained, in part, by lower quit rates among African Americans.

TABLE 1. Smoking Prevalence (Percentage) by Gender and Racial/Ethnic Group

Race/Ethnicity	Male	Female	Total
White, non-Hispanic	27.4%	23.3%	25.3%
Black, non-Hispanic	32.1%	22.4%	26.7%
Hispanic	26.2%	14.3%	20.4%
American Indian/Alaskan Native	37.9%	31.3%	34.1%
Asian/Pacific Islander	21.6%	12.4%	16.9%
Total	27.6%	22.1%	24.7%

Source: CDC 1999b.

A large majority of children experiment with smoking, yet fewer than half go on to become regular smokers. As we discuss in chapter 2, social scientists attribute much of the propensity to experiment with tobacco, as well as the propensity to become a regular smoker, to the influence of peer and parental behavior. It is widely believed, for example, that the children of smokers are twice as likely to smoke as the children of nonsmokers (but the data from multiple studies are not uniformly consistent in finding a significant association).[36] There are important socioeconomic and educational links as well: in the United States, as in most developed nations today, smoking is increasingly becoming a marker for lower socioeconomic status.[37]

Clearly, the preeminent determinant of smoking dependency in a given individual is addiction to nicotine. A wealth of evidence from biology, brain chemistry, and sociology indicts nicotine as a classic addictive substance.[38] Ironically, when the surgeon general observed in 1988 that nicotine was as addictive as heroin and cocaine, he may have been understating the case in one important respect: of all the dependency-forming substances of abuse, nicotine likely addicts the largest proportion of its users. But the question remains as to why some people can take it or leave it, while others find themselves incapable of renouncing its use. Intriguing clues are emerging from the rapidly developing field of genetic science. Recent research offers provocative evidence of a genetic explanation for as much as half of the propensity to become a smoker and half of the apparent inability of some smokers to quit.[39]

That the social context in which smoking occurs affects the amount and nature of smoking is evident in the literature on children's role modeling.[40] Intriguing new evidence on contemporary patterns of adult smoking illustrates just how influential societal norms can be. A change in the questions asked by the National Health Interview Survey (NHIS) in 1992 to determine smoking status permitted analysts to assess how many people smoke cigarettes on a nondaily basis. The conventional wisdom among experts on smoking had always been that only 5 percent or so of smokers were "chippers," "recreational" smokers who consumed only a few cigarettes per day or smoked on a nondaily basis. The NHIS data indicate that close to a fifth of all smokers do not smoke every day. Multiple possible explanations may be offered, yet there is widespread agreement that the movement to expand clean indoor air laws, prohibiting smoking in many public places and workplaces, likely has redefined smoking for a subset of smokers. These smokers have learned how to "survive" in a smoking-hostile environment by restricting their smoking to locations, and days, when it is acceptable.

This shift in the social environment in which smoking takes place is but one example of the determinants of smoking that lend themselves to conscious collective intervention. Another, of great concern within the tobacco control community, relates to the marketing of cigarettes and other tobacco products. It is an article of faith within the tobacco control community that advertising and, increasingly, other forms of marketing (ranging from sports sponsorship to distribution of paraphernalia related to cigarette brands) seduce youngsters into experimenting with cigarettes and keep hooked adults who otherwise would quit. The weight of the evidence supports this view, but there is no "smoking gun" that demonstrates it conclusively.[41] One study shows a relationship between the number of promotional items owned and smoking behavior (i.e., the more cigarette promotional items owned, the greater the likelihood of smoking).[42] Otherwise, the empirical evidence on the issue is mixed.[43]

Nevertheless, it is clear that the marketing of tobacco products is a major front in the war on smoking; notable tobacco control victories have been realized within the past few years, most recently the result of the multistate settlement concluded between the state attorneys general and the tobacco industry.[44] As a consequence of that settlement, tobacco billboards have disappeared and human subjects and cartoon characters will no longer grace the pages of cigarette ads. We discuss the specific terms of the settlement and how it came about in chapter 1.

The Objectives of Tobacco Control

Tobacco control policy has three principal objectives, all directed toward avoiding the enormous burden of disease wrought by tobacco use.

- Preventing the initiation of tobacco use by young people (the primary focus of this book)
- Helping smokers (this objective is focused mostly on adults) to quit using tobacco (or at least to reduce their risk)
- Protecting nonsmokers from the annoyance and risk posed by environmental tobacco smoke.

These three objectives are distinct in concept, though realization of any one of them (partial or complete) will often affect one or both of the other objectives.

In principle, proponents of tobacco control should and do support all three objectives. In practice, however, a vigorous national debate has emerged pitting advocates for a youth prevention focus (the first objective) against those who insist on a more comprehensive strategy, one devoted more centrally to preservation of clean indoor air (the third objective) and more explicitly to helping adult smokers quit (the second objective). We will turn to that debate in chapter 1.

To achieve these three objectives, all tobacco control (and indeed other public health) interventions can be classified into one of three broad categories, with differing levels of coerciveness (i.e., the degree to which they force behavior change): education and information interventions, incentives, and laws and regulations. Subsequent chapters will discuss each type of intervention in relation to youth smoking.

The first category, education and information interventions, encompasses all activities designed to inform the public about hazards or benefits to health and/or to persuade people to take health-enhancing behavioral action. In the case of tobacco control, disseminating the findings published in the surgeon general's reports on smoking and health educates the public about the dangers of smoking (and passive smoking) or the health benefits of quitting. Media "counteradvertising" campaigns attempt to persuade young people or adults to avoid tobacco use. Warning labels on cigarette packs and ads are intended to inform about dangers and, implicitly, to discourage use.

The second category, incentives, refers primarily to economic inducements to avoid tobacco. The most obvious and important example is an increase in a cigarette excise tax, driving up the price of cigarettes and thereby discouraging cigarette purchases by individuals who "feel the bite" of the higher price in their wallets. Other examples include differential life insurance rates (you pay more for given coverage if you smoke than if you do not) and explicit smoking cessation incentives, such as employers' rewarding workers who do not smoke with pay bonuses.[45]

The final category, laws and regulations, refers to explicit, legally binding requirements to do, or not do, something pertaining to tobacco consumption. Most notable here are clean indoor air laws, which prohibit smoking in public places, and laws stipulating minimum age of purchase, which forbid vendors from selling cigarettes to minors and minors from buying them.

Definitions

Throughout this book, we use certain terms to define various stages of smoking behavior. Despite the vast literature on all aspects of tobacco policy, there is no standard set of definitions for commonly used terms, such as *smoking, smoking initiation,* or *regular tobacco use.* While the concepts surrounding these terms are generally well understood and accepted, agreement on precise definitions is elusive. In part, this is because individual smoking patterns differ widely. One person might smoke only on weekends, while another might smoke more often but consume fewer total cigarettes. In subsequent surveys, however, one might be classified as a regular smoker, the other only as a current smoker. Thus, there is some inconsistency on what constitutes a smoker, even if the long-term patterns are unaffected by short-term definitional disparities. The 1994 surgeon general's report focuses on the number of days smoking in the past month and the number of cigarettes per day.

For this book, we use the following definitions: *Experimentation* means taking occasional puffs on a cigarette. An *ever-smoker* is anyone who has ever smoked. (Some researchers define ever-smokers as individuals who reported that they had smoked at least 100 cigarettes in their lifetime.[46] This seems too high a threshold.) A *current smoker* is someone who has smoked one cigarette within the past 30 days. A *nonsmoker,* whom we define as someone who has not smoked even one cigarette within the past 30 days, is different from a *never-smoker* (someone who has never experimented).

Since we are concerned with what leads adolescents from first use to more regular smoking and patterns of tobacco use, we are not particularly concerned with random experimentation. We are far more concerned with *smoking initiation,* which we define as a process of moving along a continuum toward becoming a heavy tobacco user. In our approach, the term *initiation* implies some intent to continue smoking, even if not on a daily basis. In this sense, our use of the term *initiation* differs from the terms presently being used. Many surveys define *current smoking* as smoking one cigarette within the past 30 days. Because the definition of current use is now common, we follow that convention, even though we do not necessarily agree that this definition represents current smoking.

By *regular smoking,* we mean that someone has smoked cigarettes in 20 out of the past 30 days. *Daily smoking* means that someone averages one or more cigarettes per day, and *heavy smoking* is defined as consuming more than half a pack per day.

Throughout the book, such terms as *cigarette smoking, tobacco consumption,* and *tobacco use* are used reasonably interchangeably. Unless the context dictates otherwise, the reader should interpret references to smoking as applying generally to other forms of tobacco use as well. (An example of a context that precludes generalization is discussion of laws that prohibit smoking in public places. Clearly this would not apply to use of smokeless tobacco.) Cigarette smoking (or just smoking) is referred to specifically in many instances primarily because it is far and away the most important source of tobacco-produced disease.

Finally, the terms *adolescent smoking* and *adolescent tobacco use* are used frequently. By *adolescent,* we mean the age-group between 12 and 17 years of age. *Preadolescents* constitute ages 11 and below. *Young adults* are those between 18 and 24 years old.

NOTES

This chapter borrows liberally from Warner 2000b. We appreciate the Institute of Medicine's permission to use this material.

1. FDA 1996.
2. IOM 1994; USDHHS 1994.
3. Because most of the programs discussed in part 2 operate to prevent adolescent tobacco use, we have segmented the chapters along common themes for the readers' convenience.
4. USDHHS 1994.
5. IOM 2000.
6. CDC 1999j.
7. CDC 2000a; National Cancer Policy Board 2000.
8. Kluger 1996. For a libertarian perspective on these issues, see Sullum 1998.
9. McGinnis and Foege 1993.
10. USDHHS 1989; Napier 1996.
11. USDHHS 1989.
12. USDHEW 1964.
13. CDC 1999b.
14. Tobacco Institute 1998.

15. Mendez and Warner 1998.

16. Mannino et al. 1996.

17. EPA 1993. See also California EPA 1997.

18. Brownson et al. 1997.

19. CDC 1999a.

20. Warner 1989.

21. World Bank 1999.

22. Murray and Lopez 1996.

23. Goodman 1994; Wagner 1971; Kluger 1996.

24. Bhonsle, Murti, and Gupta 1992.

25. As quoted in Wagner 1971, 11.

26. USDHHS 1989.

27. Tilley 1985.

28. As a sad footnote, both Bogart and Murrow died of lung cancer in their fifties, along with a plethora of other prominent smokers from the era.

29. Warner 1986.

30. Warner 1986.

31. Warner and Murt 1982.

32. CDC 1998b; NHIS 1999.

33. Ramirez and Gallion 1993.

34. Harris 1983.

35. MTF 1999.

36. USDHHS 1994.

37. USDHHS 1989.

38. USDHHS 1988; Henningfield, Cohen, and Pickworth 1993.

39. Pomerleau 1995.

40. USDHHS 1994; IOM 1994.

41. USDHHS 1989.

42. Sargent, Dalton, and Beach 2000. This is known as a dose-response relationship.

43. Chaloupka and Warner 2000.

44. National Association of Attorneys General 2000.

45. Warner and Murt 1984; USDHHS 1989.

46. Douglas and Hariharan 1994.

Part 1

Adolescent Smoking in Context

1

The Policy Context

The use and regulation of tobacco remains one of the most controversial public policy topics at all levels of government. As a result, tobacco control reveals some of the most salient tensions in American political theory: Under what circumstances can or should government limit individual freedoms to protect citizens from the consequences of their personal and lifestyle choices? Does such intervention gain greater legitimacy when directed at adolescent behavior?

Even today, when smoking is highly regulated in many states, the debate over the scope of the regulation needed to discourage adolescent smoking is far from settled. Increased adolescent smoking rates in the early 1990s (now, once again, declining) indicate that previous declines in smoking prevalence are not irreversible, particularly for youth smoking initiation. Thus, the current and future harms from tobacco products continue to raise serious public health and public policy concerns. From a policy perspective, if we can develop effective interventions that inhibit youth smoking initiation rates, we will be able to make significant progress toward reducing the morbidity and mortality costs of smoking in future years.

Historical Antecedents of Tobacco Regulation

Policy debates over controlling tobacco use are not new. Despite a few seventeenth-century colonial restrictions, significant antismoking legislation was not enacted until the second half of the nineteenth century, primarily in response to the fire hazard created by smoking and by ongoing concerns about the morality of smoking.

Before the development of sound scientific evidence showing the harms from tobacco use, smoking opponents relied on other arguments to discourage tobacco use. In 1856–57, the British medical journal *The Lancet* featured an issue in which 50 doctors expressed their views on "The Great Tobacco Question." Various doctors associated tobacco with increases in crime, nervous paralysis, loss of intellectual capacity, and vision impairment. But the editors of *The Lancet* argued that since tobacco use was so widespread, it must have some good or at least pleasurable effects. If the evil effects of tobacco were as dreadful as these doctors claimed, the journal's editors concluded, then the human race would have ceased to exist.[1]

By the late 1800s, many observers thought cigarettes were corrupt and morally repugnant. In 1884, for instance, the *New York Times* warned that smoking could "ruin the republic." Women who smoked were considered promiscuous and were warned they could become sterile, mustached, or consumptive. In the 1890s, Lucy Page Gaston led a Chicago-based antitobacco campaign modeled on the antialcohol campaign. Similarly, Henry Ford spoke out against smoking, and Thomas Edison refused to hire smokers.[2]

The moral arguments no doubt influenced public policy in the late nineteenth century. At the beginning of the twentieth century, 14 states had passed laws banning the production, sale, advertisement, or use of cigarettes within their boundaries. For example, in 1897, Tennessee adopted a statute to prohibit the sale of cigarettes. The statute was upheld by the Tennessee and United States Supreme Courts as a valid exercise of a state's police power to protect public health (*Austin v Tennessee*, 179 US 472 [1900]). In 1901, New Hampshire made it illegal for any person, firm, or corporation to produce, sell, or store for sale any form of cigarette. A 1907 Illinois law made the manufacture, sale, or gift of a cigarette punishable by a fine of not more than $100 or jail for not more than 30 days. In New York, women were forbidden to smoke in public. Progressive reformers in the early twentieth century were particularly concerned about the "demoralizing" effects of tobacco on children, leading to laws prohibiting tobacco sales (primarily cigarettes) to children under the age of 18 (or 21) in many states.[3]

Eventually, opposition to smoking on moral grounds was swept aside by the economic benefits associated with tobacco production and consumption.[4] By 1909, national cigarette sales were twice what they had been five years earlier. Cigarette smoking increased dramatically after 1930, with the greatest percentage gains during and immediately following World War II. In 1945, 267 billion cigarettes were sold, 12 percent more than in 1944, 48 percent more than in 1940, and 124 percent more than in 1930.[5] As the popularity of smoking grew, states realized that cigarette taxes were an important source of revenue, so early anti-smoking legislation was not enforced and was ultimately repealed. In fact, by 1927, all state statutes were repealed and the antitobacco movement was legally, as well as practically, moribund. The political tide did not begin to turn again until the 1960s and lacked momentum until the 1980s.[6]

The Federal Government's Role

Most of the tobacco control activity between the 1960s and 1980s (what little of it existed) emanated largely from the federal government.[7] Federal activity to regulate smoking has a mixed heritage. Congress has provided subsidies for tobacco farmers and encouraged overseas tobacco sales. It has also acquiesced in the tobacco industry's lobbying efforts to block stronger regulatory oversight. At the same time, the surgeon general's office has been a consistent moral and scientific voice against smoking, and the FDA has emerged as a strong proponent of tobacco regulation.

But even before recent federal attempts to regulate tobacco, Congress had enacted some legislation of note. Congress responded to the 1964 surgeon general's report by enacting the Cigarette Labeling and Advertising Act of 1965, requiring the first of the now familiar warning labels on cigarette packages. A few years later, Congress passed the Public Health Cigarette Smoking Act of 1969, banning all cigarette advertising from radio and television, effective January 2, 1971. The ban eliminated the need for broadcasters to provide equal time for anti-smoking advertisements. Many observers believe that the industry actually supported this legislation (albeit quietly) because the anti-smoking ads were adversely affecting cigarette sales.[8] The act also strengthened the warning labels.

In recent years, Congress gradually eliminated smoking on airlines, first by banning smoking on short flights and then by extending the ban to all domestic flights. With few exceptions, however, Congress has failed to enact any additional legislation to restrict the use of tobacco products in public places and work sites or to strengthen the federal regulatory presence.[9]

In 1992, Congress enacted the Synar Amendment, which sets compliance conditions for states seeking block grant allocations that deal with alcohol, drug abuse, and mental health. The Synar Amendment requires states to enact and enforce laws against the sale and distribution of tobacco products to persons under 18 years of age. Under implementing regulations issued by the Department of Health and Human Services in 1996, states must comply with four major provisions: (1) enact a law prohibiting the sale and distribution of tobacco products to persons under age 18; (2) enforce the laws restricting tobacco sales to minors; (3) conduct random, unannounced inspections of retail vendors for compliance with these laws, at least on an annual basis; and (4) obtain an inspection failure rate of less than 20 percent by the year 2000.[10] Despite the threat of removing funds, states have been slow to enforce this law.[11] Also in 1996, the FDA issued regulations restricting youth access to tobacco products and began entering into agreements with the states to enforce them.[12]

Federal tobacco policy is well known for its susceptibility to influence from the tobacco industry. Studies have shown a strong relationship between the level of tobacco industry contributions to individual congressional members and the probability that these members will vote against tobacco control legislation.[13] Indeed, the difficulties in codifying the 1997 settlement agreement between the states and the tobacco industry suggest that looking to Congress for tobacco control legislation is unlikely to be an effective strategy. In fact, most of the significant tobacco control action in the 1980s and 1990s occurred at the state and local levels.

Tobacco Control in the 1980s and 1990s

Beginning with the Minnesota Clean Indoor Air Act in 1975, the first of the model comprehensive statewide smoking restrictions, all states (except Alabama) and many localities have now enacted clean indoor air restrictions. Most tobacco control in the past 15 to 20 years has been accomplished at the state and local levels, although the federal Environmental Protection Agency has taken a lead role in disseminating information about the need to reduce the amount of public exposure to environmental tobacco smoke (ETS). The content of these laws varies widely, resulting in a "patchwork of smoking restrictions"[14] that apply to a large number of Americans both at work and in public places.

Laws restricting smoking in public places range from nominal restrictions (in public buildings and schools in Indiana and Kentucky) to very extensive restrictions (in many public places in Vermont). Only a few states (California, Minnesota, New York, Massachusetts, and

Utah) have enacted comprehensive clean indoor laws that restrict or prohibit smoking in a wide variety of public places, including restaurants.[15] At the local level, increasing numbers of municipalities and cities are enacting bans on smoking in restaurants, and some have enacted restrictions on tobacco advertising as well. A surprising number of businesses have voluntarily gone smoke-free.[16] A good number of drug stores no longer sell cigarettes, on grounds that health-destroying items should not be disseminated by any enterprise professionally devoted to the furtherance of good health. The sight of smokers huddled in doorways because they are prohibited from smoking inside buildings is a manifestation of the shifting balance of power between smokers and nonsmokers.

Many of the clean indoor air laws are motivated by the public's growing intolerance for routine exposure to ETS, resulting from an increasing awareness of the health dangers it presents and increasing irritation at being exposed to cigarette smoke. But these policies may have an even greater impact on society. The potential exists for restrictions and bans on smoking to play a role in changing and shaping social norms regarding smoking, to encourage current smokers to quit and discourage nonsmokers from initiating tobacco use.

Until the mid-1990s, most tobacco control policy attention was focused on reducing smoking in public places. Since then, policymakers have shifted their focus to discouraging adolescent tobacco use through various laws and strategies, which we discuss throughout this book. For instance, as we discuss in chapter 7, the predominant state and local legislative agenda in the 1990s has focused on enacting laws to restrict youth access to tobacco.[17]

The Role of Litigation

Along with attempting to control tobacco use through legislative and regulatory processes, smokers (and, most often, former smokers) have sued tobacco manufacturers to recover damages allegedly incurred from tobacco-produced diseases. For many years, the tobacco industry was invulnerable to tort litigation seeking damages.[18] With limited exceptions, juries have been reluctant to hold cigarette manufacturers responsible for the choices an adult smoker makes, and courts have not imposed strict liability[19] on the manufacturers, thus limiting the effectiveness of litigation in generating damage awards or policy changes. Until 1997, when the industry began suffering limited losses before juries, the tobacco industry's successful defense that the smoker assumes the risk of tobacco's health harms meant that litigation "contributed virtually nothing to the array of strategies employed to control tobacco use."[20] The tobacco industry's arguments on personal freedom (i.e., free choice) have resonated with juries, usually convincing them to rule against individual smokers.

Tobacco litigation scholars speak of three waves of litigation. The first two waves (the first lasted from 1954 to 1973 and the second from 1983 to 1992) were dominated by individuals suing the tobacco companies for negligence. In these cases, the litigation was intended to impose damages for harms that the tobacco industry caused to individuals. The third wave (beginning in 1994) has also included individual lawsuits, but it has been dominated by class actions (lawsuits brought on behalf of large numbers of persons who claim to have suffered common injuries) and especially by cases filed by state attorneys general to recover states' Medicaid costs for tobacco-produced illnesses. The states' litigation was initiated in 1994 to obtain damages from the tobacco industry based on the theory that the states could recover the tobacco-produced financial costs absorbed by the Medicaid program.[21] This litigation has applied novel legal theories designed to avoid the arguments on personal freedom that led to industry successes in the first two waves. The states' litigation forced tobacco companies to disclose damaging internal documents demonstrating the extent to which the industry had misled the public about tobacco's health harms. In turn, these documents began to be introduced into evidence in other tobacco litigation, and, for the first time, the industry began losing some cases.[22]

Current Policy Debates

With the preceding brief background, we can now turn to a discussion of the current policy debates over tobacco use. To begin, we must consider the outcome of the states' Medicaid litigation, which resulted in a negotiated settlement between the states and the tobacco industry. This settlement, called the Master Settlement Agreement (MSA), frames at least the short-term policy context over how to allocate the settlement funds. Both the policy response to the MSA and smoking trends will influence policy development over the longer term.

The Master Settlement Agreement and the Postsettlement
Tobacco Industry

During the summer of 1997, the tobacco industry settled the first two of
the scheduled Medicaid cases, agreeing to pay Mississippi and Florida
more than $3 billion and $11 billion, respectively, over a 25-year period.
Several months later, the industry then settled two other cases: one
with Texas for $14 billion and one with Minnesota for $6 billion. This
put pressure on the remaining states to agree to a comprehensive settlement of the litigation, which most assented to do. The terms of the
resulting settlement included payment of $368.5 billion to the states
and substantial public health measures, largely focused on actions to
reduce youth smoking. For example, the settlement required tobacco
firms to show specific reductions in teen smoking or face additional
penalties (called the "look-back provision"). The industry agreed that
the FDA could regulate nicotine and also agreed to substantial reductions in advertising and marketing. In return, the industry would be
granted broad immunity from future litigation.

Since several of the proposed settlement provisions required congressional approval, legislation was introduced by Senator McCain and
others to codify the settlement. For a variety of reasons, including
strong industry opposition and lack of support from the Republican
leadership, the legislation was not enacted, and the settlement col-
lapsed. No additional states (beyond Mississippi, Florida, Texas, and
Minnesota) settled with the industry until late 1998. By this time, the
negotiating circumstances were less favorable to the states.

On November 19, 1998, 46 state attorneys general in the United
States agreed to a $206 billion settlement with the tobacco industry.[23]
(The final amount is indexed to inflation but could be less if tobacco
sales decline.) The money from the settlement was given to states to
reimburse them for past and future health care costs associated with
smoking. There are no requirements, however, for how states must
spend the settlement funds. Faced with a windfall of billions of unre-
stricted dollars, state legislators are being pressured to spend the
money on a number of issues unrelated to smoking, from tax breaks to
improving roads. As important and politically popular as the latter
measures might be, the settlement will not maximize public health
objectives unless a significant portion of the money is used to reduce
the morbidity and mortality burdens of tobacco use. As of early 2000,

only about 8 percent of available settlement funds has been allocated directly to tobacco control programs, with only a small number of states having made comprehensive tobacco control a priority area.

Aside from the direct financial contributions to the states, the settlement requires the tobacco industry to fund a charitable foundation at $25 million per year for 10 years to support ways to reduce adolescent tobacco use and requires it to disband the Tobacco Institute (the industry's lobbying organization) and the Center for Tobacco Research. The industry also agreed to create a national public education fund for tobacco control. This fund will be administered by an independent organization, the newly formed American Legacy Foundation. This foundation was established to pursue a variety of tobacco control goals, such as reducing youth tobacco use, protecting nonsmokers from environmental tobacco smoke, and helping adult smokers to quit. The foundation will receive approximately $1.45 billion to spend toward these goals in its first four years, with the majority of funds being targeted toward youth smoking prevention, especially through mass media antitobacco campaigns. The foundation will work through states, primarily through grant mechanisms, to develop novel and effective interventions. At the present time, the foundation intends to direct its support to states that provide matching funds for the effort, which further emphasizes the importance of state investment of some settlement funds in tobacco control.

Most of the remaining public health provisions emphasize the prevention of youth smoking by restricting the industry's marketing to children. For example, the settlement

- bans the use of cartoon characters in tobacco advertising, promotion, and packaging;
- prohibits targeting youth in tobacco advertising, promotions, or marketing;
- bans all tobacco advertising outdoors and on transit systems;
- bans the distribution and sale of apparel and merchandise with tobacco brand-name logos;
- prohibits ownership of sports teams by tobacco companies;
- limits tobacco brand-name sponsorship of sports teams to one year;
- limits tobacco product placement (i.e., in the production of movies);

- limits sponsorship of events with a youth audience by tobacco companies;
- bans tobacco product sampling.

Unlike the proposed 1997 settlement, the final settlement does not contain an agreement as to the FDA's jurisdiction over tobacco products. Nor is there a "look-back provision" whereby the industry would be fined if targets for youth smoking reduction are not met. Some outdoor advertising, limited in scope, is permitted. Even so, states were able to extract some important concessions on public health issues, which may, in the long term, operate to discourage youth smoking. The restrictions on marketing and product placement are especially welcome, though the industry and the states will no doubt differ about what the terms mean and how they should operate.

Already, for instance, the industry is advertising in *Rolling Stone, Hot Rod, Sports Illustrated, Essence, Sport,* and other magazines, publications ostensibly aimed at a young adult audience (ages 18–24) but also read by adolescents under age 18.[24] After releasing its first antismoking advertising in early 2000 as part of its Truth media campaign, the American Legacy Foundation was attacked by the tobacco industry for violating the MSA by going beyond the expected education campaign and vilifying the industry instead. The attack forced the foundation to cancel some of the initial ads.[25]

These skirmishes are likely to continue as each side attempts to gain the advantage in the postsettlement environment. Still, when taken together, the restrictions on tobacco marketing and the introduction of a well-funded counteradvertising campaign may have a significant influence on youth smoking by altering the social environment in which it has been glamorized so effectively for decades.

The Postsettlement Tobacco Industry

As policymakers formulate their responses to the settlement and other aspects of tobacco control policy, it will be important to factor in how the tobacco industry will respond to the postsettlement environment. Following the settlement, the major cigarette manufacturers have taken several steps to portray themselves as responsible members of corporate society, newly committed to a good-faith effort to deal with the societal problems associated with use of their products. The hallmarks of this endeavor, according to company statements, include a bit more candor about the hazards associated with smoking, as well as engagement with the public and governmental health agencies to develop reasonable solutions to smoking-related social issues. The objectives of the companies' "new face" appear to be to regain public credibility—the cigarette manufacturers are widely regarded as corporate pariahs—and to find approaches that will minimize damage to the companies' now threatened bottom lines. The latter objective responds not only to expensive developments like the MSA but also to threats looming on the horizon, such as ongoing private class action lawsuits against the industry. Still, none of the companies explicitly admits the health consequences or addictiveness of tobacco use.

Emblematic of the companies' new campaigns is the multifaceted effort of Philip Morris (PM) to improve the firm's public image. Most visible is a series of television ads in which PM extols its commitment to aiding the needy in society—battered women, the hungry and infirm, and victims of natural disasters. Also prominent is the company's redesigned Web site, which now purportedly offers candid information and advice concerning the dangers of smoking and the firm's positions on controversial public matters concerning smoking. A senior vice president of PM announced that the company supported "reasonable" regulation of tobacco products by the FDA. To the firm's thinking, however, "reasonable" regulation did not include FDA regulation of the amount of nicotine in tobacco products.

Prominent public figures welcomed the company's "new candor" and "willingness to cooperate." For example, immediately after the new Web site was introduced, former FDA commissioner David Kessler, M.D., hailed the new openness and honesty reflected in statements on the site. After PM announced its acceptance of the idea of limited FDA regulation, President Clinton publicly congratulated PM on its constructive attitude.

Longtime industry critics reacted to both moves with skepticism borne of innumerable experiences in which industry actions, ostensibly in the interests of public health, have proven to be quite the opposite. A notable example is industry backing of state-level clean indoor air laws. Promoted as supporting the rights of nonsmokers, these watered-down versions of clean air laws included a critical flaw from the point of view of public health: they explicitly preempted stronger indoor air regulations at the local level of government. The net effect was a substantial weakening of clean indoor air protection in the states that adopted such legislation.[26]

Critical examination of PM's new moves reveals an attempt to capture a public relations victory. The industry has employed such attempts for decades but is doing so with greater subtlety now. The Web site's language, for example, is carefully and cleverly crafted to suggest that PM now accepts that cigarettes kill their consumers. In fact, the Web site does nothing of the kind, as the following PM discourse on the dangers of smoking indicates.

> Cigarette Smoking and Disease in Smokers: There is an overwhelming medical and scientific consensus that cigarette smoking causes lung cancer, heart disease, emphysema and other serious diseases in smokers. Smokers are far more likely to develop serious diseases, like lung cancer, than non-smokers. There is no "safe" cigarette. These are and have been the messages of public health authorities worldwide. Smokers and potential smokers should rely on these messages in making all smoking-related decisions.
> (<http://www.philipmorris.com/tobacco_bus/tobacco_issues/health_issues.html>)

As critics have observed, PM is merely stating the obvious: the consensus on the dangers of smoking *is* overwhelming, and smokers and potential smokers *should* rely on public health authorities in evaluating the dangers. What the words do not say, quite intentionally, is that PM accepts and concurs with the overwhelming scientific consensus. To the contrary, the firm has said that it will continue to label smoking a "risk factor" for disease and will rely on the absence of proof of causality in defending the many liability lawsuits against it.

Similarly, PM's expression of willingness to accept reasonable FDA regulation falls far short of the concessions the company signed onto in the proposed global settlement of June 20, 1997. In the statement, PM ruled regulating nicotine out of the set of reasonable regulations. The dominant bottom-line appraisal of the tobacco control community concerning the new candor from the tobacco companies is that it is nothing more than the same old public relations pitch. In most important ways, the postsettlement industry looks much the same as it did prior to the MSA.

Defining the Current Policy Debates

Even before the settlement, state officials were debating how best to prevent or reduce the harms from tobacco use, especially by discouraging adolescents from using tobacco products. With billions of dollars now available for the states to spend, that debate has taken on increased urgency. How should the settlement funds be allocated? Should they be targeted to tobacco control efforts, including prevention activities, or should they be allocated to general funds, perhaps for tax relief? Underlying this debate are several unresolved issues in tobacco control: What mechanisms work best to discourage the use of tobacco products? Should the focus of tobacco prevention and control policy be youth-centered, with a strong emphasis on reducing or eliminating smoking among school-age children, or should these efforts be more comprehensive and include strategies designed for adults, such as smoking cessation efforts? What role should harm reduction strategies play (i.e., the development of safer cigarettes)?

Tobacco control advocates are divided about how to answer these questions. The debate continues over whether tobacco control policy should be focused on adolescents or on both adolescents and adults. Even if that debate were to be resolved quickly, the second likely source of disagreement has emerged, this time over harm reduction strategies, specifically whether to encourage the development of less harmful tobacco products or to promote reduction in use as an alternative to full cessation.

Adults vs. Children
States already have laws restricting tobacco sales to people 18 years of age and under, and the federal Synar Amendment ties maintaining and enforcing such laws to the provision of block grants to combat mental illness and substance abuse. No one argues that such restrictions deprive teenagers of fundamental liberties. Even the tobacco industry claims to believe that smoking is an adult activity that should not be easily available to teenagers.[27] Therefore, some policy analysts have suggested that the focus of public policy should be to reduce teenage smoking initiation rates.[28] Others have suggested that the focus on children will undermine the broader, more comprehensive program needed to attack smoking.[29]

This debate continues to engage and roil the tobacco control community. As is usual in debates of this nature, the long-term strategic goals are shared. The differences rest largely in what actions to pursue in the short-term to achieve the broader goals. In the journal *Tobacco Control*, David Hill[30] and Matt Myers[31] reflected the tenor of the issue, with Hill suggesting the need to focus first on adult tobacco use and Myers taking the position that youth prevention and adult cessation activities should be pursued simultaneously. The title of Myers's editorial, "Adults versus Teenagers: A False Dilemma and a Dangerous Choice," is closer to our view than is Hill's emphasis on adult smoking behavior. From a practical perspective, there is no contradiction between a focus on youth and a broader effort to discourage all tobacco use. Both can be pursued simultaneously and, as will be discussed later, should be considered complementary strategies.

Arguments against Focusing on Youths
In 1996, Stanton Glantz, an influential tobacco control advocate, published an editorial in the *American Journal of Public Health* severely criticizing the focus on youth.[32] For a variety of reasons, he argued that a focus on youth would be counterproductive, would essentially be favorable to the tobacco industry by reinforcing industry depictions of smoking as an adult habit, and would shift attention away from comprehensive efforts to reduce all tobacco use. As an example, Glantz noted that the tobacco control community organized around the proposed FDA regulations on youth access to tobacco but ignored the Occupational Safety and Health Administration's attempts to regulate smoking in the workplace, despite evidence that the latter has demonstrably reduced smoking prevalence.

Glantz argued that antismoking messages aimed at children (i.e., "we don't want adolescents to smoke") reinforce the industry's message and make the tobacco industry look reasonable. According to Glantz, this actually encourages adolescents to smoke by making it alluring as a forbidden, adults-only habit. David Hill argued more recently that at-risk adolescents are most likely to reject adult anti-smoking messages and that smoking is a way to differentiate themselves from those less willing to take the risk (what he calls the "dare-to phenomenon").[33] Both Glantz and Hill believe that such messages only reinforce adolescents' natural rebelliousness against adults. Rebellious children often do the opposite of what the adult world tells them.

Glantz also expressed concern that concentrating on stopping illegal sales to minors could shift the focus away from the tobacco industry and toward the retail vendor, with no evident reduction in overall availability of tobacco products to minors.[34] Just as important, Glantz was worried that a focus on youths would displace more comprehensive, adult-oriented approaches. Glantz went on to add:

> the public health community should realize that the best way to keep adolescents from smoking is to reduce tobacco consumption among everyone. The message should not be "we don't want adolescents to smoke"; it should be "we want a smoke-free society." As the tobacco industry knows well, adolescents want to be like adults, and reducing adult smoking sends a strong message to adolescents about social norms.

Hill shares this concern, asserting that adult cessation programs are much more likely to reduce adolescent tobacco use in the long run than are efforts to prevent adolescent smoking initiation. Ultimately, they perceive the youth prevention strategy as counterproductive. Thus, they are not sanguine about the ability to achieve broader tobacco control objectives when policies and programs are constrained explicitly to target youth. Even if this would work at least partially, in their judgment it would necessarily represent an inefficient attack on such issues as adult quitting and protection of nonsmokers' rights to clean air. Confronted with the massive war chests of the tobacco industry, its top-quality legal and public relations talent, and the inherent allure of nicotine, tobacco control can ill afford less than the best possible approaches to achieving the three tobacco control objectives noted in our introduction.

From the opposite end of the political spectrum, Jacob Sullum offered arguments—based on a libertarian philosophy—against governmental tobacco control intervention, even to protect children. In his 1998 book, Sullum argued generally that smoking is not necessarily irrational (i.e., smokers derive certain pleasures from the habit); that individuals are best able to determine and assert their own preferences, even if the majority disapproves; and that the arguments in favor of government intervention (e.g., the harms from environmental tobacco smoke) are not sufficient to justify governmental intrusions into market arrangements and individual decisions.[35]

With specific regard to children, Sullum declared that the antidrug messages of the early 1990s and restrictions on advertising and marketing made tobacco more appealing by actually teaching adolescents ways in which to express their independence. As did Glantz, Sullum postulated that these restrictions and the focus on adolescents would enhance the "allure of the forbidden." In particular, Sullum noted:

> The important symbolic role of smoking suggests that adults should proceed with caution in trying to steer adolescents away from cigarettes. When authority figures condemn smoking as reckless, obnoxious, and antisocial, they may inadvertently make it all the more appealing to some teenagers.[36]

Taken together, these arguments present a quandary for antismoking advocates. How can advocates develop programs to discourage youths from smoking without using methods that unintentionally stimulate, rather than discourage, tobacco use? This is the same dilemma the tobacco industry faces in its attempts to develop messages that are ostensibly intended to discourage youths from smoking—though, it must be cynically noted, with an obviously different underlying concern. Whatever actions the industry takes to discourage youth smoking behavior will be derided by tobacco control advocates as actually encouraging the very behaviors that lead youths to smoke in the first place. Ironically, this is the precise problem that tobacco control advocates face in crafting their own antismoking messages.

Harm Reduction Strategies

A strategic division likely to dominate many coming debates about tobacco control is centered in but certain to erupt outside the community of smoking cessation experts. These experts are pondering the possibility of finding effective harm reduction strategies that fall short of smokers' completely renouncing their dependence on nicotine. Producing less hazardous cigarettes would be one such strategy. The interest in harm reduction derives from frustration with the slow pace of smoking cessation—only 3 percent of smokers quit each year—and the emergence of a plethora of new technologies for nicotine delivery, produced by both the tobacco and the pharmaceutical industries. The notion is that many smokers who find themselves unable (or unwilling) to give up nicotine might find lower-risk devices for nicotine delivery acceptable substitutes for conventional cigarettes.[37]

The harm reduction concept faces considerable opposition among public health professionals, many of whom adhere strictly to the "just say no" philosophy when it comes to tobacco. To many experts, harm reduction is the crucial new frontier in America's ongoing battle against tobacco-produced disease. It is, however, fraught with the peril that it might result in greater numbers of adolescents taking up smoking under the impression that the new cigarettes are "safer." This complicated and fascinating debate is certain to capture the attention of much of the tobacco control community as technology evolves and appropriate policy responses are contemplated. It explains why the second general objective of tobacco control—helping adult smokers to quit—was modified in our consideration of tobacco control objectives in our introduction by the phrase "or at least to reduce their risk."[38] An Institute of Medicine (IOM) committee is studying the scientific base for evaluating the harm reduction potential of new technologies in nicotine delivery.

Arguments for Focusing on Youth

As we noted in our introduction, the premise underlying this book is that there is a need for a comprehensive and coherent research and policy strategy on ways to discourage tobacco use. A balanced program directed at all population groups is likely to be more effective than a program targeted at adults or adolescents alone. We recommend a comprehensive strategy with distinctive, well-defined components. Those components could include three prongs: one directed largely toward adolescents, one directed toward young adults (ages 18–24), and one directed toward adults. Each component would have different emphases. For example, an adult-oriented campaign might focus on cessation and expanded restrictions on smoking in public places and work sites. Taken together, however, each component of the comprehensive program would have direct and indirect smoking reduction benefits for the entire population. For the reasons set forth shortly, we focus our analysis on the adolescent component. In our "Conclusion and Recommendations," we return to the theme of developing a comprehensive strategy.

Because the debate over the youth vs. adult strategy has become so contentious in the tobacco control community, we feel compelled to explain in greater detail why it is reasonable to focus this study on preventing youth smoking. Such an approach seems logical if we are to break the seemingly endless cycle of youthful experimentation, addiction, and subsequent long-term use, disease, and death.

In the early to mid-1990s, tobacco control efforts began to focus on discouraging youth tobacco use. At that time, the strategy was based on the thinking that taking steps to reduce adolescent experimentation with tobacco products would eventually dramatically lower tobacco's morbidity and mortality costs. Thus, it seemed natural to concentrate resources on school-based and other youth programs targeted at reducing youth smoking initiation rates.[39] Policymakers had already begun to crack down on adolescent alcohol use and proceeded to apply the same stringency to prevent the sale of tobacco to minors. We also know that legislators are more inclined to enact antitobacco legislation that protects children.[40] For these reasons, a strategy focusing on reducing youth access to cigarettes was pursued by state and local governments, and few tobacco control advocates opposed this approach at that time. As we noted in our introduction, the youth prevention orientation evolved in the mid-1990s in large part as a political strategy: preventing smoking by children is a nearly universally lauded objective, with even the tobacco industry now paying lip service to this goal.[41]

There is much to be said in favor of the positions articulated by both Glantz and Sullum. Yet their positions do not present an altogether compelling argument that should dissuade policymakers from focusing on youth tobacco use. The rate of increase in adolescent smoking seen in the early 1990s began before the shift in policy focus to youths and might have increased more rapidly absent such policies.[42] Moreover, the recent decline in teen smoking rates may be related to the youth-oriented policies developed in the mid-1990s, including increasing prices. Just as important, there are compelling philosophical and pragmatic arguments favoring a youth-oriented antismoking campaign.

The primary argument in favor of focusing on adolescents remains the potential for changing their smoking behavior—before they become addicted; at transition states when intervention may prevent or limit the shift from occasional to routine use; and shortly after they become addicted, when some adolescents begin to express a desire to quit. Because of these factors, there is a potentially large gain from concentrating resources on reducing youth access to tobacco products and determining what additional approaches would be effective in reducing teenage smoking initiation rates.[43] Stopping a lifetime of tobacco use before it starts seems at least as important as postaddiction cessation interventions for adults. If one generation's cycle of tobacco addiction could be reduced substantially, the next generation might be less likely to start smoking in large numbers. As a practical matter, reducing youth smoking initiation rates will not only lower long-term morbidity and mortality costs, it will serve to increasingly marginalize tobacco use within society.

A second argument is that both politicians and the public are more likely to tolerate restrictions on youth tobacco use and on smoking in public places that are frequented by adolescents. From the perspective of many tobacco control advocates, a youth-centered strategy permits a foot in the legislative door to achieve broader objectives by dressing them in prevention clothing. For example, the call for a large tax increase to discourage youth smoking would, if adopted, also decrease smoking by adults. A media antismoking campaign would reach adults both directly and indirectly, the latter by adults' awareness of the changing attitudes and behaviors of young people with regard to smoking. It is certainly reasonable to call for smoke-free indoor environments in locations frequented by young people, such as schools, malls, and sporting events; adults work and play in those settings as well. Banning tobacco billboards has an effect on its ostensible target, youth, and on adults too. In this way, the youth prevention strategy engages in and capitalizes on the art of the possible. In addition, paternalistic policies are more widely tolerated toward children than they are toward adults. Sullum recognizes this, saying that "emphasizing children is an effective strategy for gaining support from people who might be uneasy about a broader assault on smoking."[44] But Sullum's response is that we should enforce existing laws against tobacco sales to minors, rather than expanding governmental intervention. Sullum's response is no doubt necessary, yet it is hardly sufficient given the extent of the problem and the need to consider new strategies for discouraging adolescents' initiation of tobacco use.

A third reason why policymakers should focus on adolescents is that it is not entirely clear how accurately adolescents understand the consequences of nicotine addiction. Among high school smokers who say they will definitely not be smoking 5 years later, 41.6 percent smoke half a pack per day, and 31.9 percent smoke a full pack per day. Five years later, 81.2 percent of those smoking half a pack per day still smoke, along with 86.6 percent of those smoking a full pack per day.[45] Any doubts in the empirical evidence should be resolved in favor of protecting children. Paternalism is justified to prevent adolescents from becoming addicted, even if similar arguments directed against adults might be inappropriate because the government should generally be wary of intervening to prevent harm to oneself. In our "Conclusion and Recommendations," we address this issue at greater length. Suffice it to say at this point that we are dubious that adolescents accurately understand the nature of the risks and the addictiveness of tobacco products, especially given recent evidence that teens are particularly vulnerable to becoming addicted.[46]

While an exclusive concentration on youth smoking may not be advisable, it seems important as a matter of social policy to do everything reasonable to discourage youths from using tobacco products. To be sure, it is unrealistic to expect that enactment and implementation of youth access restrictions can eliminate teen smoking, especially since demonstrated reductions in illegal sales to minors may not affect their overall cigarette consumption.[47] Zero tolerance is not realistic and should not be the primary policy objective. For one thing, the history of tobacco outlined in our introduction suggests that such an approach would be futile. For another, the availability of cigarettes to adolescents may not be significantly affected by the reduction of illegal sales to minors. They may be able to obtain cigarettes from other sources (e.g., family members and older adolescents). Nonetheless, reducing illegal sales to minors will, at a minimum, make it more difficult for teens to obtain tobacco products.

Our Assessment

The division of the tobacco control forces into the two strategic camps reflects their terrain: the leadership of the youth prevention strategy comes from national "establishment" organizations, including the American Cancer Society, the American Heart Association, the National Center for Tobacco-Free Kids, and the new American Legacy Foundation. The leader of these national organizations appears to be the National Center to Campaign for Tobacco-Free Kids, funded largely by the Robert Wood Johnson Foundation and the American Cancer Society. The Campaign for Tobacco-Free Kids was organized to be a national resource center for youth smoking, with a focus on legislative advocacy for children. Savvy in the ways of Washington and replete with financial resources and congressional lobbying experience, these organizations believe that the most effective results ultimately must be achieved with a national strategy, which must necessarily be youth-oriented.

In contrast, proponents of a more comprehensive approach derive support from state and local organizations, including local chapters of the major health voluntaries, tobacco control divisions of state and local units of government, grassroots tobacco control organizations, and the American Medical Association. The leadership of this school consists of individuals who have fought the tobacco wars in the trenches of state and local politics, directing state ballot initiatives to raise cigarette excise taxes and dedicate revenues to tobacco control and heading campaigns to ban smoking in restaurants and other public places within cities and counties.

Our view of this debate is straightforward—and, we hope, not too simplistic. Policies designed to discourage adolescents from using tobacco products are important for several reasons. First, politicians respond to arguments about protecting children.[48] Thus, policies designed to reduce youth smoking are likely to reach a receptive political audience. As we discuss in chapter 7, the trends in enacting youth tobacco restrictions support this analysis. This, in turn, may provide tobacco control advocates with a mechanism to achieve political goals that would not otherwise be attainable through a more general population-based approach to legislators.

Second, in contrast to Sullum's pure libertarian arguments, we believe that there is ample reason why government should act to discourage youth tobacco use. Even if one accepts Sullum's precepts that tobacco use is rational and that smokers derive certain pleasures from its use, tobacco, in fact, is a product that is deadly when used as intended—both to those who consume it and to those who must endure secondhand smoke. It follows that government should not condone its use and should use its powers to make it as difficult as possible for youths (and adults) to smoke in public or for adolescents to purchase the product. One need not ascribe to a prohibitionist approach (which we reject) to suggest that some products are so harmful that governmental neutrality is not appropriate. In making this argument, we recognize that many legal products may cause harm. For example, cars can be deadly, especially when operated by drunk drivers. Nevertheless, tobacco is responsible for so much more harm than any other legal product when used as intended that we see little danger of a slippery slope leading to calls to similarly restrict automobile use. When the ban on television and radio advertisement of tobacco went into effect, similar fears were raised about a slippery slope, but nothing has been banned since then. At least on a symbolic level, government's willingness to help establish norms that discourage youths from smoking seems an entirely defensible strategy. Just as public policy seeks to marginalize illicit substance use, it is appropriate for government to design policy mechanisms to marginalize tobacco use. By analogy, government restricts many behaviors that may be offensive to the community, even if they are not harmful to individuals. For instance, laws forbidding nude dancing in public have been uniformly upheld against challenges based on the First Amendment. Surely, if government need not remain neutral regarding such activities—harmless though offensive to many people—it should not remain neutral with regard to both harmful and offensive behaviors, such as smoking in public places.

Third, Glantz is perhaps correct that a focus on adolescents reinforces both their sense of rebellion and the industry's message that tobacco is for adults only. But that does not seem to be an adequate reason to abandon attempts to discourage youth smoking behavior. What may be required are more creative and subtle attempts to address the reasons why adolescents smoke and to develop messages directed at them. This does not mean that we should abandon efforts to reduce adult smoking behavior. As Glantz and others have observed, the two strategies are intimately related. In our view, however, we cannot confront adolescent tobacco use merely by ignoring the problem. Adolescence is a time of experimentation and a time when sporadic smoking becomes habitual. The more we can discourage teen tobacco initiation rates and routine smoking, the lower future smoking-related mortality and morbidity costs are likely to be.

Finally, we need to understand better why most adolescents do not become regular smokers (even though most experiment). As much as we can learn from the literature addressing the determinative factors predicting why youths smoke, we can learn just as much from assessing why the majority of adolescents never smoke or do not advance beyond occasional tobacco use.

There is, to be sure, no magic bullet for reducing adolescent tobacco use. Efforts to do so are likely to require a process of trial and error, along with a long-term commitment of resources and energy. For example, new research is emerging on the role of genetics in becoming a regular smoker, in the difficulty of quitting, and in possible vaccines against nicotine addiction. It will take many years before we know whether these avenues of research can lead to an effective antidote to tobacco use.

Glantz and Sullum raise important challenges for activists working in youth smoking prevention. Measures against youth smoking may have unintended effects by unwittingly encouraging some young people to initiate smoking. Of course, the same measures may dissuade or deter other young people from the same behavior. Empirically sound policy analysis is therefore required to determine the ultimate impact of any specific intervention. Unfortunately, the literature evaluating effective policies for reducing teen smoking initiation rates is limited.[49] As a consequence, we lack adequate data evaluating the effectiveness of many newer approaches for discouraging adolescent tobacco use. Much of this book evaluates the relative merits of different policy approaches and illuminates innovative ways of discouraging adolescent tobacco use.

Conclusion

An important policy issue is to determine where and how to allocate antitobacco resources, given the current legislative and regulatory environment. Policymakers now have an incentive to become more active in tobacco control, as the policy environment has changed considerably within the past few years. Unquestionably, the current state of regulatory, judicial, and legislative pressure on the tobacco industry represents a concentrated and unprecedented assault on a legal product. Even so, tobacco remains an alluring, addictive substance that adolescents continue to use.

We believe that previous calls for tobacco control efforts that are youth-centered remain relevant and critically important as we move into the twenty-first century. As we discuss in part 2 of this book, a number of interventions and strategies deserve further consideration, dissemination, and evaluation. The resources available through the settlement with the tobacco industry provide an unprecedented opportunity to invest in youth tobacco control. Thus, we strongly advocate that this opportunity be seized and that significant state resources—along with other resources—be devoted to expanding, improving, and evaluating tobacco prevention and control activities among youth. In fact, one of our purposes is to assist state officials in deciding how to allocate their tobacco settlement funds. This book is not designed to evaluate options among competing uses of funds outside of tobacco control (e.g., tax relief vs. public health) but will be useful for assessing what we know about various tobacco prevention strategies and how funds allocated for tobacco control might be spent.

It is possible that the recent IOM and CDC recommendations favoring comprehensive programs including both adults and children will lead to a consensus among tobacco control advocates. If so, this will be a welcome development. Tobacco advocates need to move beyond the fragmentation that ensued during the wars over the McCain Bill.

NOTES

For the historical review in this chapter, we have borrowed liberally from Jacobson, Wasserman, and Anderson 1997.
1. Wagner 1971; Kluger 1996.
2. Wagner 1971; Kluger 1996; Sullum 1998.
3. IOM 1994.
4. Critics argue that the current antismoking movement is no less animated by moral fervor than its predecessors.
5. Wagner 1971.
6. For greater detail about the historical development of antismoking sentiment, see Sullum 1998, especially 143–59.
7. See Jacobson, Wasserman, and Anderson 1997 for additional details.
8. Kagan and Vogel 1993.
9. Siegel et al. 1997.
10. USDHHS 1996a.
11. DiFranza and Rigotti 1999.
12. USDHHS 1996b.
13. Siegel et al. 1997; Samuels and Glantz 1991; Bearman, Goldstein, and Bryan 1995.
14. Rigotti and Pashos 1991.
15. California also curbs smoking in bars.
16. Jacobson and Wu 2000.
17. Jacobson and Wasserman 1999; CDC 1999i.
18. Schwartz 1993; Annas 1997. For a recent review of tobacco litigation, see Jacobson and Warner 1999.
19. Strict liability means that an industry bears responsibility for its products regardless of whether it was negligent (i.e., at fault).
20. Rabin 1991, 494.
21. Moore and Mikhail 1996; Kelder and Daynard 1997.
22. Most of those cases are either on appeal or still in progress, so we do not know whether the tobacco industry will be forced to pay large damage awards.
23. National Association of Attorneys General 2000.
24. Turner-Bowker and Hamilton 2000; Sanchez and Goldberg 2000.
25. Teinowitz 2000.
26. Jacobson and Wu 2000.

27. See   <http://www.philipmorrisusa.com/DisplayPageWithTopic.asp?ID=56> (accessed June 7, 2000).

Philip Morris's home page stresses that the company makes "adult products." The tobacco link also indicates that cigarettes are for adults, particularly that smoking is an "adult choice." Links to the youth prevention page also indicate that Philip Morris is against adolescent smoking. See these other industry Web sites for additional examples of the portrayal of smoking as an adult activity: <http://www.rjr.com/TI/Pages/TIcover.asp>; <http://www.brownandwilliamson.com/8_yspc.html> (both accessed June 7, 2000).

28. IOM 1994; USDHHS 1994; Jacobson and Wasserman 1999.

29. Glantz 1996.

30. Hill 1999.

31. Myers 1999.

32. Glantz 1996.

33. Hill 1999.

34. See also Levy and Friend 1999.

35. Sullum 1998, 177–80.

36. Sullum 1998, 250.

37. Warner, Slade, and Sweanor 1997; Warner 2000a.

38. Interested readers should consult the provocative literature emerging on the subject: Tobacco dependence 1998; Ferrence et al. 2000.

39. Brownson et al. 1995.

40. Jacobson, Wasserman, and Raube 1993.

41. Brown & Williamson 2000; Philip Morris 2000.

42. Cigarette prices declined in the early 1990s relative to inflation, a factor that might have stimulated the increasing adolescent smoking rates.

43. Brownson et al. 1995; Hine et al. 1997.

44. Sullum 1998, 252.

45. USDHHS 1994.

46. Kandel et al. 2000; Laux 2000.

47. IOM 1994; Rigotti et al. 1997; Levy and Friend 1999.

48. Jacobson, Wasserman, and Raube 1993; Sullum 1998.

49. IOM 1994; Feighery, Altman, and Shaffer 1991; Jason et al. 1991; Jason et al. 1996a, 1996b.

2

Trends in Youth Smoking

Despite the ever increasing information on the adverse health effects of using tobacco products, adolescents continue to experiment with and use tobacco at stubbornly high rates. These rates have remained high during what has otherwise been a remarkable transformation in the nation's smoking behavior over the past 30 years. As we noted in our introduction, from 1963 until 1997, the prevalence of smoking among adults declined from 45 percent to 25 percent. This decline represents profound changes in social attitudes toward smoking, in civil norms that increasingly find smoking in public places to be unacceptable behavior, and in the willingness to challenge a powerful and creative industry.

Unfortunately, these declines among adults have not been replicated among adolescents. During the early 1990s, for example, teen smoking rates rose while adult rates declined or remained stable. Since 1996, however, adolescent tobacco use has also been declining. Teenage smoking rates are of particular concern because considerable research has shown that few people initiate smoking behavior once past their teenage years.[1] By age 18, nearly 90 percent of the people who will ever smoke routinely have already become or are in the process of becoming habitual smokers.

The purpose of this chapter is to synthesize and present information concerning youth smoking behaviors from a variety of sources and topics. Data on youth smoking behavior and trends are abundant. Although the outlines of these trends will be familiar to tobacco control experts, summarizing what we know about trends in adolescent tobacco use will establish a context for the remainder of the book and will introduce those not as familiar with these trends to the underlying dynamics of tobacco use. This synthesis of the relevant data is intended to provide readers with current smoking data and trends in youth smoking from the past 25 years, as well as to indicate the sources of youth smoking data for further inquiry. For comparative purposes, we also describe available data on adolescent use of illicit substances and alcohol.

Overview

Data Summary

For people just interested in the bottom-line facts of teen smoking, the American Legacy Foundation issued the *Teens and Tobacco Fact Sheet* as part of its Truth media campaign. Here, we adapt their fact sheet and supplement it with additional facts.[2] This list presents a good snapshot of adolescent smoking behavior.

- Every day, 3,000 young people in the United States become regular smokers, and more than 6,000 adolescents try their first cigarette.[3] That represents more than one million U.S. youth each year.
- Nearly 13 percent of middle school students and nearly 35 percent of high school students currently use tobacco. Smoking among high school seniors reached a 19-year high of 36.9 percent in 1996.[4]
- Nearly 20 percent of youth aged 12–17 describe themselves as current smokers (defined as one cigarette during the past 30 days).
- Forty-one percent of youth aged 18–25 smoke, an increase of 7 percent since 1994.
- Eighty-nine percent of adult daily smokers began before they turned 19.
- Eighty-six percent of teens who smoke prefer one of the three most heavily advertised brands: Marlboro, Camel, or Newport.
- Marlboro, the most heavily advertised brand, constitutes almost 60 percent of the youth market but only about 25 percent of the adult market.
- Popular youth cigarette brands are more likely than adult brands to be advertised in magazines with high youth readerships.
- Each year, the five largest tobacco companies in the United

States earn an estimated $480 million in profit from cigarettes sold to people under the age of 18.

- Between 1989 and 1993, when advertising for the Joe Camel campaign jumped from $27 million to $43 million, Camel's market share among youth increased by more than 50 percent, while its adult market share did not change.
- Over 5,000,000 youths under 18 alive today will ultimately die from tobacco use if current trends continue.

Trends

The overall trend lines indicate that adolescent smoking behaviors (for both initiation and daily use) have not changed considerably over the past 35 years (fig. 1). After peaking in 1975, adolescent tobacco use declined steadily until 1991. Between 1991 and 1996, adolescent smoking rates substantially increased, before beginning a steady decline in 1996 (through the present). Among twelfth graders, prevalence rates for ever smoking, current smoking (smoking at all in the past 30 days), daily use, and smoking more than half a pack per day have declined since 1997 (fig. 2); for eighth and tenth graders, the declines date from 1996. While the declines are not large, the downward trend is a welcome development after steep increases in the early to middle years of the 1990s. Adult smoking rates declined steadily from 1979 through 1999 (fig. 3).

Adolescent drinking, marijuana use, and cocaine use also increased during the 1990s. Yet in contrast to teen smoking behavior, adolescent use of these other substances had declined markedly during the 1980s (fig. 4). Even though illicit drug use also increased during the early 1990s, tobacco is the only major substance that is more widely abused by adolescents today than 20 years ago.

Several national surveys track youth smoking patterns, and thanks to reasonably standard data collection and analytic measures, comparisons between surveys and across years are possible. In general, these data show increases in smoking prevalence for all adolescent groups. Data from the Monitoring the Future (MTF) survey show that greater percentages of twelfth graders tried smoking for the first time (thus becoming ever-smokers), were current smokers (had smoked in the past 30 days), were smoking daily, or were smoking more than half a pack a day in the 1990s than in the previous decade (fig. 2).[5] A CDC survey reported a 73 percent rise in the number of

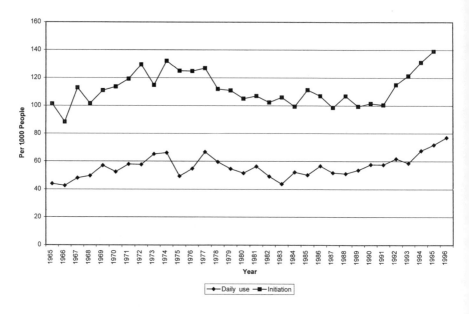

Fig. 1. Adolescent tobacco use

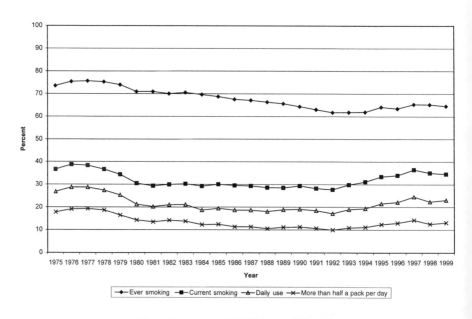

Fig. 2. Frequency of smoking, twelfth grade

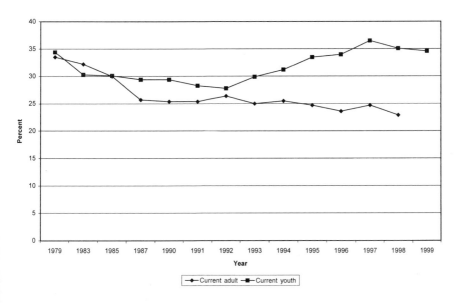

Fig. 3. Adult and youth current smoking, selected years. (Data from Johnson, O'Malley, and Backman 1999, 2000.)

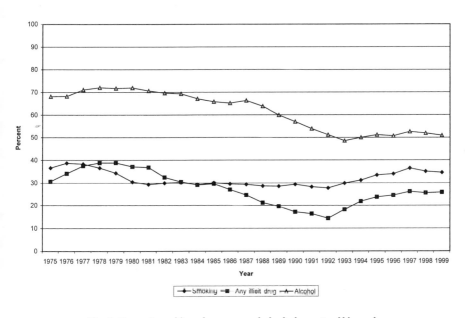

Fig. 4. Current smoking, drug use, and alcohol use, twelfth grade

adolescents who first became daily tobacco users during the 1990s, and the same survey estimated that adolescents experimenting with their first cigarette every day increased by 50 percent from 1988 to 1996.[6] Thirty-day adolescent prevalence rates were 34.6 percent in 1999, down from 36 percent in 1997, but up from 28 percent in 1991.[7] The average age of first experimentation with tobacco dropped from 15.9 in 1994 to 15.4 in 1995.[8]

On a more encouraging note, the MTF 2000 survey found that declining youth tobacco use, first observed in 1996, accelerated between 1999 and 2000.[9] Although the youth smoking rates have not yet returned to their pre-1990s level, the downtrend is encouraging.

Other trends emerged in the 1990s. In 1999, almost 35 percent of U.S. high school twelfth graders were current cigarette smokers.[10] According to a CDC analysis of the 1997 Youth Risk Behavior Surveillance System (YRBSS) survey, 70.2 percent of high school students had tried smoking cigarettes, and 35.8 percent of those students became daily smokers.[11] Further, 4.1 million adolescents aged 12–17 were current smokers in 1998.[12] In the past, more boys smoked than girls, but now adolescent females smoke at the same level as their male counterparts.[13] The dramatic decreases in smoking rates of African Americans seen during the 1980s were somewhat reversed in the 1990s, although they remained lower than the rates for whites and Hispanics (fig. 5). African American teens continue to smoke at a lower rate compared to whites, but cigarette use rose among this group more than 50 percent between the late 1980s and 1997.[14] Smoking prevalence is also increasing rapidly among younger adolescents and is significantly higher among youth who have dropped out of school.[15] Younger students who smoke are at less advanced stages of smoking and smoke less intensely than older smokers,[16] but young adolescent smokers are more likely to become addicted smokers than are those who begin smoking at a later age.

Smoking initiation is largely a youth phenomenon with lasting effects. The National Household Survey on Drug Abuse (NHSDA) reports that the median age of experimentation with cigarettes is 14.5 years, and nearly 25 percent of adolescents surveyed have reported smoking a whole cigarette by age 13.[17] Data from the National Health Interview Survey (NHIS) indicate that for successive 10-year birth cohorts from 1885 to 1989, smoking prevalence peaks by the age of 30, with the most dramatic increases (indicating initiation) occurring between the ages of 10 and 20.[18] Cigarettes are by far the drug most commonly used daily by teenagers.[19] Compared with other substances,

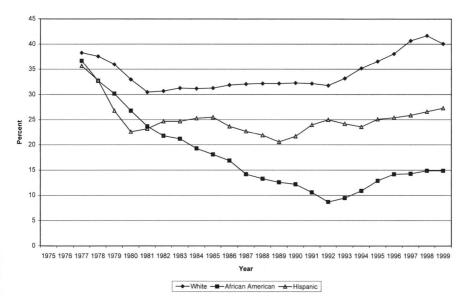

Fig. 5. Smoking by race, twelfth grade

tobacco is also consumed in much heavier dosages likely to cause lasting health harms.

Organization of the Chapter

In the remainder of this chapter, we first describe the primary data sources of youth smoking trends. We define common data measures and variables and explain our methods. Data on current incidence and prevalence of smoking, as well as trends for the past 25 years by demographic characteristics, follow. We then describe factors influencing adolescent tobacco use trends and discuss adolescent use of cigars and other noncigarette tobacco products. We conclude with a discussion of trends in adolescent use of alcohol and illicit substances.

Definitions

In this chapter, we use the following definitions, drawn from the major surveys cited below.[20] *Experimental smoking* is ever trying a cigarette in one's lifetime. *Current smoking* is smoking at least one cigarette in the 30 days preceding the survey. *Daily smoking* constitutes smoking every day in the 30 days preceding the survey.[21] *Heavy smoking* constitutes half a pack or more per day. *Initiation* means the process of beginning to move through the various smoking stages.

Data on Adolescent Tobacco Use

To understand the nature and extent of problems related to adolescent tobacco use, policymakers must be aware of both the prevalence and the incidence of adolescent smoking. Prevalence is a measure of all adolescents who smoke at a given point in time. Incidence represents the number of new smokers in any given time period. Therefore, prevalence trends are affected both by the number of new smokers and by adolescent smoking cessation patterns. Although adolescents are not quitting smoking in significant numbers, many among current smokers do not go beyond the experimentation stage.

Data Sources and Measures

There are a variety of sources of smoking data; some are adolescent-focused, and others include adolescents in a larger sample. The YRBSS survey provides data on several smoking behaviors: age of initiation; experimentation, regular use, and pattern of use; smoking cessation; and smokeless tobacco use.[22] Likewise, the Teenage Attitudes and Practices Survey (TAPS) is adolescent-focused. A survey sponsored by the American Legacy Foundation, called the National Youth Tobacco Survey, also concentrates specifically on youth tobacco trends. In contrast, the MTF survey, conducted by the Institute for Social Research at the University of Michigan, provides data on general adult trends in smoking and on youth smoking trends specifically. The National Household Survey on Drug Abuse, which asks respondents about current and past experiences with a variety of drugs, is an example of a survey that includes adolescents (ages 12–17) in its sample but is not specifically adolescent-focused.

Fortunately, there is remarkable parity in measures and methodology used in the surveys applicable to teen smoking, facilitating comparisons across studies. The most common measures include incidence, prevalence by smoking stage, and smoking intensity. These data are often further subdivided by sociodemographic categories, such as gender, ethnicity, age, and grade, to facilitate analysis. With some exceptions, most of the surveys are cross-sectional. A cross-sectional survey is essentially a snapshot of smoking activity at one particular period of time. In cross-sectional surveys, individual respondents are not tracked from year to year, as they would be in longitudinal surveys. For understanding smoking behavior, longitudinal data are preferable because they provide more insight into the various transitions between smoking stages. The trends data presented in this chapter represent cohorts, or specific age-groups, for the years of the survey.

Methods

The data and data trends presented in this chapter are available through previously published materials and ongoing publicly available surveys. We did not collect primary data. The source for most graphs is MTF data from 1975 to 1999. MTF is the most authoritative data source regarding adolescent smoking and is widely cited by policymakers, researchers, and the broader public health community. MTF data also allow for comparisons of different age-groups and for analysis of transition states (i.e., movement from nonsmoker to smoker and from experimenter to routine smoker). Furthermore, the large sample size of annual data spanning more than two decades facilitates discussions of smoking behavior trends. Additional sources are cited for comparison purposes where appropriate.

Incidence of Adolescent Smoking Behavior

The progression from nonsmoking to contemplation to experimentation to regular smoking has been the subject of extensive research, which we summarize in chapter 3. The first step in this progression is experimentation—the act of trying a cigarette for the first time. By asking respondents the age at which they first smoked a whole cigarette, or in some cases the age at which they first took a puff or two, researchers can measure smoking incidence.

Incidence Data

Incidence data furnish an estimate of the number of people who try smoking or who begin to smoke daily, weekly, or less frequently in any given year. Incidence data also provide the best indicator of changes in adolescent behavior over time. In a sense, this measure acts as a gauge of the smoking environment from year to year. The incidence data cited here come from the NHSDA, based on interviews conducted between 1994 and 1997. Incidence was there defined as the number of youths who experimented with tobacco over the total number of those surveyed who had not already initiated tobacco use.[23] The 1994–97 survey data also included age of first use of cigarettes and age of first daily use of cigarettes.

The number of new adolescent smokers in the United States increased from the 1980s through 1996. For instance, the number of minors who initiated smoking was 1,929,000 in 1988 but jumped to 2,441,000 in 1995. In 1988, the number of minors who began smoking daily was estimated at 708,000. By 1996, that figure had nearly doubled, at 1,226,000.[24] The NHSDA data confirm that initiation is largely an activity of minors. Of the persons who first smoked a cigarette in 1995, nearly 80 percent were under 18 years old, and 66.2 percent of the people who became daily smokers in 1996 were under 18 years old.[25] As these figures make plain, the morbidity and mortality implications of reducing youth initiation rates are immense (which supports the focus on youth prevention activities). The CDC concluded that "if the incidence of initiation had not increased during 1988–96, approximately 1,492,000 fewer persons aged less than 18 years would have been daily smokers by 1996."[26]

There is remarkable consistency in the rate of initiation across the decades for the 12–17 age-group. Initiation has never dropped below 10 in 100 per year and has never reached above 15 in 100 per year. Among persons aged 12–17, the analyses indicate that from 1965 to 1977 and from 1988 to 1996, the incidence of initiation of first use increased by 25 percent and 30 percent, respectively.[27] Between 1977 and 1988, the rate of initiation was relatively unchanged. Between 1992 and 1996, the rise in the rate of initiation was particularly steep.

Over the period from 1983 to 1996, first daily use increased by over 75 percent, nearly doubling.[28] Increases in the incidence of daily use of cigarettes in the mid-1980s preceded by several years the increases in initiation, which started in the early 1990s. Perhaps the higher visibility of regular smoking and the greater number of daily smokers created an environment of heightened curiosity, provided expanded opportunities to smoke, and created a perception of increased prevalence and normalcy of smoking, which in turn led to increases in initiation rates. During the 1990s, adult smoking rates remained virtually unchanged.

At the same time, smoking rates for ages 18–24 rose from 24.8 percent in 1995 to 28.7 percent in 1997.[29]

Not only are more kids lighting up, but they are initiating smoking at earlier ages. Results from the 1997 YRBSS survey indicate that ninth graders (32 percent) and tenth graders (27.5 percent) were significantly more likely to have smoked a cigarette before the age of 13 than either eleventh graders (22.2 percent) or twelfth graders (18.6 percent). This may partly be explained by an overall increase in the incidence of smoking initiation, but it also indicates a possible trend toward earlier smoking uptake.[30] According to an analysis of YBRSS data, those who initiate tobacco use at a younger age smoke more cigarettes per day than those who initiate use at an older age.[31] Since researchers also believe that early initiators have a more difficult time quitting than later initiators,[32] this trend is important for policymakers to understand.

Prevalence of Youth Smoking

As we noted earlier, prevalence is a measure of the number of smokers at a given time. The prevalence of smoking is integral to discussions concerning the mechanisms by which adolescents procure cigarettes (e.g., "bumming" them from friends or peers), how they view smoking (perceived prevalence and social norms), and the rate at which they progress through the various stages of smoking. Prevalence can be measured by asking questions concerning smoking behavior in the past week, month, year, or ever in one's lifetime. Data on the number of people who smoke every day and the intensity of smoking behavior (how much one smokes per day) also provide important contextual information for considering what tobacco control interventions to undertake.

One caveat with regard to interpreting prevalence data is particularly important. Adolescents' reporting of their smoking behavior may not be accurate, as they may either underreport or overreport their actual smoking activity. In one study, students reported ever smoking at one phase and never smoking at another.[33] This means that the true number of ever-smokers, current smokers, and daily smokers may be greater (or smaller) than reported.

As adolescents pass through different stages of smoking, their "reported smoking status should be regarded from a developmental point of view and not as a static event."[34] Questions used to determine prevalence can capture an adolescent's smoking stage, but not the direction he or she is heading or how long he or she has been or will be at that stage. For example, a response to the question "Have you smoked within the last 30 days?" would be "No" if the individual had smoked 31 days prior. If the individual answered "Yes," he or she would be labeled a current smoker even if it were the first and last cigarette. Therefore, the number of current smokers reported by any study may contain respondents ranging from those who have smoked only once and will never again to those smoking more than 100 times in the past 30 days. Because these trajectories are so important to the natural history of tobacco use, the paucity of longitudinal data that thoroughly track specific individuals is a serious limitation of existing research.

The MTF project has been collecting data on smoking prevalence since 1975 for high school seniors and since 1991 for eighth and tenth graders. The subsections that follow show the changes in prevalence for lifetime, 30-day, and daily smoking over the past 25 years.

Prevalence of Ever Smoking

Students who initiate smoking, even once, become ever-smokers, meaning that they have ever smoked in their lifetime. The prevalence of ever-smokers has hovered around 70 percent for twelfth graders since 1975[35] and, as expected, is lower for tenth graders and lower still for eighth graders. Just under half of students leaving middle school throughout the 1990s had tried smoking, according to the MTF survey.[36] Significantly lower numbers are reported by the 1997 NHSDA for comparably aged adolescents.[37] However, data from the 1998 NHSDA follow the same pattern as MTF data for age, with a higher percentage of older students than younger students having tried smoking.[38] These surveys indicate that a majority of adolescents leave high school with at least some experience with smoking.

Prevalence of Current Smoking

Many of the data sources also contain survey information concerning contemporary adolescent smoking behavior. In the literature, this is referred to as current smoking, 30-day prevalence, or past-month smoking, and it measures whether the survey respondent smoked at least one cigarette in the 30 days preceding the survey.[39] Current smokers are considered more at risk than ever-smokers for advanced stages of smoking, but their numbers have declined recently.[40] In 1998, approximately 4.1 million adolescents aged 12–17 were current smokers,[41] down from 4.5 million in 1997.[42]

For all age-groups, 30-day prevalence is somewhat lower than lifetime prevalence, suggesting that many students do not progress from trying one cigarette to somewhat more regular smoking. MTF data show remarkable declines after 1976 in the percentage of twelfth graders smoking within the 30 days preceding the survey. From 1980 to 1992, the percentage of seniors reporting current smoking hovered around 30 percent. The MTF study reported sharp increases in current smoking for eighth and tenth graders beginning in 1991 and for twelfth graders starting in 1992. But MTF data from 2000 show substantial declines from 1996 figures in smoking in the past 30 days for eighth and tenth graders.[43] Nevertheless, these data indicate that 15 percent of eighth graders, 24 percent of tenth graders, and 31 percent of twelfth graders smoked at least one cigarette during the past 30 days.

Last thirty days or current smoking prevalence rates for adolescents vary markedly by survey. For example, in 1990, adolescents reported smoking at least once in the last 30 days at rates ranging from 9.2 percent from the California Tobacco Survey (CTS)[44] to 15.7 percent from the TAPS (in 1989) and 29.4 percent from the MTF survey. More current data are as variable. The disparities in 30-day smoking rates for given years translate into visible differences in smoking trends over time as reported by the MTF survey, the NHSDA, and the NHIS.[45] No survey reported declines in 30-day prevalence in the mid-1990s, and both the CTS and the MTF survey showed increases. The low numbers reported by the CTS most likely reflect the influence of California's youth tobacco control campaign (discussed in chapter 4), along with the influence of more restrictive clean indoor air laws. It may also reflect being a local sample in a state with a different social and ethnic mix and the second lowest smoking rate in the nation. In view of differences between these surveys, the common upward trend is probably more reliable than any given cross-sectional estimate in any of the surveys.

Prevalence of Daily Smoking

MTF data concerning the prevalence of daily smoking and smoking more than half a pack a day show similar trends as the lifetime and 30-

day data. Those who smoke frequently[46] or daily are fewer in number and tend to be older.[47] Those who smoke more than half a pack a day are even rarer. In 1999, 13.2 percent of twelfth graders smoked more than half a pack per day. We can ascertain a trend starting in the early 1990s of increased daily smoking, which is consistent with trends in 30-day smoking rates and first-time and daily initiation rates.[48]

Yet the stability in the rates of adolescents smoking half a pack a day will indicate that the upward trend in the number of adolescent smokers may not, as some researchers have found, result in heavier smoking over time. In addition, it may suggest more experimenters and changes in transition patterns that have not so far been detected in research findings. This would be consistent with the recent observation that adult smoking data show a sizable (nearly 20 percent) and growing proportion of nondaily smokers.[49]

Prevalence Data by Subgroup

Consistent with trends in other subgroup smoking behaviors, there have been overall increases in smoking prevalence for all levels of smoking in this decade, regardless of socioeconomic status (SES) or parents' education level. Disparities in smoking rates by parents' education level have lessened since 1975. Figures from 1998 show that the differences in the proportion of smokers among twelfth graders were minimal, which means that twelfth-grade students at all SES levels are smoking at approximately the same rate. For eighth graders, however, smoking rates vary by SES, with children of families with higher SES smoking far less than children of families with lower SES.[50]

The percent of blacks and whites in the twelfth grade who had smoked in the past 30 days in 1977 were comparable, at 37 percent and 38 percent, respectively, according to MTF data. However, the percentage of twelfth-grade African American smokers dropped dramatically over the next 15 years to 11 percent in 1991, while the prevalence for whites remained high (at 32 percent in 1991).

Reversing the trends of the 1980s,[51] it appears as if all major subgroups (whites, Hispanics, African Americans, boys, girls, eighth graders, tenth graders, and twelfth graders) experienced increased smoking prevalence between 1991 and 1996.[52] The smoking behaviors of these groups were similar in 1977 but varied by the late 1980s, until the unified upward trend starting in the early 1990s.

Updated to 1999 in the National Youth Tobacco Survey, the low smoking prevalence observed among African American youth prior to the early 1990s is no longer apparent in middle school. These middle school trends presage increasing high school and adult smoking rates among African Americans. A CDC report summarized these trends: "current cigarette smoking prevalence among middle school black students was similar to rates among white and Hispanic students and . . . cigar use prevalence among middle school black students was significantly higher than among white students."[53]

In contrast, the proportion of African American adults who smoke is slightly higher than the proportion of white adults who smoke.[54] The smoking behavior of different groups may change during the transition from adolescence to adulthood—specifically, whites may reduce smoking or quit at a greater rate than do African Americans. African Americans may initiate smoking at older ages than whites, which may suggest why adult African American smoking rates are higher than those of whites while adolescent rates are the opposite. With the increases in current smoking by African Americans and whites, adult prevalence rates will probably increase, but disproportionately, so that in the next few years we may see considerable growth in adult African American smoking rates.

Another aspect of disparate smoking rates across subgroups is economic disadvantage. Several studies of low-income families have found low smoking prevalence rates.[55] In particular, these studies suggest that the very poor smoke less but that lower-than-average income groups smoke more than higher-than-average income groups. Perhaps SES, parental education levels, and disposable income, rather than racial differences, can account for some of the disparities in smoking rates.

Adolescents who are not in school or who have been placed in alternative educational settings are particularly at risk of tobacco use. These students are at risk for being expelled or dropping out of regular high school. In a recent YRBSS survey of alternative high school students, the CDC reported that this subgroup is more likely to use cigarettes and cigars than a comparable regular high school population.[56] For example, 90.8 percent of the subgroup had ever tried cigarettes, while 64.1 percent reported smoking during the past 30 days. They were also more likely to use smokeless tobacco and smoke cigars than were the comparable high school age-group. As we detail in chapter 3, this subgroup is also at high risk of alcohol and illicit substance use.

Prevalence Data by Age

Despite disparities in reported percentages of current smokers across the surveys, there is general agreement on smoking prevalence by age-group. The NHSDA reports 30-day prevalence at 8 percent for 12–13 year olds, 18.2 percent for 14–15 year olds, and 29.3 percent for 16–17 year olds.[57] Similar trends are reported by the CTS[58] and the YRBSS[59] and MTF surveys.[60]

As teens reach late adolescence and enter into young adulthood, their current smoking rates approach adult-level smoking rates. One reason for this may be that so few adolescents and young adults quit. Although current smoking rates peak in the twenties, adolescent current smoking rates are as high or higher than rates in other segments of the population.[61] The percentage of current adult smokers as compared to the percentage of adolescent smokers is shown in figure 3. The figure shows distinctly that adult smoking rates are continuing to decline just as adolescent smoking rates are continuing to increase. This suggests that we are having greater success in adult cessation than in preventing youth initiation and that reduced teen initiation rates in the 1980s led to lower adult smoking rates thereafter. Much of the subsequent adult decline represents the aging-out of smokers from their peak smoking years. A result of the higher smoking rates seen in the mid-1990s will probably be increases in current smoking rates for adult populations in the next decade (2000–2009), suggesting the policy need to provide incentives for youth and adult smoking cessation.

Prevalence Data by Gender

MTF data show that twelfth-grade males' 30-day smoking prevalence actually slowly increased for most of the 1980s (from 27 percent in 1981 to 29 percent in 1991) before more rapidly increasing in the 1990s. By contrast, 30-day prevalence for twelfth-grade females was declining in the 1980s (from 33 percent in 1980 to 26 percent in 1992) before increasing. Since 1991, the percentage of male and female smokers has been relatively equal.[62]

Cessation

As we noted earlier, prevalence data are influenced by the number of new smokers, current smokers, and those who quit smoking. A number of regular adolescent smokers attempt to quit each year. Nearly three-quarters of smokers reported in the TAPS data (1989) that they had seriously considered quitting.[63] Between 1976 and 1989, more than 40 percent of high school seniors who were current smokers reported wanting to stop smoking. During the same time period, between 25 percent and 40 percent of those trying to stop smoking found they could not.[64]

The consequences of even small increases in youth smoking prevalence are still quite large to society because of the low cessation rates in adolescence. A large number of adolescent smokers seem to believe that they will not smoke in the future, even though adolescent quit rates are rather low. Among high school seniors, 31.9 percent of those smoking a pack or more a day, 41.6 percent of those smoking about half a pack daily, 60.6 percent of those smoking one to five cigarettes daily, and 84.8 percent of those smoking less than once a day thought they "probably" or "definitely" would not be smoking in five years.[65] Rather than succeeding at quitting within five years, one study estimates that for white males and females born between 1975 and 1979, only 50 percent of smokers will have quit by ages 33 and 37, respectively. The study further estimates that a male adolescent who initiates smoking now may smoke for 16 to 20 years; a female adolescent, for 20 to 30 years.[66] Among seniors who reported smoking one to five cigarettes a day, twice as many as the number who had quit smoking were smoking with the same intensity or consuming more cigarettes five to six years later. Among people who had been smoking about half a pack of cigarettes a day in their senior year of high school and people who had been smoking a pack or more a day, respectively three and four times as many as had quit were still smoking as much or more five to six years later.[67]

Factors Influencing Adolescent Tobacco Use Trends

Perceptions

Youths' perceptions of smoking are also captured in the data. The MTF survey asks respondents whether they believe that smoking a pack or more a day is harmful; whether or not cigarettes are easily accessible; and the extent to which they disapprove of people who smoke more than a pack of cigarettes per day.[68] Analysis of MTF data reveals a relationship between lifetime tobacco use and disapproval of smoking. As smoking increases, disapproval decreases (measured among twelfth graders from 1975 to 1999 and among eighth and tenth graders from 1991 to 1999). Similarly, as more adolescents smoke, the perceived risk of smoking also declines. In short, when adolescent smoking rates are increasing, both disapproval and perceived risk decline. When adolescent smoking rates are decreasing, disapproval and perceived risk increase. Nonetheless, disapproval of smoking has remained high for all age-groups through the years, with at least 65 percent or more strongly disapproving of smoking more than one and a half packs per day. Awareness of the risks of smoking has increased since 1975.

Sources for Adolescent Access to Tobacco Products

Most adolescents believe that cigarettes are readily available,[69] even though it is illegal for minors to purchase or be sold cigarettes in virtually every state.[70] A vast majority of eighth graders (around 70 percent) and tenth graders (around 88 percent) believe that cigarettes are "fairly easy" or "very easy" to obtain.[71] Cigarettes are perceived to be easier to obtain than other drugs, such as marijuana. This relationship is maintained in use rates, with a greater percentage of adolescents using cigarettes than marijuana, but with a smaller percentage using cigarettes than alcohol.[72]

In one study, 83 percent of ever-smokers reported not usually buying their own cigarettes; also, adolescents with best friends who smoke are significantly more likely than others to report getting cigarettes from other smokers.[73] It appears that experimenters rely on friends, peers, and family members to supply cigarettes.[74] Not surprisingly, older adolescents are more likely to purchase their own cigarettes than are their younger counterparts.[75] This pattern is independent of smoking status (although smoking status and age are highly correlated).

That friends play a vital role in smoking, as, at the very least, suppliers of cigarettes, is supported by the literature on risk factors (described in greater detail in chapter 3). Some observers suggest that as adolescents progress to higher use rates, they cannot depend so heavily on the generosity of friends and must take cigarettes from home or attempt to purchase them.[76] That is why 25 percent of current smokers in the 1999 YRBSS survey (down from 30 percent in 1997) had purchased their own cigarettes in the last 30 days[77] and why over 80 percent of addicted smokers in the CTS reported their usual source as the store.[78] Adolescents overwhelmingly purchase cigarettes from retailers, either from liquor stores or gas stations or from large stores, such as supermarkets; only a small percent from 1990 to 1996 reported getting cigarettes from vending machines.[79] Determining where adolescents purchase cigarettes and then denying access by means of enforcement is an important tobacco control policy concern.

Adolescent Use of Other Tobacco Products

In addition to cigarettes, policymakers need to be aware of adolescent use of other tobacco products, such as cigars, bidis, and smokeless tobacco (fig. 6). Shifting from cigarettes to these other tobacco products would not necessarily present any public health gains, though smokeless tobacco is less harmful than cigarettes.

Cigars

The use of cigars by the adolescent population appears to mirror their rise in popularity among adults earlier this decade. According to the results of the NHSDA, an estimated 6.9 percent of the population 12 years old and older reported smoking cigars within the past month in 1998; this represents a significant increase from the 1997 rate of 5.9 percent.[80] In a 1996 national survey of youth from age 14–19 conducted by the Robert Wood Johnson Foundation, 26.7 percent admitted having smoked a cigar in the past year. Males (at 37 percent) were more than twice as likely as females (at 16 percent) to report smoking cigars.[81]

More recent data from a survey of middle school and high school students in Florida indicate that cigar use may be declining.[82] Several significant declines were reported for the percentage of males, whites, and total adolescents smoking cigars within the past month in populations at junior high age.[83]

The adolescents who appear most likely to experiment with cigars are those who have already initiated some other form of tobacco use. Cigarette smokers and smokeless tobacco users were both more than three times as likely to have reported smoking a cigar than were nonusers of tobacco, and they were respectively nine and seven times more likely to report cigar use than were nonusers in a survey by the

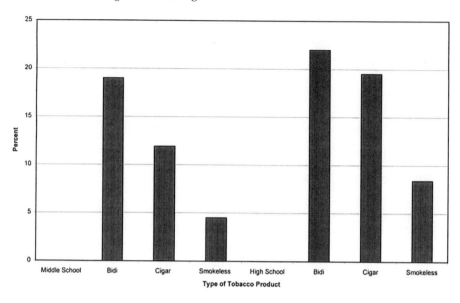

Fig. 6. Current tobacco use, 1999

Massachusetts Public Health Department (1996–97).[84] Marijuana users (using in the past 30 days and ever) are between six and eight times as likely to report cigar smoking.[85]

These findings indicate that cigar use and use of other tobacco products and marijuana overlap. The same students who are experimenting with cigars are also experimenting with other forms of tobacco and other drugs, while other students are refraining from experimentation with these substances altogether. Among students who had ever purchased their own cigars, more than half reported that they were "never" or "rarely" questioned about their age.[86]

Bidis

Bidis are filterless, flavored, hand-rolled cigarettes that deliver three times the carbon monoxide and nicotine and five times the tar of regular cigarettes.[87] Addiction to nicotine may occur more rapidly to regular smokers of bidis because of their higher nicotine content as compared to cigarettes. However, adolescents believe them to be safer, as well as easier to buy, than cigarettes.[88]

At this time, bidi use is somewhat lower than cigarette use, but we are in the early stages of bidi experimentation; predicting an upward trend in their use seems reasonable. Approximately 16 percent of adolescents use bidis currently, though national data remain sketchy. In a survey of inner-city youth, 40 percent of seventh through twelfth graders indicated that they had ever smoked a bidi, and 16 percent said that they were current bidi smokers. Surprisingly, 8 percent of those surveyed had smoked 100 or more, which suggests that bidi use may be a substitute for cigarette smoking.[89] The National Youth Tobacco Survey found that high school students' use of bidis and similar products equals that of smokeless tobacco use.[90]

However, researchers assessing the Massachusetts Tobacco Control Program conducted a follow-up survey of Massachusetts youth and found that bidi use was much lower among the general adolescent population.[91] In this survey, ever use was 7.8 percent, while current use was under 1 percent. If confirmed by subsequent analyses, these results suggest that the bidi phenomenon is less extensive than currently believed, though its concentration in minority communities is worrisome.

Of particular interest to those concerned with reducing youth tobacco consumption is the finding that bidis are considered by adolescents to be safer, better tasting, more flavorful, and easier to buy than cigarettes. Adolescents in this survey also indicated that they smoked bidis "just to try it" or because "my friends smoke them."[92] That bidis have been reported to be substitutes for cigarettes or marijuana[93] for some adolescents indicates that education about the health effects of bidis should be integrated into existing smoking and drug prevention interventions.

Because bidi use is a relatively recent phenomenon in the United States, much of what we know either comes from scholarship concerning India or is anecdotal. Given the magnitude of its adoption by adolescents, bidi use merits considerable attention and research.

Smokeless Tobacco

Smokeless tobacco is also referred to as snuff, chew, dip, or spit tobacco. The use of smokeless tobacco is not nearly as common as cigarette use (for either adolescents or adults).[94] Data from the 1998 NHSDA indicate that approximately 3.1 percent of the population aged

12 and older were current smokeless tobacco users (as measured by 30-day prevalence rates), a percentage that has been stable since 1991.[95] The 1998 rates of current adolescent use were 6.9 percent in middle school populations and 6.7 percent in high school populations (including 8.8 percent for twelfth graders).[96] However, survey data from Florida from 1998 and 1999 indicate some significant declines in then current use of smokeless tobacco among middle school students and insignificant declines among high school students.[97] MTF data from 2000 show significant declines in use of smokeless tobacco, dropping by 45 percent among eighth graders, 42 percent for tenth graders, and 38 percent among twelfth graders.[98]

Data from the 1989 and 1993 TAPS found that 12.7 percent of 12–18 year olds had experimented with smokeless tobacco[99] and that 4 percent had become daily users between baseline and the 4-year follow-up period.[100] Males and whites use smokeless tobacco at higher rates than do females and other ethnicities.[101] Smokeless tobacco use has been considered a rural problem, but recent data indicate that it is almost as common in suburban and urban populations.[102]

Unlike cigarette use, which is associated with less physical activity, two studies found that smokeless tobacco use could be predicted by participation in organized sports.[103] As with cigar and bidi smoking, smokeless tobacco use is associated with other substance use. In one study, smokeless tobacco users of all ethnicities were more likely to smoke cigarettes or marijuana and to drink alcohol.[104]

As is the case with cigarettes, research indicates that smokeless tobacco is often purchasable by youth. Two studies from Florida report that adolescents were able to purchase smokeless tobacco 32–35 percent of the time,[105] with similar findings in California.[106] In all likelihood, these studies actually underestimate availability, because individuals can make repeated purchases once they find a merchant who does not require proper identification.

Adolescent Substance Use

Since 1990, adolescent consumption of alcohol and illegal drugs has increased, though consumption of these substances remains significantly below the levels of 20 years ago. This is a different pattern than for adolescent tobacco use, though trends seemed similar during the early 1990s.

Illicit Drugs

A report from the 1997 NHSDA indicates that current smokers, aged 12–17, are 12 times more likely to use illicit drugs and 23 times more likely to drink heavily than are noncurrent smokers.[107] Of current smokers in 1997, 19.8 percent had used an illicit drug other than marijuana in the past month, compared to only 1.6 percent of noncurrent smokers. This confirms findings from studies discussed in chapter 3 linking cigarette use with other drug use and suggests that some students are experimenting concurrently, or perhaps even simultaneously, with drugs, alcohol, and cigarettes. Figure 4 shows trends in current smoking and any illicit drug use by high school seniors, based on MTF data. The decreases in use starting in the 1980s began reversing for current smoking, any illicit drug use, and any illicit drug use other than marijuana in 1992.

The parallel trends across different substances are especially noteworthy. They may indicate that drugs are often used in combination, with the implication that successful reduction in use of one drug may lead to reduction in other drug use. Another interpretation is that some important underlying factors are driving all of these substance abuse trends. Unfortunately, we do not really know what these factors are or how we might change them.

Figure 7 illustrates the magnitude of these trends, using annual data from the MTF survey of self-reported adolescent substance use. The survey asked students in grades 7–12 whether they had used tobacco or other substances during the previous month. Cocaine use is far less common than the other three behaviors targeted in the survey. It is therefore plotted on a different scale, using the secondary axis labeled on the right-hand side of figure 7.

As is shown in the figure, adolescent substance use has widely fluctuated over the 1980s and 1990s. Especially significant for policy, smoking is the only form of adolescent substance use that was more prevalent in 1998 than it was in 1980.

Swings in the reported prevalence of cocaine use are especially marked. The initial rise in adolescent use likely reflects the dramatic decline in cocaine prices, and accompanying increase in availability, that began during the early 1980s. Casual cocaine use by adolescents subsequently declined, despite continued reductions in cocaine market prices. These trends appear to reflect the greatly increased social stigma

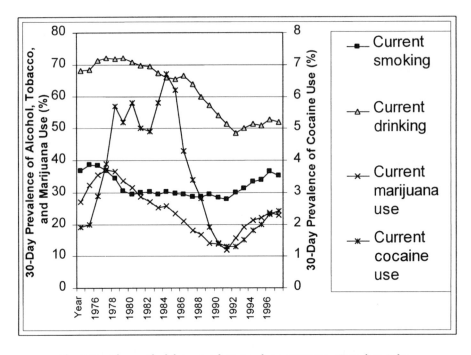

Fig. 7. Prevalence of adolescent substance abuse, 1976–96. (Data from Johnson, O'Malley, and Bachman 1999, 2000. Annual prevalence estimates, various years.)

associated with cocaine use, focused prevention efforts, and the more vigorous law enforcement activity of the late 1980s and early 1990s.[108]

The MTF data also suggest that adolescent substance use became more prevalent during the 1990s. Marijuana and tobacco use show the largest prevalence increases in the 1990s, though marijuana use remains more than 15 percentage points less prevalent than it was in 1980. Reasons for the increased prevalence are not fully known. At any point in time, individual factors, such as family income, grades, and truancy, strongly predict which adolescents are most likely to use illicit substances. Over time, however, patterns of adolescent substance use changed much more rapidly than did individual risk factors known to influence substance use.

Alcohol Use

The MTF data presented in figure 7 also show important patterns in adolescent alcohol use. The prevalence of adolescent drinking declined by almost 20 percentage points between 1986 and 1993. Indirect evidence, such as reduced youth involvement in road fatalities, also suggests declining alcohol use.[109] This sharp drop coincided with several policy initiatives that discouraged adolescent alcohol use. The 1984 Federal Uniform Drinking Act authorized the Department of Transportation to withhold a portion of federal highway funds to states that maintained minimum drinking ages below the age of 21. By 1988, all 50 states had raised the minimum drinking age to meet federal requirements.[110] By examining the timing of these policy initiatives in different states, researchers have shown that as the minimum age for drinking rises from 18 to 21, adolescent alcohol consumption declines.[111]

Many analysts suggest that youth consumption would have declined even further if alcohol excise taxes had been increased to keep pace with inflation in recent years. Correcting for inflation, excise taxes on beer and liquor are substantially lower than they were during the 1950s and represent a smaller fraction of consumer prices.[112] At least one study suggests that alcohol taxes are far below the levels necessary to compensate for alcohol's social costs.[113]

Communicating Risks

There is strong evidence that adolescents are sensitive to the perceived risks and social stigma in their decisions about marijuana and cocaine use.[114] Changes in the prevalence of self-reported substance use are linked with the proportion of teens reporting that marijuana and cocaine bring health and other risks. In this study, use trends were also highly correlated with changes in the proportion of adolescents who report that they would disapprove of regular users. As news coverage of drug issues and antidrug advertisements declined during the early 1990s, there was a proportionate rise in drug use.

As described in Michael Massing's *The Fix,* government antidrug efforts strongly emphasized adolescent marijuana use during the early 1980s.[115] These public policies were complemented by parent and community groups that also focused on adolescent marijuana use. Ten years later, policymakers placed less emphasis on this issue, as other social problems—such as adult crack addiction and HIV infection among injection drug users—rose to public prominence.

It is also possible that marijuana has become more widely used in the wake of stronger policy measures against youth drinking. Although the available empirical evidence is mixed, many analysts suggest that alcohol and marijuana are economic substitutes.[116] This means that if the price of one of these substances is raised, buyers will purchase more of the other. If so, increased barriers to alcohol use (such as enhanced law enforcement or higher prices) are likely to encourage some compensating increase in marijuana use.[117]

Noting that alcohol is more addictive than marijuana and that alcohol is more closely related to criminal violence and road fatalities, some commentators suggest that less stringent marijuana enforcement may have unintended, yet desirable, effects if such policies reduce the overall level of alcohol use.[118] The point of such analyses is not to encourage any form of adolescent substance use. Rather, the point is to highlight the unintended (and sometimes undesirable) consequences of substance-specific policies that affect interrelated drug-using behaviors.

Conclusion

Despite a decade of close attention to discouraging youth tobacco use, rates of adolescent tobacco use are higher now than a decade earlier, virtually erasing previous progress in reducing such use. This is puzzling because the rise occurred despite reduced adult tobacco use and decreased use of illicit substances among adolescents. To understand why these trends are occurring, we need to focus on the factors that predict and explain adolescent tobacco use. That is the subject of chapter 3.

NOTES

1. USDHHS 1994.
2. CDC 2000a.
3. CDC 1998b.
4. MTF 1997, 1998, 1999; MMWR (2000).
5. This figure combines data from the Monitoring the Future survey and the NHIS. The rates of current smoking reported by other surveys are different, so it is not possible to generalize trends across all surveys. However, upward trends were reported in most surveys.
6. CDC 1998b.
7. Johnston et al. 1999.
8. SAMHSA 1998.
9. Johnston, O'Malley, and Bachman 2000.
10. Johnston et al. 1999. For a recent review of adolescent tobacco use trends, see Giovino 1999.
11. CDC 2000.

12. SAMHSA 1999.

13. Johnston, O'Malley, and Bachman 1998b.

14. CDC 1998a.

15. Greene, Ennett, and Ringwalt 1997; CDC 1999e.

16. Pierce et al. 1998a.

17. USDHHS 1994; CDC 1998a; CDC 1996c.

18. Pierce and Gilpin 1996.

19. Johnston, O'Malley, and Bachman 1998b.

20. Anda et al. 1999.

21. The YRBSS survey adds a category of frequent smoking, which is smoking on 20 of the past 30 days.

22. Marcus et al. 1993.

23. "Respondents completed the questionnaire that included questions about cigarette use. To estimate age of first use, respondents were asked, 'How old were you the first time you smoked a cigarette, even one or two puffs?' To estimate age of first daily use, respondents were asked, 'How old were you when you first started smoking cigarettes every day?' The year of initiation of first use and of first daily use were calculated by subtracting each respondent's date of birth from the interview date and then adding the age of first use or first daily use. Estimates of the number of new smokers for a given year during 1965–1995 (for first use) and 1965–1996 (for first daily use) were calculated by combining data on all respondents and applying sample weights; age-specific estimates for any given year used only data for persons in the respective age ranges during the year" (CDC 1998b).

24. CDC 1998b.

25. CDC 1998b.

26. CDC 1998b.

27. CDC 1998b.

28. Researchers estimate that 1,226,000 persons less than 18 years of age became daily smokers in 1996 (CDC 1998b).

29. CDC 1999f.

30. CDC 1998a.

31. Everett et al. 1999.

32. Breslau and Peterson 1996.

33. Abernathy 1997.

34. Abernathy 1997.

35. Johnston, O'Malley, and Bachman 1999.

36. Johnston, O'Malley, and Bachman 1999. YRBSS data are for students in the ninth through twelfth grades. Lifetime prevalence for whites was 71.1 percent for whites, 66 percent for African Americans, and 76.3 percent for Hispanics.

37. Lifetime prevalence percentages for 16–17 year olds in 1996 and 1997 were 52.5 percent and 56.3 percent, respectively. For 18–20 year olds in 1996 and 1997, 64.3 percent and 65 percent, respectively, reported ever smoking (SAMHSA 1998).

38. SAMHSA 1999.

39. USDHHS 1994; Johnston, O'Malley, and Bachman 1996.

40. See chapter 3 for a full discussion, and see particularly Rowe et al. 1996 and Patton et al. 1998b.

41. SAMHSA 1999.

42. SAMHSA 1998.

43. Johnston, O'Malley, and Bachman 2000. NHSDA data indicate declines after 1997 (from 19.9 percent to 18.2 percent) (SAMHSA 1998, 1999).

44. The California Tobacco Survey is part of an evaluation of the California Tobacco Control Program.

45. Nelson et al. 1995.

46. Among the surveys, only the YRBSS measures frequency, which it defines as smoking on 20 of the past 30 days preceding the survey.

47. Johnston, O'Malley, and Bachman 1999b; CDC 1991.

48. CDC 1998b; Johnston, O'Malley, and Bachman 1998b.

49. Mendez and Warner 1998.

50. Giovino 1999.

51. Nelson et al. 1995. The MTF data indicate a slow increase in smoking prevalence in males over this decade, which differs from other results reported in Nelson et al. 1995.

52. Johnston, O'Malley, and Bachman 1999.

53. CDC 2000a.

54. CDC 1999f; Feigelman and Lee 1995. Fiegelman and Lee (1995) attribute low rates of smoking cessation in African American populations to earlier initiation of smoking in this group, which has been found to be related to lowered cessation rates in other studies (Breslau and Peterson 1996).

55. Epstein, Botvin, and Diaz 1998a, 1998b; Farrell, Danish, and Howard 1992; Epstein et al. 1999.

56. CDC 1999e.

57. SAMHSA 1999.

58. Pierce, Gilpin, Emery, Farkas, et al. 1998.

59. CDC 1998a.

60. Johnston, O'Malley, and Bachman 1999b.

61. SAMHSA 1999.

62. Johnston, O'Malley, and Bachman 1999b.

63. Allen et al. 1993.

64. USDHHS 1994.

65. USDHHS 1994.

66. Pierce and Gilpin 1996. To be classified as a smoker, the respondent had to have smoked more than 100 cigarettes in his or her lifetime.

67. USDHHS 1994. The actual figures are as follows: For those smoking 15 cigarettes, 56 years later 29.6 percent had quit and 61.6 percent were smoking as much or more. For those smoking about half a pack a day, 56 years later 18.8 percent had quit and 67.7 percent were smoking as much or more. For those smoking more than one pack a day, 56 years later 13.2 percent had quit and 69.2 percent were smoking as much or more. These data come from the Monitoring the Future project.

68. The actual questions are "How much do you think people risk harming themselves (physically or other ways) if they . . . ?" "How difficult do you think

it would be for you to get each of the following types of drugs, if you wanted some?" and "Do you disapprove of people who . . . ?" The data discussed earlier pertain to cigarette data only: see <http://health.org/pubs/monito/table6.htm>.

69. Johnston, O'Malley, and Bachman 1998b.

70. Johnston et al. 1999.

71. Johnston et al. 1999.

72. Johnston, O'Malley, and Bachman 1998b.

73. Pierce, Gilpin, Emery, Farkas, et al. 1998.

74. Pierce, Gilpin, Emery, Farkas, et al. 1998.

75. Pierce, Gilpin, Emery, Farkas, et al. 1998; Johnston et al. 1999.

76. Pierce, Gilpin, Emery, Farkas, et al. 1998c.

77. CDC 2000b.

78. Pierce, Gilpin, Emery, Farkas, et al. 1998c.

79. Pierce, Gilpin, Emery, Farkas, et al. 1998c.

80. SAMHSA 1999.

81. CDC 1997a.

82. CDC 1999a.

83. CDC 1999a.

84. CDC 1997a.

85. CDC 1997a.

86. CDC 1997a.

87. CDC 1999b.

88. CDC 1999b.

89. CDC 1999b.

90. CDC 2000a.

91. Unpublished results by Biener, E-mail message to the Society for Research on Nicotine and Tobacco, February 3, 2000.

92. CDC 1999b.

93. CDC 1999b.

94. Hu et al. 1996; CDC 1998c.

95. SAMHSA 1999.

96. CDC 1999a; Johnston, O'Malley, and Bachman 1998b.

97. CDC 1999a.

98. Johnston, O'Malley, and Bachman 2000.

99. An experimenter was defined as someone who used smokeless tobacco but not regularly. Regular users reported having started using smokeless tobacco on a regular basis.

100. Tomar and Giovino 1998.

101. Hu et al. 1996; SAMHSA 1999; Tomar and Giovino 1998; CDC 2000a.

102. Sussman et al. 1993; Tomar and Giovino 1998.

103. Hu et al. 1996; Tomar and Giovino 1998.

104. Hu et al. 1996. All odds ratios were significant except for the interaction of use with drinking in the African American population.

105. CDC 1995; CDC 1996a.

106. CDC 1996b.

107. SAMHSA 1998.

108. Caulkins and Reuter 1998; Kleiman 1993.

109. Kenkel 1993; Chaloupka, Saffer, and Grossman 1993; Cook and Moore 1994; Dee and Evans 1997.

110. Bachman, Johnston, and O'Malley 1990.

111. Chaloupka, Saffer, and Grossman 1993.

112. Kenkel 1993; Chaloupka, Saffer, and Grossman 1993; Cook and Moore 1994; Dee and Evans 1997.

113. Manning et al. 1989.

114. Bachman, Johnston, and O'Malley 1990; Bachman et al. 1988.

115. Massing 1998.

116. Pacula 1998; Chaloupka and Laixuthai 1997.

117. Boyum and Kleiman 1995.

118. Boyum and Kleiman 1995.

3

The Social Context of
Adolescent Smoking

Why do some children and adolescents initiate smoking when most are aware that tobacco use is harmful and may result in early death? Interventions to prevent youth smoking must start with this basic puzzle. Clinical and policy interventions must confront the underlying dynamics that lead some children and adolescents to experiment with or to initiate regular smoking while others avoid tobacco use altogether. Clinicians, tobacco control advocates, and policymakers should be aware of the processes that lead most adolescents who become routine smokers to continue to use tobacco into adulthood while a smaller group ceases continued use.

This chapter considers these matters in some detail to frame the social context in which youth tobacco use emerges and how tobacco control policy toward adolescents must operate. Among the questions we will address are: Which young people are especially likely to initiate smoking and at which ages? Which young people appear most resistant to tobacco use? How and why do adolescents move through the different stages of smoking behaviors? What can policymakers, tobacco control advocates, and clinicians learn from these examples?

Our primary interest in this chapter is to review existing research regarding adolescent tobacco use.[1] In doing so, we describe the considerable progress researchers have made in understanding individual risk factors and social influences on smoking initiation and on critical transitions from nonsmoking to experimentation to regular smoking to cessation. We examine the complex interactions between individual characteristics, personal behaviors, and the social influences associated with adolescent smoking, focusing on how those factors affect smoking decisions at the various stages of smoking behavior.

The literature presents a myriad of risk factors associated with youth smoking, often working in conjunction with each other (see table 2). Adolescents do not make choices or decisions regarding tobacco use in a personal vacuum. Policymakers and tobacco control advocates must be aware that the reasons adolescents smoke are as varied as teens themselves. Another caveat is that the studies are for the most part performed on white, middle-class, suburban, usually school-based samples—a fact that has obvious implications for their application to the general adolescent population.

The studies we synthesize in this chapter vary in types of analyses performed, which are largely dependent on the type of data collected.

TABLE 2. Association of Risk Factors with Youth Smoking

Factors	Association
Sociodemographic	
Age	Yes
Gender	No
Ethnicity/race	Yes
Acculturation	Yes
Family structure	Yes
Parental socioeconomic status	Yes
Personal income	Yes
Urban/rural residence	Undecided
Environmental	
Parental smoking	Yes
Parental attitudes	Yes
Sibling smoking	Yes
Peer smoking	Yes
Peer attitudes and norms	Yes
Family environment	Yes
Attachment to family/friends	Yes
Availability of tobacco	Undecided
Behavioral	
School factors	Yes
Risk behavior	Yes
Lifestyle	Yes
Personal	
Stress	Yes
Coping	Undecided
Depression/distress	Yes
Self-esteem	Yes
Attitudes toward smoking/smokers	Yes
Knowledge of health effects	Undecided
Personal health concerns	Yes

Source: Tyas and Pederson 1998.

Most studies use a cross-sectional design, but several provide longitudinal data on adolescent smoking initiation. A cross-sectional study is equivalent to a snapshot at one point in time. In a longitudinal study, participants are followed over a period of time. Longitudinal studies more accurately describe how and when (and perhaps why) adolescents progress from one stage to another. Unless otherwise noted, the characteristics of adolescents discussed here are meant to connote associations and correlations with cigarette smoking rather than causal links. This means that the existing research is suggestive of how the various factors influence smoking behavior rather than concluding that particular factors cause tobacco use. It is nearly impossible to separate any one factor from the other forces influencing adolescent smoking behavior.

Overview

Adolescent smoking behavior is a dynamic process that changes over time. For most adolescents, attitudes toward smoking change at different ages, and decisions to smoke or not smoke are made at multiple times during adolescence. For most youth, there is no one point where a permanent decision regarding tobacco use is irrevocably made. In fact, the "nonsmoking adolescent population" is a more complex, diverse group than that name might imply. Some are people who will never smoke, some may be susceptible to smoking in the future or are currently experimenting at low levels, and others are former experimenters or regular smokers.

We now know a fair amount about the reasons adolescents smoke and the characteristics of adolescent smokers. In the years since the 1994 surgeon general's report and the publication, in the same year, of the IOM's *Growing Up Tobacco Free*, a substantial body of research has emerged to provide greater insight into these reasons and, at times, how they might interact with each other. Recent research adds considerably to our understanding of how the various factors influence decisions to initiate tobacco use. Yet our understanding of the causes of the progression through other stages of smoking behaviors is relatively inferior to our knowledge of relationships between the risk factors and smoking. Despite the gaps in our knowledge, the following points reasonably describe the social context of adolescent smoking.

- Peer influences play a critical role both in decisions to smoke and in transitions to more intense smoking. Peer influences become stronger as adolescents age.
- Parental and familial attitudes toward smoking, smoking status, and cigarette advertising are influential in adolescents' decisions to smoke or not. That there are substantial factors influencing tobacco uptake outside the realm of adolescents' control must be recognized.
- Such factors as susceptibility, peer influence, and parental smoking status apply to all adolescent subgroups.
- The social environment changes rapidly as adolescents age, including more extensive exposure to experimentation with cigarettes and other drugs. As a result, attitudes and intentions toward smoking and images of smokers change over time.
- There is strong evidence for continuation of smoking once initiation has occurred. It is of great importance to reduce the number of new smokers and delay transitions from experimental to regular smoking.
- Few smokers become ex-smokers in adolescence. Although cessation is frequently attempted, indicating that some adolescents are not committed to lifetime smoking, it is rarely successful. Youth often underestimate how difficult it is to quit or may not have the ability to plan and accomplish cessation. Also, few adolescents understand the range of cessation interventions available for assistance.
- Nonsmokers tend to make friends with fellow nonsmokers, and smokers do the same. Friends offer other friends cigarettes, and smokers use other drugs more than nonsmokers. Smoking changes an adolescent's attitudes toward both tobacco use and its accompanying health hazards. This, in turn, can influence self-image. Because smoking alters peer networks, it may also influence other social, academic, and health outcomes.
- Adolescent beliefs about smoking and smokers help shape tobacco use decisions. Adolescent smokers treat smoking as a normal and acceptable social activity. Both smoking and nonsmoking adolescents overestimate the prevalence of smoking among their peers and among adults. That most adolescents do not smoke is not well known by other teens.
- Adolescents do not necessarily understand the true risks of tobacco-related diseases. The harms may be too remote to per-

sonalize or comprehend fully or to expect the risks to apply to them.[2]

Throughout our work on this book, we have closely monitored media coverage of adolescent smoking. A constant refrain adolescents offer when asked why they smoke is "because it's cool." As one reporter put it: "If coolness is everything, then it follows that the only way to get kids not to smoke is to make smoking not cool. And how do we do that?"[3] As our discussion of the factors influencing adolescent smoking suggests, this is hardly all there is to it. Even so, policymakers and advocates must grapple with the reality that a deadly activity seems cool to many adolescents.

Organization of the Chapter

A vast amount of research has been conducted examining why adolescents use tobacco. The story we tell is necessarily complex, for no simple answer explains smoking behavior. If there were a simple answer, the debate over how to invest in tobacco control interventions would be straightforward.

In the remainder of this chapter, we focus on the dominant individual characteristics and social factors that influence youth tobacco use. Although a myriad of factors might be described, four different factors emerge from the literature as being the major influences: (1) peer smoking behavior, (2) parental smoking and other familial influences, (3) individual susceptibility to smoking (meaning an intention to smoke in the future or lack of a firm commitment not to smoke in the future), and (4) personal beliefs, attitudes, and self-image. Two of the most powerful and most consistent predictors of an adolescent's smoking status are whether he or she has any friends who smoke and whether his or her parents or siblings smoke. Adolescents' decisions to smoke may also be influenced by their intentions to smoke in the future, how common they perceive smoking to be, and how they view smoking, other smokers, and themselves as smokers. Media influences—while an ostensibly important social influence on youth smoking behavior—are reviewed in chapter 4. For the reader's convenience, we here discuss each factor separately, although the factors operate simultaneously and interact with one another to shape an individual's tobacco use decisions.

The influence and importance of each of these four factors varies across the different stages of adolescent smoking behavior. In this chapter, we illustrate the influence of each type of factor both on the transition from nonsmoking to smoking initiation or experimentation and on the intensification of smoking as adolescents move from casual or occasional use to regular or habitual use. An understanding of the factors related to smoking susceptibility, experimentation, and initiation is crucial to the success of primary prevention programs (those programs aimed generally toward discouraging youth tobacco use). An understanding of what influences movement to another stage is crucial for secondary prevention and cessation programs (those programs aimed at specific inidividuals at risk of tobacco use). Understanding why a 12 year old and a 17 year old may have different opinions about and experiences with tobacco is central to developing interventions to inhibit movement to more intense smoking and to enhance cessation possibilities.

After considering the four primary factors that affect adolescent tobacco use, we turn in this chapter to a review of the literature on the association of adolescent smoking with other types of risk-taking activities and problem behaviors. For example, adolescents exhibiting signs of stress or depression are more likely to be smokers than are nondepressed adolescents. This chapter concludes with a summary and a discussion of the relative importance of peer versus familial influences on adolescent smoking. Subsequently, in part 2 and the "Conclusion and Recommendations" of the book, we consider the policy implications and potential interventions that emerge from this review.

Peer Smoking

Most adolescents are heavily influenced by their peers and by perceptions of what is acceptable and unacceptable within peer groups. A vast body of research confirms the importance of peer influences on the decision to begin smoking and on transitions between stages. Gravitating toward peers with similar smoking behaviors is called *peer selection*. This is a different concept from *peer influence*, which describes how an individual's attitudes and behaviors are affected by a group. But determining whether peer influences actually cause others to use tobacco is notoriously difficult.

Peer Influence

The smoking status of friends has been found by researchers to be a strong—perhaps the strongest—predictor of the smoking status of all adolescent groups.[4] In fact, smoking and friendships are reinforcing, suggesting an important social significance to tobacco initiation.[5]

Responses to the Teenage Attitudes and Practices Survey (TAPS) of 12,100 adolescents in 1989 and 1993 provide insight into adolescent thinking about tobacco use. For youths aged 14–18, having any best friends of either sex or a boyfriend/girlfriend who smoked was the strongest and most consistently significant predictor of whether an adolescent used tobacco.[6] However, it is important to recognize that if one likes to smoke, he or she might simply choose friends who also smoke (though establishing a causal link is difficult).[7]

Having friends or peers who smoke not only is a good predictor of an individual's smoking behavior but is seen by researchers as an integral part of the process of initiation and progression toward routine smoking.[8] Friends and peers play an active role in promoting cigarette smoking throughout adolescence. Tobacco initiation by one student has the potential to trigger smoking initiation among close friends.[9] As smoking increases in visibility within one's peer group and in the school at large, adolescents are often encouraged to contemplate experimenting with tobacco within a social environment where tobacco is increasingly prevalent and visible. This provides greater opportunities (in part through cigarette offers from peers) and pressures for nonsmokers to experiment with tobacco use.[10]

The number of cigarette offers experienced by an adolescent is related to both experimental and regular smoking.[11] Just as important, the number of cigarette offers can also predict the transition from nonsmoking to experimenting and that from experimenting to more intense smoking.[12] As all children get older, they are more likely to have been offered cigarettes, and the more times an adolescent is offered cigarettes, the more times he or she is likely to smoke. Cigarette offers from friends may influence adolescents in three ways: first, implicit in the offer of a cigarette is peer pressure to smoke; second, it sends a powerful message that it is socially acceptable to smoke (that it does not have to be done alone); and third, it may raise an adolescent's awareness about smoking and perception of smoking prevalence (i.e., it may make them think more adolescents smoke than actually do).

In all likelihood, smokers involved in offering cigarettes to others play an active role in changing the new initiators' perceptions of smoking. Along with the offer of a cigarette, the smoker may add pro-smoking propaganda (either explicitly to encourage smoking behavior or implicitly in the message of social acceptability).[13] Another potential consequence of this process is to erode an adolescent's defenses to refuse cigarette offers. For instance, adolescent girls participating in a focus group who had previously tried cigarettes were less likely to have a good response or counterargument to the pro-smoking arguments made by their peers than were those who had not smoked before.[14] In this sense, peer influence operates both to encourage initiation and to discourage attempts to refuse the offer or to quit at a later time.

Peer pressure to use tobacco starts early. Adolescents from sixth to tenth grade who have tried cigarettes are more likely to know people[15] or to have friends[16] who have tried smoking than are their nonsmoking peers. Smoking status has also been found to be related to the number of times in a week sixth and eighth graders saw their friends who smoke.[17] The relationship between smoking status and number of friends seen in a week suggests that meetings with peers provide opportunities for smoking episodes through promotion of smoking behaviors and cigarette offers. This is a disturbing finding for two reasons (already noted in chap. 2): adolescents are experimenting with tobacco at younger ages, and the earlier the age of initiation, the harder it is to quit smoking. As a result, strategies need to be developed to disrupt the formation of smoking peer groups during the middle school years.

Peers transmit not only smoking behavior but also attitudes and beliefs about smoking. The mere fact that few adolescent smokers suffer visible health consequences may counteract public health messages about the harms associated with tobacco use. Adolescents are notorious for an attitude of invulnerability (i.e., "it won't happen to me"). Those who initiate tobacco use at early ages consequently show increased susceptibility to ongoing and future tobacco use and decreased expectations of the negative health consequences from smoking.[18] This suggests that concurrent with their adoption of smoking, adolescents deny or ignore the health harms of smoking and adopt views on smoking that are consistent with the behavior (as we discuss in greater detail later in this chapter).

Fortunately, peer influence is not unidirectional when it comes to smoking initiation, which helps explain in part why many adolescents do not use tobacco products. Cigarette offers are not always accepted. Some students who have developed multiple refusal skills are successful at avoiding smoking initiation when offered a cigarette.[19] Friendships in a nonsmoking clique can be protective against smoking, by insulating nonsmokers (in nonsmoking cliques) from the influence of a few smokers (in their own, smoking clique).[20] Friendships among adolescents who hold negative attitudes toward smoking can be protective against smoking initiation and can reinforce existing doubts about using tobacco. In one study, fourth and fifth graders who were concerned about their friends' smoking were at decreased risk of smoking.[21] In another study, more than 25 percent of 14–15 year olds had actively influenced their peers not to smoke, while only 2.7 percent reported having tried to get someone to smoke.[22]

Social Groups and Peer Selection

It seems that group formation is an important aspect of adolescent decisions about tobacco use. In turn, cigarette smoking plays a meaningful role in group formation and culture. Smokers tend to associate with other smokers, in essence forming smoking cliques; and nonsmokers tend to associate with other nonsmokers.[23] Several studies show that peers actively seek out groups of friends with similar smoking behaviors and attitudes.[24] For example, members of a nonsmoking group believed their friends to have negative views of smoking, while members of a smoking group believed their friends supported smoking.[25] This is strong evidence of peer influence, with similarity of attitudes about smoking producing similarity of smoking behaviors (either nonsmoking or smoking) within groups.

Peer smoking and friends' approval of smoking influence whether an adolescent will experiment with tobacco and also whether he or she will progress toward regular or current smoking.[26] Exposure to friends who smoke facilitates the progression to the next stage of smoking through increased intention to smoke in the future, perceived peer approval of smoking, and decreased expectations of adverse health problems. Early experimenters may gravitate toward other experimenters, contributing to the strong association between having friends who smoke and the transition to regular smoking.[27] Hence, peer selection plays an important role in explaining whether an adolescent will make the transition to more frequent smoking.

Peer groups among adolescents change frequently. Over a two-year period in one longitudinal study, more than half of high school adolescent smokers and nonsmokers changed peer groups (about 55 percent in each group).[28] But what is most interesting about the movement among peer groups is how consistently adolescents remained in either a smoking or a nonsmoking group. Thus, 70 percent of smokers remained within predominantly smoking peer groups, and 75 percent of nonsmokers remained within predominantly nonsmoking peer groups. In short, the individuals in a peer group change, but the smoking status of the peer group remains generally fixed.[29]

Perceptions

As we discuss later in this chapter, individual beliefs, perceptions, and attitudes are important in understanding what messages might be more well received than others. In fact, an important research question is whether adolescents' perceptions of peer cigarette use predicts adolescents' smoking status better than does actual peer use.[30] Interestingly, two studies found that adolescent tobacco use is more closely associated with perceptions of peer smoking than with actual use rates and that actual use rates only weakly explain adolescent smoking behavior. Because adolescents perceive their friends' behavior to be more similar to their own than it actually is, they estimate their friends' smoking behavior as being similar to their own[31] and may change behavior to match their friends'.

These findings support other studies indicating that children who smoke overestimate the prevalence of smokers more than do nonsmoking children,[32] but there is also a dimension of cognitive dissonance (two contrary attitudes existing simultaneously) in these results. If people believe that smoking is safe or socially acceptable, they have psychological reasons to overstate the perceived prevalence of tobacco use.[33] Taken together, these results indicate that clinicians, tobacco control advocates, and policymakers must address how early adolescents form perceptions of how many adolescents smoke and about the known health harms from tobacco use.

Parental Smoking and Other Familial Influences

While quite important in forming an adolescent's view of the social acceptability of smoking, peer influences do not tell the whole story of why an adolescent chooses whether or not to use tobacco. Parental and familial influences also play a significant role in shaping an adolescent's perceptions of tobacco use.

Children of smoking parents enter adolescence and the contemplation stage of smoking with a decade of knowledge, attitudes, and justifications gleaned from parental and sibling smoking behavior. It is no wonder that students with parents or siblings who smoke are more likely to smoke.[34] For example, parental smoking status during the seventh grade can be a significant predictor of initiation, experimentation, and regular smoking in twelfth grade.[35] An analysis of the TAPS data from 1989 and 1993 found a strong parental influence on adolescent smoking behavior.[36]

Despite some findings questioning the importance of parental influence relative to other factors,[37] the consensus in the literature is that there is a significant association between parental smoking status and adolescent smoking behavior.[38] There is also a consensus that immediate parental influence wanes in later adolescence as best friends become a more significant factor.[39] As a result, one important question (which we address later in this chapter) is the relative influences of parents versus peers in adolescent smoking decisions.

Having a sibling or other nonparental family member who smokes is also associated with smoking initiation.[40] Indeed, smoking can be and often is a family affair. One study found that 40 percent of third through sixth graders initiated smoking with a family member. Also, 46 percent got their first cigarette from a family member and tried smoking because a family member smoked.[41]

Parental Smoking Status

The relationship between parental smoking status and initiation of smoking is particularly evident and important in late childhood and early adolescence, where parental authority and behavior modeling is strongest.[42] Parental smoking status also remains a significant influence in the transition from experimentation to regular smoking.[43] Adolescents may be more likely to try smoking if either parent smokes and to experiment further if they do not perceive parental disapproval of smoking.

The smoking status of parents is a measure of parental influence because of the assumption that adolescents imitate their parents' behaviors. For instance, the smoking behavior of children of ex-smokers is similar to that of children of current smokers and significantly different from children of never-smokers.[44] Even if parents do not actively tolerate adolescent smoking or if children do not duplicate their parents' behavior, having cigarettes easily available in the home certainly facilities adolescent experimentation. Cigarettes just lying around can easily be taken by a teen who wishes to experiment.

Parental Attitudes and Support

Regardless of parents' smoking status, parental attitudes play a role in an adolescent's smoking behavior. Researchers have found a relationship between parental attitudes toward smoking and the transition from nonsmoking to experimentation.[45] Parental smoking is usually construed as at least tacit approval for an adolescent's own tobacco use patterns and conveys an important message about tobacco's social acceptance. For example, adolescent never-smokers were most likely to report parental disapproval of smoking;[46] ex-smokers and current smokers reported the least parental disapproval. More important, smoking by parents increased adolescents' perceived parental approval of smoking.[47] Not surprisingly, current smokers were most likely to have parent or sibling smokers in their families, followed by ex-smokers, then experimenters, then nonsmokers.[48] Adolescents may be more likely to try smoking if either parent smokes and to experiment further if they do not perceive parental disapproval of smoking.

Parenting style is closely related to parental smoking status in affecting a child's choice to smoke or ability to resist smoking. Parenting style also influences a child's self-esteem, academic performance, and other more general risk factors for adolescent smoking initiation. Authoritative parenting, defined as being nurturing and responsive as well as "exercising firm, assertive control without being permissive or intrusive,"[49] appears to be associated with increased self-esteem, self-regulation, positive work orientation, and resistance to peer pressure. In turn, these characteristics have all been found to discourage smoking in third and fifth graders.[50]

Parental support for children facilitates coping and academic competence and reduces deviant behaviors, including tobacco use, in part by acting as a buffer against stress.[51] Thus, parental support helps to develop positive coping skills and to lessen negative reactions to stress from deviant attitudes and peer affiliations, which reduces the risk of drug use.

Parents' smoking status and the degree to which parental behavior is authoritative are independent risk factors for children's smoking, meaning that they each play a separate role.[52] Parental smoking status (whether currently smoking or having ever smoked) and family characteristics in general (e.g., parenting style, family structure, and family closeness and conflict) are also independent explanations for adolescents' smoking behavior.[53] The relationship developed between parents and children is influential in smoking initiation, but not more so than whether or not the parent has ever smoked.[54]

Interventions that inform parents about the messages that their own smoking behavior or tolerance for smoking send to children should be emphasized. Even if parental influence wanes toward the end of adolescence, a consistent parental message opposing smoking can be an important factor contributing to a child's decision not to use tobacco. As we will discuss in our "Conclusion and Recommendations," program interventions, such as smoking cessation or physician counseling, should involve parents and families, not just adolescents.

Parental Policies on Smoking at Home

Several studies analyzing national survey data indicate that voluntary restrictions on smoking in the home can reduce teen tobacco initiation and smoking rates. These surveys, which control for parental and sibling smoking behavior, suggest that complete smoking bans in the home have greater effects on adolescent smoking than partial bans (smoking is allowed in some places at some times) or no restrictions at all.[55] Another study found similar results for middle-school and high school experimenters, but no effects on current high school smokers.[56] The plausible implication of these studies is that voluntary restrictions on smoking at home can lower experimentation rates, particularly among younger children. More research will be needed to confirm these results, especially the use of longitudinal surveys, but "Adoption of a smoke-free home . . . sends a message to family members that smoking is not condoned, while the lack of such . . . may send the opposite message."[57]

Adverse Childhood Events

Research from a variety of fields has begun to assess the importance of adverse childhood events (e.g., child abuse and neglect, divorce) on a range of adolescent behaviors, including tobacco use. This research consistently links adverse childhood events with high-risk, problematic behaviors, such as illicit substance and alcohol use, high-risk sexual conduct, and tobacco use. The most comprehensive analysis to date clearly demonstrated a close relationship between adverse childhood experiences and adolescent smoking behavior.[58] The study found that children exposed to adverse experiences or growing up with a substance-using family member have a substantially increased risk of early smoking initiation and subsequent heavy smoking.

Likewise, family structure adversely affects a range of adolescent behaviors. For example, there is an association between single-parent families or families including stepparents, low academic orientation, and future drug use, including tobacco use.[59] Being in such a household greatly increases the likelihood that adolescents will engage in a range of high-risk behaviors. Increased family conflict, common during adolescence, also influences the transition from experimental smoking to regular smoking.[60] For the same reasons, there may be a direct relationship between single-parent families, including those resulting from divorce, and experimentation with cigarettes.[61] Adolescents living in single-parent families are more likely to be involved in tobacco use than are adolescents living in two-parent households.[62]

Parental Education and Income

For many years, the conventional wisdom has been that adults with more education are smoking less, while smoking rates for adults with less education have not declined. Thus, it was widely assumed that adolescents from families with low parental education levels would also smoke more than those from families with higher levels of parental education.[63] But as we detailed in chapter 2, the conventional wisdom may not be accurate for adolescents.

The evidence on the effects of parental education and income shows differing results for adult and adolescent tobacco use. Some studies have found that low parental education levels are associated with increased smoking initiation rates and earlier experimentation by offspring.[64] However, data from the large Teenage Attitudes and Practices Survey (TAPS) in 1993 did not indicate a relationship between a respondent's smoking status and the degree of education his or her parents had attained. Adolescents living below poverty levels were less likely to be regular smokers, which suggests that the parents' income may be the more relevant variable in assessing adolescents' risks of smoking.[65] Yet adult smoking has increasingly become associated with lower levels of income and education as more educated individuals have quit.

Adolescent smokers are more likely to have divorced parents and to report low family incomes and are more likely to live in poor communities in specific regions of the country. These differences in social background are important for understanding the social context of adolescent tobacco use. On average, adolescent smoking is associated with lower scores on standardized tests. Nevertheless, the differences are largely beyond the reach of tobacco control policy and go to the heart of social policy concerns across a wide variety of domestic policy issues.

Some economists appeal to an alternative explanation for higher rates of smoking (or lower rates of quitting) in groups with low socioeconomic status, one that suggests that the rate differences (from those of groups with higher socioeconomic status) are rational. The explanation relates to the economist's notion of "discounting": poorer people may discount the future more heavily than do more affluent people. In turn, poorer people will be more likely to prefer consumption today (to satisfy immediate desires) over investments today for future return (which they may see as not very likely). The reason is that poorer people perceive their futures as bleaker than do the affluent—as more dependent on continued work to pay the bills, less likely to include leisure time and the rewards of an enjoyable retirement (vacation trips, etc.), and quite possibly shorter. Since the prospects for a well-funded and lengthy retirement are lower for the disadvantaged, it is quite rational of them to be less concerned with (to discount more heavily) the future than are those for whom the future promises good health, relaxation, and enjoyment. This, in turn, means that the immediate rewards of smoking are more compelling for disadvantaged people.

Susceptibility to Tobacco Use

Regardless of peer or parental influences, it is at least arguable that an adolescent would not experiment with cigarettes absent some susceptibility to tobacco's allures. *Susceptibility* is a term used to describe a person's self-reported intentions to smoke in the future. Susceptibility can be measured by whether an adolescent has a strong commitment not to smoke, is ambivalent toward smoking in the future, or is strongly committed to smoking in the future.[66] Measuring an adolescent's future intentions to smoke may be a surrogate measure for vulnerability to pro-smoking forces, such as peers who smoke and tobacco advertising.

Intentions to smoke are also related to age. Younger adolescents, particularly those exposed to the Drug Abuse Resistance Education (DARE) program, generally say that they have no intentions of using tobacco in the future. But as they age, many adolescents become less resolute about their intentions. This helps explain why the rate of smoking initiation seems to increase over time, with 3–7 percent initiating at age 11, rising to around 20 percent by age 15.[67] One longitudinal study found that 90 percent of 10-year-old nonsmokers were nonsmokers at age 12 but that only 67 percent of those who were nonsmokers at age 14 were still nonsmokers at age 16.[68] In the space of a year, those who have become experimenters can double or even triple.[69]

During the stage when adolescents contemplate experimenting with tobacco, children who are found to be susceptible to future smoking are between 80 percent and 400 percent more likely to initiate smoking than are those who had a strong commitment not to smoke. For third and fifth graders in this stage, susceptibility is a powerful predictor of future experimentation.[70]

Susceptibility is also a relevant risk factor in later adolescence, when more students are contemplating initiation or progressing to more routine tobacco use. For example, a future intention to smoke can predict the transition from trying cigarettes in seventh grade to becoming a more routine smoker in twelfth grade.[71] Similarly, student susceptibility to future smoking can predict the transition from never smoking to experimenting in 12–18 year olds.[72] Once adolescents initiate smoking, they have greater intentions to smoke in the future, which puts them at increased risk of further experimentation.[73] That the increase in the number of youths who have experimented with cigarettes peaks around the age of 15 or 16 is most likely a result of the fact that a majority have already become experimenters by that age.

The transition to regular smoking is also modified by the level of commitment not to smoke. An analysis of the TAPS data suggests that susceptibility to future smoking may be a better predictor of the transition from experimentation to regular smoking than is friends' smoking status.[74] Adolescents at an earlier stage of experimentation but without a strong commitment not to smoke were as likely to develop into established smokers as were adolescents at the next later stage of experimentation with a strong commitment not to smoke.[75] The lack of commitment not to smoke was a significant predictor of progression to established smoking in older adolescents but not in younger ones.[76]

Such findings highlight the importance of preferences and values in shaping actual behavior. Because preferences and values matter, altering adolescent intentions to use tobacco is an important element of prevention policy. There is also a strong self-selection concern. Early initiators are those with the strongest preferences to smoke, a fact borne out by trends showing that early initiators are less likely to quit during adolescence. This creates a troublesome and intertwined relationship between susceptibility and initiation. Once an adolescent initiates tobacco use, regardless of previous intentions not to smoke, future intentions are likely to move toward an expectation of continued smoking.

Transition Stages

Developing mechanisms to discourage youths from initiating experimentation with tobacco has received considerable public policy attention. Disrupting the transition stages to more routine smoking has received less policy attention but is no less important. If the transition to greater smoking intensity can be interrupted, fewer adolescents will become adult smokers.

There are three major predictors of the transition to regular smoking: an adolescent's smoking history, age, and friends' smoking status. Once adolescents have become occasional smokers, it is likely they will either remain occasional smokers or progress to regular smoking; there is little probability that they will become ex-smokers.[77]

Not surprisingly, prior smoking is strongly associated with current smoking and predictive of future smoking.[78] The implication of this is that forays into smoking generally lead only in one direction— toward more regular smoking. The longer adolescents smoke, the more likely they are to make the transition to regular smoking. Thus, adolescents who start smoking early relative to their peers would be more likely to have made the transition to regular smoking earlier than their peers.

Two simultaneous trends seem to be at work. First, older adolescents progress more quickly to established smoking than their younger counterparts.[79] This may be evidence of what some have called "transition acceleration,"[80] which describes the increased likelihood of progression from one stage of smoking to another as one gets older. One study, for instance, measured adolescent occasional smokers at two-year intervals,[81] finding that the probability of remaining an occasional smoker decreased from 41 percent between ages 10 and 12, to 35 percent from ages 12 to 14, to 26 percent by ages 14 to 16. At the same time, the probabilities of occasional smokers progressing to regular smoking substantially increased each time over the same time sequences (from 3, to 17, to 45 percent).

Second, early initiation of smoking behavior is a strong predictor of regular smoking in later adolescence.[82] In one study, students initiating tobacco use before age 12 were more likely to have made the transition to regular smoking than were those initiating after age 12. Among current smokers, those initiating before age 12 were more likely to be heavy current smokers (smoking more than five cigarettes a day) than were current smokers initiating smoking after age 12.[83] Those who had initiated before age 11 were four times more likely to be daily smokers than were those initiating after age 11.[84]

As early adolescent smokers get older, therefore, the tendency is to progress to more routine smoking rather than toward cessation. These findings are particularly significant because research on adult cessation rates indicates that early initiation of smoking reduces the likelihood of quit success.[85]

Biomedical Influences

An emerging area of research is in biomedical markers of adolescent tobacco use. According to recent research, tobacco use is a response to both genetic and social (environmental) factors .[86] Clearly, genetic factors play a role in susceptibility to nicotine dependence, but little is known about why some adolescents become addicted to nicotine while others do not progress to regular tobacco use.[87] While it is highly unlikely that researchers will find a tobacco addiction gene, such research can illuminate the relationship between genetic and social factors influencing smoking and thus help to clarify the types of interventions that might be effective. Nonetheless, it may be difficult to separate socialization and genetic influences in the smoking behaviors of adolescents.

Some researchers have found evidence of genetic influence on smoking behaviors in adult and adolescent populations, respectively, but they also found significant environmental influences.[88] One study found a large genetic contribution to cigarette use in adult twins but also found that individual environmental risk factors are important.[89] Other studies suggest the importance of genetic influences on lifetime and current smoking.[90] For instance, one study found a genetic component to nonsmoking in adult populations that came of age at a time when smoking was more socially acceptable and more prevalent.[91] This suggests that even in a pro-smoking environment, there may have been genetic protection from smoking initiation. Some studies have failed to find a genetic association with smoking initiation.[92] This means that social influences play a significant and independent role in an adolescent's decision to smoke, even if a genetic predisposition exists.

Tobacco addiction and the ability to quit smoking show genetic components as well, though there has been little research in the area as compared to other drugs.[93] Smokers lacking a fully functioning, genetically variable enzyme that metabolizes nicotine smoked significantly fewer cigarettes than did smokers with normally functioning enzymes.[94] They are, in effect, protected against becoming nicotine-dependent heavy smokers.

Just as important, researchers have recently found a relationship between a certain genetic makeup and the ability to stop smoking, suggesting that some individuals may find it easier to quit than others.[95] Understanding genetic protections against becoming dependent on nicotine or in facilitating smoking cessation would be useful in devising more effective smoking cessation interventions.

Beliefs, Attitudes, and Self-Image

Adolescent tobacco use involves a set of choices that are deeply influenced by attitudes toward smoking, which are no doubt heavily influenced by parents and peers. Perhaps more important, an adolescent's smoking decisions revolve around self-image. Determining how adolescents view smoking, smokers, and themselves is invaluable in explaining their motivations for smoking behavior and in predicting which adolescents are likely to experiment with tobacco.

Surprisingly, adolescent smokers and nonsmokers may not differ in certain aspects, as both ever-smokers and nonsmokers in sixth grade agreed that smoking affects appearance, smoking can be addictive, smoking can be influenced by the social environment, smoking affects health, smoking creates a false image, and secondhand smoke affects people. Certainly, anecdotal reports based on interviews with adolescents confirm that they are well aware of tobacco's health risks. Research suggests, however, that adolescents often underestimate these risks (i.e., they may not fully understand or comprehend the risks) and usually deflect any such risk by arguing it will never happen to them.[96]

Attitudes toward Smokers and Nonsmokers

Beliefs about the positive and negative aspects of smoking often change throughout adolescence. Fifth-grade students in one study had many more negative perceptions of smokers than of nonsmokers, many more positive perceptions of nonsmokers than of smokers.[97] Two years later, the students' views of smokers and nonsmokers were much less clear-cut; both positive and negative characteristics were assigned to smoking and nonsmoking. Positive characteristics that had been associated with nonsmokers in fifth grade but that were associated with smokers in seventh grade included being successful, good-looking, and cool. Smokers were considered uncool (negative) among fifth graders, whereas nonsmokers became uncool by seventh grade.[98] During this period, both smoking behaviors and perceptions of coolness may change as a result of adopting more adult-associated roles and changes in one's self-image. Adolescents often want to be more adultlike. When smoking is associated with positive attributes of being an adult, adolescents may equate positive characteristics to smoking.

It is of particular concern that positive beliefs about smokers among nonsmokers may increase the likelihood of smoking later in adolescence. Believing in fifth grade that smokers were healthy or good in sports increased the risk of smoking in ninth grade 7.5 and 3.8 times, respectively.[99] Nonsmoking fifth graders who characterized nonsmokers as "trying to act cool" (but not in fact cool) or as "uncool" were 4 times more likely to be smokers in ninth grade than were nonsmokers with positive views of nonsmokers.[100] The same study found that among seventh graders, perceptions of smokers as independent or good-looking were significant predictors of smoking in ninth grade. This indicates that the characteristics associated with smokers and nonsmokers (from cool to independent and good-looking) change with age and may increase or decrease in value over time.[101]

In short, as kids move through adolescence, their perceptions change so that smoking becomes cool to them. When they are younger, smoking is very unattractive to them. These changing perceptions may help explain why some school-based interventions (e.g., the DARE program), described in chapter 4, have only short-term positive results with little long-term success. These interventions are effective with younger children, in part because the interventions reinforce existing attitudes about smoking and other drug use. But as adolescents age and their perceptions about tobacco use change, the earlier interventions are at odds with new beliefs.

Transitions through smoking stages may also affect adolescents' views of smoking and smokers. A never-smoker is likely to feel very differently about being around smokers than does a regular smoker. Current smokers aged 14–18 have expressed more positive beliefs and attitudes toward smoking (e.g., that cigarettes relieve stress, aid in relaxation, and decrease boredom) than have nonsmokers.[102] Smokers have expressed more positive attitudes about other smokers. For example, smokers were up to 35.3 times less likely than nonsmokers to dislike being around people who were smoking.[103]

It seems clear that the social environment influences adolescents' attitudes and beliefs as well. Thus, peer and parental influences help shape adolescent attitudes and beliefs about tobacco use. Take also the impact of movie stars on adolescents. Based on preliminary evidence, one study concluded that smoking by movie stars on and off camera encourages adolescent smoking behavior.[104] As an example, according to numerous media reports, adolescents responded favorably to the glorification of smoking in the movie *Titanic*. Adolescents positively viewed the youthful actors' smoking as an expression of rebellion against social mores.

Self-Image

Adolescence is a time of vulnerability about one's self-image. At the same time, adolescents tend to be consumed by changes in their self-image. It stands to reason, therefore, that how adolescents perceive tobacco in relation to their self-image plays an important role in smoking behavior. In particular, smoking initiation may be motivated by adolescents' beliefs about themselves in relation to their beliefs and attitudes about smokers.

Teens may smoke because their self-image matches the smoker image: in this sense, smoking is consistent with an adolescent's own self-image.[105] Or they may value the image of a smoker more than their own self-image and hence smoke to improve their self-image.[106] That older adolescents' self-image is more closely aligned with the smoker image puts them at increased risk of using tobacco.[107]

Smoking initiation is considered to be more likely for those whose self-image is similar to the image they have of smokers.[108] Adolescents tend to describe themselves more positively than they describe smokers. Yet teens often report reasons for smoking that are positive[109] and find in smokers positive characteristics that correspond to the model that teens want to cultivate—namely, the smoker image. So how can adolescents describe smokers in a positive light and yet describe themselves in a more positive way than they do smokers? The dissonance can be rectified if one takes into account that there are also negative attributes associated with smokers (unhealthy, etc.). Adolescents might wish to be more like they perceive smokers to be—that is, cooler, more sociable, and so on—while holding an overall more negative image of a smoker than of themselves. In effect, these people wish to be like smokers without actually smoking. Since some adolescents initiate smoking to improve their self-image, it may seem counterintuitive that as they progress through the stages of smoking, they report lower self-esteem.[110]

There may be significant differences in self-image between the genders. Girls may be more likely than boys to hold a self-image that is similar to a smoker image and to smoke to boost their self-image.[111] Valuing the smoker image above one's own self-image may say more about girls' self-esteem than about how girls value tobacco use. In addition, adolescent girls who believe that smoking curbs appetite, is an effective method of weight control, and enhances appearance are at increased risk of smoking initiation.[112] Some researchers have found that smoking as a weight-control strategy is almost exclusively present in white female adolescent populations,[113] though boys have also expressed weight concerns.[114]

Adolescents' dependence on smoking as a coping mechanism and self-medication device for weight control has particularly serious implications for cessation interventions in this population, especially since weight-control problems are more immediate than tobacco-produced health problems in this age-group. Weight concerns may lessen an adolescent's interest in contemplating quitting or in successfully completing a cessation program. Breaking through this barrier presents an important challenge, especially for reaching adolescent girls.

Perceived Health

Another factor influencing adolescent attitudes toward smoking is how adolescents perceive the health consequences of tobacco use. As the importance adolescents place on their health status increases, the likelihood that they will smoke decreases.[115] Adolescents choosing healthful lifestyles and thereby developing positive health-status images may be protected from initiating smoking. Conversely, those with negative perceived health status are more likely to use tobacco products.[116]

Perception of one's health status is both directly and indirectly related to participation in sports. Participation in sports reduces the likelihood that an adolescent will experiment with smoking.[117] The more sports an adolescent plays, the less likely he or she is to be a regular smoker, experimental smoker, or ever-smoker. Physically active adolescents are less likely to smoke.[118]

Rebelliousness and Risk-Taking Behaviors

While some of the appeal of tobacco use is emulating the behavior of others, researchers have also found an association between self-reports of rebelliousness and smoking. Rebelliousness, in fact, is a strong predictor of smoking behavior.[119] Increased levels of rebelliousness predict smoking initiation. As self-reported levels of rebelliousness increase, so does the intensity of smoking (from never smoking, to experimenting, to current smoking).[120] Adolescents cite "daring" and "independent" as characteristics of smokers whom they choose to emulate.[121] It is possible that with progression through the stages of smoking, adolescents self-report as more rebellious[122] because they have adopted a smoker's image.

Closely related to rebelliousness, risk-taking behaviors are often pursued in adolescence. Youth smoking arises within a web of social relations that foster many types of experimentation, along with predictable behavioral risks. Given this social context, youth smoking arises from some of the same family, peer, and community influences that are important to other high-risk behaviors, such as sexual risk taking, crime, and violence, as well as the initiation of harmful alcohol and illicit substance use. Risk takers may form an image of themselves that either includes existing cigarette smoking behavior or encourages them to take up smoking. In a recent study, researchers found that they could predict smoking status of students who described themselves as risk takers.[123]

The discussion of risk-taking behavior is particularly apropos to smoking because of the health risks involved with nicotine addiction. In one study, smokers perceived themselves at no greater risk of dying from smoking-related diseases than did nonsmokers.[124] Smoking may be an attractive behavior to risk takers because they do not perceive themselves as susceptible to its negative consequences. Risk taking is often accompanied by a strong preference for current over future well-being, which would provide another reason for risk taking to be associated with adolescent tobacco use.

Social Competence

In the section on parental influences, we noted the importance of familial support in providing adolescents with a sense of competence about their own abilities. Competence can be categorized as academic capability, physical appearance, social acceptance, behavioral conduct, and athletic ability.[125] In general, children with higher levels of competencies are less likely to experiment with tobacco use or to intend to smoke in the future than are children displaying lower levels of competencies. Reduced self-esteem, poor work orientation, and substandard academic performance are associated with progressively passing through the various stages of smoking (intention, initiation, experimentation, regular use).[126] Adolescents who believe in their decision-making skills and competencies and who have knowledge of refusal skills are less likely to smoke in the future.[127]

Adolescents who perceive themselves to be relatively competent academically are less likely to experiment with cigarettes.[128] Low academic achievement and orientation are associated with increased tobacco initiation[129] and frequency of smoking.[130] For students with low academic orientation, studies report figures of 1.5 to 5 times greater risk of intending to smoke or initiating smoking.[131] Students with high grades are less likely to be current or lifetime smokers than are students with lower grades.[132] Low academic orientation is also associated with an increased number of drug offers and pro-drug beliefs.[133] This provides additional support for finding a higher prevalence of smoking behavior in the milieu in which low academic achievers find themselves.

Although there are many reasons to expect low academic achievement to be associated with smoking, this relationship has special implications for prevention and cessation efforts. If smokers, on average, are more alienated from school and have lower levels of academic performance, they may be less susceptible to didactic or school-based tobacco prevention and cessation interventions.

Perceived Prevalence

An important aspect of how adolescents form beliefs and attitudes toward tobacco use is their estimate of their peers' smoking behavior. This is known as their perceived prevalence, which refers to adolescents' estimation of the commonality of smoking among their peers. Perceived prevalence may contribute to adolescents' understanding of social norms if they believe that smoking among their peers is more common than it actually is.

Several researchers have found that adolescents tend to overestimate by as much as 50 percent the number of their peers and the number of adults who smoke.[134] Adolescents may overestimate smoking prevalence because they believe that they are acting in similar ways as others or that others are acting in ways similar to their own behavior, or they may do so simply to justify their own smoking status.[135] Teens who smoke estimate smoking prevalence to be somewhat higher than nonsmokers do, though, as we noted earlier, nonsmokers also overestimate it.[136] A perception that smoking is a common behavior may act to encourage some teens to begin smoking, and a higher perceived prevalence of smoking encourages the transition from initiating to experimenting with cigarettes.[137] These perceptions help predict future smoking, whether adolescents are asked to estimate adult or peer smoking rates.[138] Overestimating smoking may influence girls more than boys to initiate smoking. One study found that girls who thought that approximately half of their peers smoked in seventh grade were more likely to smoke in ninth grade than were boys who estimated the same prevalence.[139]

Thus, expectations of existing social norms contribute to the promotion of adolescent smoking. This may be because adolescents use smoking prevalence as a support for their own smoking behavior or because they initiate smoking to conform to this distorted norm. Inflated prevalence estimates promote adolescent smoking—and substance use in general—regardless of their validity.[140] It is therefore imperative that school- and community-based interventions convey accurate information about tobacco use in the community.

Adolescent Smoking and Other Risk-Taking Activities and Problem Behaviors

Adolescents who use tobacco often participate concomitantly in other risk-taking behaviors, such as alcohol consumption and illicit drug use. Problem behaviors (e.g., binge drinking, substance use, missing school, or fighting) are least prevalent among nonsmokers and most prevalent among adolescents who initiate smoking at early ages. Smoking is a powerful indicator for adolescent problems of clinical and policy concern.

Adolescent tobacco use is especially strongly linked with other substance use. Data from the most recently available Youth Risk Behavior Surveillance System surveys from 1997 indicate that current smokers (those smoking at least once in the 30 days preceding the survey) were more likely to report ever using or currently using other substances than were only experimental smokers or nonsmokers. As the reported number of cigarettes smoked in the past 30 days increased, the likelihood of other drug use rose.[141] Also, there appears to be a complementary relationship between adolescent smoking and adolescent alcohol use: over 90 percent of regular adolescent smokers surveyed used alcohol.[142] These patterns suggest that cigarette smoking is initiated in a multidrug environment and that increased commitment to cigarettes occurs within the context of further drug experimentation and experience. It seems probable that adolescents are using drugs in combination and that adolescent consumption of alcohol, illicit drugs, and tobacco may be complementary.

Stress, Emotional Distress, and Depression

When interviewed by various media about their tobacco use, a constant adolescent refrain is the need to relieve stress. Almost every news article or broadcast about teen smoking focuses on how they smoke to relieve the stress and pressures of adolescence. They perceive the act of cigarette smoking as a calming influence during emotionally turbulent times.

Yet the influence of stress, emotional distress, and depression on adolescent tobacco use is difficult for researchers to assess.[143] Longitudinal studies have not found a strong causal relationship between depression and smoking initiation, but there are strong indications in cross-sectional studies that smoking and depression may be reciprocal.[144] Smoking does not cause depression, but people suffering from it smoke to gain some relief from the depressive symptoms. In this context, smoking is a possible self-medication process for feelings of depression.[145] Indeed, the potential link between depression and smoking, especially among young women, is well established, particularly since depressive symptoms are important obstacles in smoking cessation among adolescents and other patient groups.[146]

Recent research confirms the importance of peer group formation as influencing smoking patterns in this subgroup. For example, adolescents displaying psychiatric problems who did not have smoking peers were not at increased risk for smoking initiation.[147] But adolescents with psychiatric problems who reported that most of their friends smoked carried a threefold increase in risk for tobacco initiation.[148] Consistent with the importance of peer group formation, the relationship between depression and the transition to regular smoking is stronger in later adolescence than in early adolescence.[149]

Conclusion

Despite ongoing research into why some adolescents use tobacco while others are able to refrain from its allure, there is no simple answer to the questions raised at the beginning of this chapter. As a general proposition, the four groups of factors discussed in this chapter explain the various influences and how they interact to shape an adolescent's tobacco use decisions. At best, the research paints a general portrait of why some adolescents smoke and points the way to more effective tobacco control interventions.

Nevertheless, we can identify a variety of reasons why some adolescents never try cigarettes although most do.[150] Adolescents at decreased risk for smoking initiation are high academic achievers, are interested in their health, play sports, select nonsmoking peers, have parents who disapprove of smoking, show few signs of depression or negative self-image, and do not display conduct/behavioral problems. Preferences and values also play a strong role. Adolescents who display the strongest intentions not to smoke are the least likely to become regular smokers.

Youth who reach the contemplation stage of tobacco use without having formulated a strong negative belief about cigarettes, a more positive self-image of themselves than that of a smoker, or a strong intention or commitment not to smoke are vulnerable to experimenting with tobacco products. The implications of smoking initiation at a young age are twofold: adolescent smokers are more likely to make the transition to regular smoking,[151] and they are less likely to make successful quit attempts than are people who start smoking later in life.[152] Adolescents, especially smokers, underestimate the health risks and addictive nature of smoking and overvalue its social normalcy. Young initiators may find themselves developing a smoker image and becoming a member of a clique associated with smoking.

Interactions among the Explanatory Factors

As we noted earlier, the factors that explain adolescent tobacco use do not act in isolation. Rather, they interact in myriad ways to influence adolescent smoking behavior. The interactions between peer and parental influence have received considerable attention.

The Peer vs. Parental Influence Problem

Most researchers agree that peer influence factors are the strongest predictors of smoking initiation, but there have been some mixed results concerning parental influence factors. One study, using lifetime smoking status as a measure, found that adolescents aged 12–14 were equally likely to smoke whether they had a parent who had ever smoked or a best friend who smoked.[153] Other observers argue that parental influence in the form of smoking behavior precedes peer influence and that prior inclination to smoke (largely based on parental influence) predisposes youths to seek out smoking friends.[154]

A point in favor of peer smoking status as a stronger influence on smoking behavior, some researchers argue, is that parental influence has not extended to adolescent smoking behavior when parents quit smoking.[155] One hypothesis is that during adolescence, bonds with peers strengthen while bonds with parents weaken, suggesting that at the age when they are initiating smoking, peers may have more direct influence than parents.[156] Furthermore, parental influence seems to be strongest among adolescents who are nonsmokers,[157] but it is uncertain whether this is because they actively influence their children not to smoke or because fewer children of nonsmokers smoke due to lack of exposure. It is possible that smoking parents' influence may be simply that they provide access to cigarettes.[158] Making cigarettes available may amount to passive consent or even parental encouragement to smoke.

Reconciliation is possible if one looks at how influence is determined by the different studies. Adolescent smokers report getting cigarettes from home (if a sibling or parent smokes) and from peers and initiating tobacco use both at home and with friends.[159] The associations between peer and parental smoking behavior and smoking initiation can be determined readily by questionnaire but can only serve as a proxy for direct influence. Tapping the heart of the influence question is speculation about whether susceptible adolescents seek out smokers for friends or smoking behavior is transmitted after friendships form.

The primary lesson to be learned from this debate, even if it is unresolved, is that adolescents do not try cigarettes in a vacuum. The number and prominence of smoking friends and family members contribute to an individual's smoking environment and to the decisions about smoking that he or she must make. The presence of smokers in an adolescent's life provides both justifications and opportunities for smoking and may affect how he or she perceives access to cigarettes. Smokers can influence perceptions of being a smoker in society and of the acceptability of smoking in the presence of other smokers. Smoking by peers and admired role models implicitly undermines antismoking messages that emphasize the adverse social and health consequences of tobacco use. Further research is needed to determine to what extent parental behaviors and characteristics influence peer selection, which is a well-established risk factor for tobacco use.

Learning more about causal relationships between these factors is crucial to our understanding of adolescent smoking initiation. The dearth of longitudinal studies documenting the transition process is disappointing, considering the overall number of studies that have been conducted. Knowledge of the psychological state of adolescents smoking their first cigarette or of the mechanisms by which adolescents first enter the domain of ever-smokers is of particular import to the development of programs aimed at primary smoking prevention. It is important to gain greater understanding of how the factors interact with one another to influence an adolescent's use of tobacco.

NOTES

1. Even though correlations do not necessarily imply causality, they are important for what they might suggest about causal relations and for shaping policy interventions.

2. See, e.g., Slovic 2000; Viscusi 2000.

3. Swartz 1999.

4. These risk factors do not differ dramatically across white, ethnic, and minority populations (Tyas and Pederson 1998). Some minor differences are worth noting, however. African Americans seem to be less influenced by the smoking status of their close friends (Urberg, Degirmencioglu, and Pilgrim 1997) and belong to less homogeneous (in terms of smoking status) cliques than do whites (Ennett, Bauman, and Koch 1994). See Stanton and Silva 1992; Distefan et al. 1998; Epstein et al. 1999.

5. Charlton, Minagawa, and While 1999.

6. Wang, Fitzhugh, Westerfield, and Eddy 1995.

7. Norton, Lindrooth, and Ennett 1998.

8. Flay et al. 1994; Rowe et al. 1996.

9. Lucas and Lloyd 1999.

10. Yet experimenters and smokers are more likely to be offered cigarettes than are nonsmokers, another example of how smoking and friendships are reinforcing (Charlton, Minagawa, and While 1999).

11. Flay, Hu, and Richardson 1998.

12. Flay, Hu, and Richardson 1998.

13. Lucas and Lloyd 1999.

14. Lucas and Lloyd 1999.

15. Urberg, Degirmencioglu, and Pilgrim 1997.

16. Pederson, Koval, and O'Connor 1997.

17. Pederson, Koval, and O'Connor 1997; Pederson et al. 1998.

18. Flay et al. 1994.

19. Charlton, Minagawa, and While 1999. See also, Epstein, Griffin, and Botvin 2000.

20. Ennett, Bauman, and Koch 1994.

21. Iannotti, Bush, and Weinfurt 1996.

22. Stanton and McGee 1996.

23. Ennett and Bauman 1994; Urberg 1992; Engels et al. 1997; Pederson et al. 1998.

24. Engels et al. 1997; Thrush, Fife-Schaw, and Breakwell 1997; Fergusson, Lynskey, and Horwood 1995.

25. Thrush, Fife-Schaw, and Breakwell 1997.

26. Urberg, Degirmencioglu, and Pilgrim 1997; Engels et al. 1997; Flay, Hu, and Richardson 1998; Flay et al. 1994.

27. Fergusson, Lynskey, and Horwood 1995.

28. Engels et al. 1997.

29. Engels et al. 1997.

30. Bauman et al. 1992; Iannotti, Bush, and Weinfurt 1996.

31. Urberg 1992; Urberg, Shyu, and Liang 1990.

32. Urberg, Shyu, and Liang 1990. See the "Perceived Prevalence" section of this chapter for further discussion.

33. Akerlof and Dickens 1982.

34. Pederson, Koval, and O'Connor 1997.

35. Flay, Hu, and Richardson 1998.

36. Wasserman et al. 1998.

37. Although acknowledging that "there is little doubt that parenting behavior influences adolescent development," Distefan et al. (1998) surprisingly found no significant parental predictors of adolescent tobacco use in analyzing the TAPS data. This finding is consistent with studies cited in the 1994 surgeon general's report (USDHHS 1994).

38. Tyas and Pederson 1998.

39. Urberg, Degirmencioglu, and Pilgrim 1997.

40. Pederson, Koval, and O'Connor 1997.

41. Greenlund et al. 1997.

42. Flay, Hu, and Richardson 1998; Pederson et al. 1998; Jackson et al. 1998.

43. Flay, Hu, and Richardson 1998.

44. Bauman et al. (1990). Another important aspect of parental influence, in the form of family conflict or disruption of the family unit (single-parent households), may contribute to underestimates of parental influence if researchers remove it from analysis. For example, Flay et al. (1994) excluded responses from adolescents from single-parent families, a group at increased risk for smoking.

45. Flay, Hu, and Richardson 1998.

46. Pederson, Koval, and O'Connor 1997.

47. Flay et al. 1994.

48. Pederson et al. 1998.

49. Jackson et al. 1997.

50. Jackson et al. 1997.

51. Wills and Cleary 1996.

52. Jackson, Bee-Gates, and Henriksen 1994.

53. Bailey, Ennett, and Ringwalt 1993.

54. Bailey, Ennett, and Ringwalt 1993.

55. Farkas et al. 2000; Wakefield et al. 2000.

56. Proescholdbell, Chassin, and MacKinnon 2000.

57. Farkas et al. 2000.

58. Anda et al. 1999. This study used a retrospective cohort design.

59. Ellickson and Hays 1992.

60. Flay, Hu, and Richardson 1998.

61. Patton et al. 1998b; Turner, Irwin, and Millstein 1991.

62. Pederson et al. 1998.

63. Wang et al. 1998; Pederson et al. 1998; Harrell et al. 1998.

64. Harrell et al. 1998; Pederson et al. 1998.

65. Wang et al. 1998.

66. Jackson 1998; Flay, Hu, and Richardson 1998; Distefan et al. 1998.

67. Stanton and Silva 1992; Aloise-Young, Hennigan, and Graham 1996; Escobedo et al. 1993.

68. Fergusson and Horwood 1995.

69. Tschann et al. 1994; Flay et al. 1994.

70. Jackson 1998. Susceptibility may be a stronger predictor of smoking status than is the number of friends who smoke, because the prevalence of smoking is so low in this age-group.

71. Flay, Hu, and Richardson 1998.
72. Distefan et al. 1998.
73. Flay et al. 1994.
74. Distefan et al. 1998.
75. Choi et al. 1997.
76. Choi et al. 1997.
77. Fergusson and Horwood 1995.
78. Patton et al. 1998a, 1998b; Flay et al. 1994.
79. Distefan et al. 1998; Choi et al. 1997.
80. Fergusson and Horwood 1995.
81. Fergusson and Horwood 1995.
82. McGee and Stanton 1993; McGee, Williams, and Stanton 1998.
83. McGee and Stanton 1993.
84. McGee, Williams, and Stanton 1998.
85. Breslau and Peterson 1996.
86. Swan 1999.
87. Hebert 1999.
88. Carmelli et al. 1992; Han, McGue, and Iacono 1999.
89. Hettema, Corey, and Kendler 1999.
90. Carmelli et al. 1992; Han, McGue, and Iacono 1999.
91. Carmelli et al. 1992.
92. Sabol et al. 1999; Lerman et al. 1999.
93. Benowitz 1992.
94. Pianezza, Sellers, and Tyndale 1998.
95. Lerman et al. 1999.
96. Pederson, Koval, and O'Connor 1997.
97. Dinh, Sarason, and Peterson 1995.
98. Dinh, Sarason, and Peterson 1995.
99. Dinh, Sarason, and Peterson 1995.
100. Dinh, Sarason, and Peterson 1995.
101. Dinh, Sarason, and Peterson 1995.
102. Wang, Fitzhugh, Cowdry, and Trucks 1995.
103. Wang, Fitzhugh, Cowdry, and Trucks 1995.
104. Distefan et al. 1999.
105. This is called self-consistency, meaning that teens may begin to smoke because their self-image is similar to their image of most smokers. Thus, smoking is viewed as consistent with self-image.
106. This is called self-enhancement, which refers to the teen's desire to smoke because the smoker's image is more positive than the self-image. Aloise-Young and Hennigan 1996.
107. Dinh, Sarason, and Peterson 1995.
108. Aloise-Young and Hennigan 1996.
109. Sarason et al. 1992.
110. Pederson et al. 1998; Aloise-Young and Hennigan 1996.
111. Aloise-Young, Hennigan, and Graham 1996.
112. Tomeo et al. 1999; French et al. 1994; Crisp et al. 1999.
113. Camp, Klesges, and Relyea 1993; Klesges, Elliott, and Robinson 1997.

114. Tomeo et al. 1999.

115. Thorlindsson, Vilhjalmsson, and Valgeirsson 1990; Pederson et al. 1998.

116. Thorlindsson, Vilhjalmsson, and Valgeirsson 1990. Holmen et al. 2000.

117. Escobedo et al. 1993.

118. Thorlindsson, Vilhjalmsson, and Valgeirsson 1990.

119. Pederson et al. 1998; Koval and Pederson 1999.

120. Koval and Pederson 1999.

121. Sarason et al. 1992.

122. Koval and Pederson 1999; Pederson et al. 1998.

123. Flay, Hu, and Richardson 1998.

124. Greening and Dollinger 1991.

125. Dolcini and Adler 1994.

126. Jackson, Bee-Gates, and Henriksen 1994.

127. Epstein, Griffin, and Botvin 2000.

128. Lifrak et al. 1997.

129. Distefan et al. 1998.

130. Lifrak et al. 1997. Low academic achievement is also correlated with greater impatience in weighing current and future needs. Impulsiveness is a key risk factor for all forms of substance abuse.

131. Distefan et al. 1998; Jackson, Bee-Gates, and Henriksen 1994.

132. Bailey, Ennett, and Ringwalt 1993; Pederson et al. 1998.

133. Ellickson and Hays 1992.

134. Tuakli, Smith, and Heaton 1990; Botvin et al. 1992.

135. Urberg 1992; Urberg, Shyu, and Liang 1990; Botvin et al. 1992.

136. Botvin et al. 1992; Bailey, Ennett, and Ringwalt 1993.

137. Flay, Hu, and Richardson 1998.

138. Botvin et al. 1992.

139. Botvin et al. 1992.

140. Iannotti, Bush, and Weinfurt 1996.

141. Everett et al. 1998. Other drug use that was measured included alcohol, marijuana, and cocaine. Students were asked whether they had ever used any of these substances and, if so, whether they had used any of these substances in the past month. Students were also asked if they had had five or more drinks on at least one occasion in the past month.

142. Pederson et al. 1998.

143. Pederson et al. 1998.

144. Wang et al. 1996. Wu and Anthony (1999) claim that there is an association between smoking and subsequent depressive symptoms but that depressed mood is not associated with a subsequent decision to use cigarettes.

145. Patton et al. 1998a.

146. Anda et al. 1990; Floyd et al. 1993; Borrelli et al. 1996.

147. Patton et al. 1998a.

148. Patton et al. 1998a.

149. Stein, Newcomb, Bentler 1996.

150. Johnston, O'Malley, and Bachman 1998b.

151. Fergusson and Horwood 1995; Fergusson, Lynskey, and Horwood 1995; Derzon and Lipsey 1999.

152. Breslau and Peterson 1996.
153. Bauman et al. 1990.
154. Males 1995.
155. Stanton, Lowe, and Silva 1995.
156. Flay et al. 1994.
157. Stanton, Lowe, and Silva 1995.
158. Stanton, Lowe, and Silva 1995.
159. Greenlund et al. 1997.

Part 2

Strategies for Adolescent Smoking Prevention and Control

Prevention And Cessation

As we demonstrated in part 1, a large body of research shows that, at the present time, very few people initiate smoking or become habitual smokers after their teen years. In the United States, nearly 9 out of 10 current adult smokers (89 percent) started their habit before age 19. By this age, most youth who are going to smoke have already become or are in the process of becoming habitual smokers. That is why a great deal of policy and programmatic attention has been directed at youth smoking in the United States.

In this chapter, we synthesize and comment on the growing literature regarding efforts to discourage youth from smoking. We describe a number of strategies for youth smoking prevention and control, and we summarize the state of the science regarding the impact or effectiveness of each strategy. The 1994 reports on youth smoking by the U.S. surgeon general and the Institute of Medicine (IOM) are particularly valuable resources.[1] We summarize material from these earlier reports but focus on studies and strategies that have emerged since.

We limit our review to youth-oriented prevention and control strategies and to cigarette smoking, recognizing that adult interventions and the use of other tobacco products (smokeless tobacco and bidis) also deserve similar attention. Since very few tobacco intervention studies include cost analyses, we cannot offer specific advice regarding the costs of various interventions and the likely returns on these investments. Nonetheless, this chapter should be quite useful to tobacco control advocates and policymakers, as well as to community organizations, in deciding what types of interventions to conduct.[2]

We first describe the published research regarding tobacco prevention interventions. Then we discuss current adolescent tobacco cessation efforts. Next we discuss promising and innovative prevention strategies that warrant further implementation and rigorous evaluation, including recent comprehensive efforts ongoing in several states. At appropriate points throughout the chapter, we also discuss related efforts at reducing adolescent use of illicit drugs.

In general, the studies we review have shown mixed results. But some recent innovations and early results from the newly developed comprehensive programs suggest reasons for optimism that prevention strategies can be effective if sufficient resources are invested and if the programs are sustained over time. Even more important, recent research suggests considerable synergies when interventions are combined. This seems particularly applicable to ongoing comprehensive efforts in several states.

Prevention Activities

In response to the problem of adolescent smoking, policymakers and researchers have devised a wide range of disease prevention and health promotion activities to reduce tobacco use. In public health, primary prevention has the goal of preventing a disease or negative health condition before it emerges. In the case of tobacco use, primary prevention has the goal of preventing or impeding youth from initiating tobacco use. Primary prevention activities in the area of youth smoking include school-based educational interventions, community interventions, mass media/public education campaigns, tobacco advertising restrictions, youth access restrictions, tobacco excise taxes, and brief office-based clinical interventions.

In contrast, secondary prevention has the goal of minimizing negative health outcomes by changing the course of a disease or health condition through early detection and subsequent treatment. In the case of youth tobacco control, the aim of secondary prevention efforts is to identify youth who already are using tobacco products and to help them quit. While primary prevention efforts attempt to target youth before they have tried cigarettes or are engaged in the behavior, secondary prevention activities are aimed at those who are already smoking. Because of the number of regular or habitual smokers among youth—especially among older adolescents—secondary prevention is an important activity in youth tobacco control. Secondary prevention activities include direct restrictions on smoking in public and private places, office-based clinical interventions, and other tobacco cessation interventions.

School-Based Educational Interventions

Early attempts to discourage youth tobacco use focused primarily on educational interventions in elementary and secondary schools. This strategy has shown promising short-term results in some settings, but one concern is a lack of evidence that any impact is sustained over a longer period of time.

Elementary and Secondary Levels
A large number of school-based programs for tobacco use prevention have been implemented during the past three decades. Most of these efforts target elementary school and/or middle school students. As described in the IOM report on youth smoking, the majority of these programs have tended to be based on one of three main approaches. The first approach is based on an *information deficit model,* or *rational model.* In this approach, the program provides information about the health risks and negative consequences of tobacco, most often in a manner intended to arouse concern or fear. Many of the early education interventions in youth tobacco control (before the mid-1970s) were based on this model. The primary premise of this approach is that youth are generally misinformed about the risks of smoking and that educating them about the health and social determinants of smoking will provide a deterrent. Programs based on this model have generally been found to be ineffective in deterring initiation or reducing volume among current smokers, although many programs either were not evaluated or were assessed only on short-term impact.

The second major approach to youth tobacco prevention programs is based on an *affective education model.* In this approach, the program attempts to influence beliefs, attitudes, intentions, and norms related to tobacco use, with a focus on enhancing self-esteem and helping to clarify what the individual values. This type of prevention program emphasizes the factors within an individual that influence tobacco use decisions, recognizing that lack of knowledge about the harms and addictive nature of tobacco is not the only factor associated with smoking initiation. The content themes across many of these programs include enhancing self-esteem and self-image, developing stress management techniques, clarifying values, improving decision-making skills, and assisting in goal setting. Evaluation findings for this type of intervention generally have suggested a weak or insignificant impact.

The third approach to tobacco prevention is based on a *social influ-*

ence resistance model. In this approach, the program recognizes and emphasizes the social environment (e.g., peer and parental influence and other social factors discussed in chap. 3) as a critical factor in tobacco use. As such, this type of intervention focuses on building skills needed to recognize and resist influences that might encourage adolescent tobacco use, including recognition of advertising tactics and peer influences, communication and decision-making skills, and assertiveness.

The results of many individual evaluations and meta-analyses[3] of tobacco and other drug prevention programs strongly suggest that programs based on the social influence resistance model are the most effective of the three approaches. The IOM report concluded that evaluations of school-based prevention programs have "consistently demonstrated that a brief school intervention that focuses on social influences and teaches refusal skills can have a modest but significant effect in reducing the onset and level of tobacco use."[4] For example, a meta-analysis of smoking prevention program evaluations published between 1974 and 1991 found that social influence programs could account for reductions in smoking between 5 and 30 percent (with the upper range given as the highest estimate of program performance under "optimal" conditions only).[5] Other meta-analyses of controlled studies of drug use prevention programs for youth reported that interactive programs and those led by peers that addressed the social influences of substance use were most effective.[6] These findings were echoed by another meta-analysis suggesting that interactive peer interventions for middle schoolers are superior to noninteractive, didactic programs led by researchers or teachers.[7]

Similarly, a different meta-analysis of smoking prevention programs for adolescents found that the effects of interventions with a "traditional" or "rational" orientation were small and often insignificant. In contrast, those interventions with a social reinforcement orientation (i.e., interventions focusing on the development of skills to recognize and resist social pressures) had the largest effects in terms of attitude and behavioral change.[8] Although not all social influence interventions have been successful, a wide body of literature suggests that this approach has the best track record overall.[9]

One particular intervention that has received a great amount of attention is the Drug Abuse Resistance Education, or DARE, program. Taught by uniformed police officers, DARE combines the building of self-esteem, the development of resistance skills, and information about the negative effects of drug use and violence.[10] Project DARE is the most prevalent school-based drug prevention program in the country and is typically offered to students during the last year of elementary school. Despite DARE's popularity and proliferation, few positive long-term results regarding tobacco and other drug use have been revealed in numerous individual or combined program evaluations.[11]

The long-term impact of school-based educational interventions is of concern. It appears that the effects tend to dissipate with time, generally persisting in the range of one to four years. The IOM report stated that "while the results of more than 20 research studies have shown that school-based prevention programs alone have consistently delayed onset of smoking, lasting effects have only been demonstrated at 2-year follow-up."[4] Program "boosters," or subsequent interventions (e.g., telephone contacts, additional classroom discussion, or providing published materials), appear to enhance the staying power of the intervention effects, although the most appropriate content of and timing for these booster sessions is not known.[12] In a recent Dutch study, a social influence approach was combined with a booster consisting of additional published materials provided six months and then nearly two years later. The combined social influence and booster interventions reduced the onset of smoking among eighth and ninth grade nonsmokers at 18-month follow-up more than did a social influence intervention alone or no intervention among a control group.[13] Aside from booster programs as part of the health curriculum, we found no U.S. studies dealing directly with older adolescents. At the present time, there does not appear to be much tobacco prevention activity at the high school level.

CDC has recently recommended two school-based interventions based on successful evaluations. The first, the Life Skills Training (LST) curriculum, recognizes the multiple pathways leading adolescents to experiment with tobacco and drugs using a social influences model and a *personal risk factors model.* The program de-emphasizes information concerning the long-term physiological effects of smoking in favor of imparting information concerning the immediate negative effects, both socially and physically, and accurate peer prevalence estimates.[14]

The LST program is targeted at students in grades 6–9 but would ideally be implemented starting in the sixth or seventh grade with boosters in following years. In total, the program consists of 30 lessons spread over three academic years—15 in the first year, 10 in the next, and 5 in the third. At the conclusion of the program, students should be able to demonstrate knowledge concerning the development of self-image; identify misinformation concerning tobacco, alcohol, and marijuana use; describe the health consequences of smoking; show effective communication and coping skills; show media literacy; and demonstrate relationship-building skills.

The LST program significantly reduced cigarette, alcohol, and marijuana use as compared to a control group.[14] At least twelve major evaluations of LST have been conducted with a variety of implementers and student populations, with results of reductions in cigarette use of up to 87 percent being reported.[15]

The second program recommended by CDC, Project Toward No Tobacco Use (Project TNT), trains seventh graders in resistance skills. Its comprehensive approach is designed to address simultaneously the variety of risk factors influencing tobacco use. The fundamental theory of the program is that adolescents can resist using tobacco if misunderstandings about the social normalcy of smoking can be corrected, if they have the skills to resist seeking social approval by smoking, and if they can understand the physical consequences of smoking.

Project TNT consists of 10 core lessons of approximately 40–50 minutes in length, which are intended to be taught over a two-week interval. There are also two follow-up lessons. At the end of the program, students should be able to describe the health consequences of smoking; accurately estimate peer smoking prevalence; show effective peer refusal, communication, and coping skills; demonstrate media literacy; identify self-esteem building activities; and advocate strategies for no tobacco use.

According to the CDC, Project TNT reduced both the initiation and daily and weekly use of cigarettes and smokeless tobacco as compared to a control group. These results were confirmed in one- and two-year follow-up evaluations.[16]

However, a long-term randomized trial in Washington State found no significant differences between the experimental and control districts in terms of smoking at two years post high school. The school-based intervention under study was based on a social influences model which started in third grade and continued with follow-up components through twelfth grade. The disappointing results of this intensive intervention and well-designed trial suggest that new approaches to school-based tobacco prevention need to be created.[17]

College Level
Recent evidence indicates a disturbing increase in smoking behavior among college students, suggesting the limits of school-based preven-

tion efforts at the elementary and secondary levels. In recent years, the prevalence of smoking on college campuses has increased nationwide. Based on longitudinal data from 130 college campuses, the prevalence of self-reported smoking in the past 30 days increased from 22.3 percent in 1993 to 28.5 percent in 1997.[18] A subsequent survey at 119 colleges confirmed these results, finding that 38.1% smoked a cigarette during the previous year.[19] A study by the University of Minnesota found that tobacco use among first-year students increased by 150 percent between 1992 and 1998.[20]

Recent results from the Monitoring the Future project reveal a trend toward increased cigarette use among young adults (ages 18–24) in general.[21] This increase is believed to reflect the rise in smoking that occurred among adolescents earlier in the 1990s. Significantly, a study of four universities found that 10 percent of smokers had their first cigarette and 11 percent started smoking on a regular basis after high school.[22] Besides the risks posed by smoking, young adults who smoke cigarettes are also at a higher risk for binge drinking and the use of marijuana, cocaine, and LSD.[23]

A number of interventions aimed at preventing tobacco, alcohol, and other drug abuse have been implemented in both urban and rural colleges and universities, although few have undergone rigorous evaluation and few are perceived as being effective by those implementing them.[24] Nonetheless, it has been argued that "college might be an opportune time to intervene to prevent transition from occasional smoking to regular nicotine-dependent smoking, and a time to teach occasional and regular smokers why and how to quit."[18] Indeed, there is evidence that a college-based intervention against smokeless tobacco can be successful.[25] In this instance, an intervention to educate athletes about the harms from smokeless tobacco led to greater cessation rates than among the control group. Significantly, the effect of the intervention was greater among more frequent users.

These trends raise the possibility that there is an emerging increase in smoking initiation among older teenagers and young adults. If so, this may indicate that a successful strategy to reduce young adolescent smoking may result in delaying or deferring tobacco use until older adolescence or young adulthood. It may also mean that policymakers and tobacco control advocates must begin to pay more attention to the young adult population. We return to the implications of these issues in our "Conclusion and Recommendations."

School-Based Prevention of Illicit Drug Use
Schools not only must be concerned with adolescent tobacco use but also must act to prevent illicit substance use. The most widely used drug prevention strategies are similar to those described earlier for preventing tobacco use, with similar results.[26]

Drug prevention programs for older adolescents are often focused on improving academic skills. Many are also aimed at creating a sustained relationship with adult advisors or mentors who can provide social and emotional support while reinforcing appropriate social norms regarding substance abuse and other high-risk behaviors.[27] Such intense interventions are costly to implement, but they are also likely to influence a wide range of outcomes and risk behaviors of substantial policy concern. Thus, they are likely to be both more expensive initially and more cost-effective in the long term than many competing interventions that are more narrowly focused and less ambitious in their intended effects.

Summary of School-Based Programs
A large number of individual evaluations and review articles regarding educational interventions to reduce youth tobacco use have been published. A wide range of evaluation results from experimental and quasi-experimental studies suggest that some of these educational programs resulted in a significant short-term reduction in smoking, a delay in initiation, or a desirable change in attitudes toward tobacco use. Programs that embrace a social influences model tend to be the most effective, especially when enhanced by an extensive community-based health education program. The recent literature confirms but does not greatly expand on the 1994 reports of the surgeon general and the IOM. Perhaps more surprisingly, there is not a welter of new evaluations of school-based programs: either such programs have not changed very much or previous findings have discouraged scholars from exploring these programs any further.

Many of the guidelines for developing and implementing school-based tobacco prevention programs previously issued by the National Cancer Institute (NCI) and CDC are still relevant and worth considering.[28] CDC's updated recommendations include (1) developing and enforcing a school policy on tobacco use; (2) providing adolescents with information on the short- and long-term physiologic and social consequences of tobacco use and on the social influences and peer norms concerning tobacco use; (3) incorporating refusal skills training;

(4) providing smoking education from kindergarten through twelfth grade, with the most intensity in middle school and boosters in high school; (5) training teachers to implement each program; (6) encouraging families to participate in the school-based programs; (7) providing smoking cessation services for all students and school staff who use tobacco; and (8) evaluating tobacco use prevention programs regularly.[29]

Community Interventions

The increased understanding of the combined effects of environmental, social, and cultural conditions on tobacco and other substance use has resulted in an emphasis on interventions that include comprehensive, community-based approaches.[30] By labeling these approaches comprehensive, we mean that they include multiple systems, institutions, or learning channels simultaneously and employs multiple intervention strategies (i.e., education, incentives, regulation). In general, community interventions have numerous components and involve the use of resources to influence both individual behavior and community norms or practices related to discouraging adolescent tobacco use. This activity includes the involvement of families, schools, community organizations, churches, businesses, the media, social service and health agencies, government, and law enforcement. Intervention strategies are generally focused on making changes in both the environment and individual behavior. Although community interventions take a variety of shapes, common elements among them include a shared emphasis on altering the social environment or social context in which tobacco products are obtained or consumed and a shared goal of creating a social environment that is supportive of nonsmoking or cessation.[31] Some of the components of community interventions, such as mass media campaigns and youth access restrictions, are also implemented as stand-alone interventions.

An increasing number of communities are attempting to influence youth tobacco use with multiple-component interventions. While there are only a few published reports of rigorously designed evaluations, the available research results are encouraging in many cases.[32] For example, a longitudinal study reported that a community intervention involving mass media, school-based education, parent education, community organizing, and health policy components in some of the 15 communities in the Kansas City metropolitan area was effective in reducing tobacco, alcohol, and illicit drug use. Regarding tobacco use, a significantly lower rate of smoking was observed in the intervention group at six months and at two years (the rates for smoking in the last month were 19 percent in the program group vs. 29 percent in the control group).[33] In addition, the results of a randomized trial conducted in rural Oregon communities demonstrated a reduction in the prevalence of weekly cigarette use in communities exposed to the intervention (which focused on key social influences of smoking and included media advocacy, antitobacco activities for youth, and family communication activities).[34]

Evaluation results for numerous other community interventions are available and have been reviewed in several places.[35] For example, in the Class of 1989 Study, which was part of the Minnesota Heart Health Program, youth from the intervention communities had a 40 percent lower smoking prevalence rate after three years, with a significant reduction being maintained over a six-year period.[36] This intervention involved school-based activities (which were also taking place in the control community) plus community activities, including risk-factor screening, adult smoking cessation, and smoking policy changes at school and other community facilities.

The results from the Midwestern Prevention Project—which focused exclusively on youth—were also positive.[37] This six-year, longitudinal intervention study was implemented in 50 middle and junior high schools in the Indianapolis and Kansas City areas. While the intervention here was school-based, many intervention activities focused on the broader social and community environments in which youth live. The focus of the intervention activities and policy changes—which took place in schools and through the media, parents, and community organizations—was on building resistance skills among youth and environmental support for not smoking or using drugs. The results showed that, at the two-year follow-up mark, the rate of increase in smoking was 1.5 times greater in the control schools than in the program schools.[38]

School-based programs and community interventions involving parents, mass media, and community organizations appear to have a stronger impact over time when they work in tandem, rather than as separate, stand-alone interventions.[39] Mobilizing parents and community elements outside of the school (including the media) enhances school-based interventions and increases the potential for a lasting behavioral impact.[40] This finding is particularly important for states to consider in allocating tobacco control funds, since it suggests that various interventions are more effective when initiated as part of a comprehensive strategy. It also indicates the importance of involving communities in tobacco control activities.

COMMIT

An important community-based intervention, the Community Intervention Trial for Smoking Cessation (COMMIT), was the largest community intervention regarding smoking cessation prior to Project ASSIST (described shortly). Funded by NCI, COMMIT involved 11 different programs implemented in 22 communities, with each intervention community paired with a control community. The hypothesis was that the implementation of a clear intervention delivered through multiple community groups and organizations, dependent on limited external resources, would increase smoking cessation among adult smokers and reduce smoking prevalence.[41] Although the efforts of COMMIT focused on adult heavy smokers, the goals of this initiative also included increasing the influence of existing policy and economic factors that discourage smoking and increasing social norms and values that support nonsmoking. As part of a community-wide program, COMMIT interventions took place in school classrooms, at clinics and hospitals, at work sites, and in mass media campaigns.[42]

Evaluations of COMMIT suggest that this community intervention had an impact on light to moderate smokers but was unsuccessful in modifying the behavior of heavier smokers.[43] Unfortunately, COMMIT efforts aimed at youth have received little evaluative attention.

One study examined the impact of tobacco taxes, public smoking ordinances, laws regulating youth access, and exposure to tobacco messages (both for and against tobacco use) in 21 of the 22 COMMIT communities.[44] These researchers found that tax increases (discussed in chap. 6), exposure to tobacco education in schools, and policies restricting youth access to tobacco (discussed in chap. 7) were associated with decreased smoking and a lesser intention to use cigarettes among ninth graders. The authors also observed that the frequency of exposure to antitobacco advertisements was associated with an increased likelihood of smoking. This counterintuitive finding was not statistically significant in some of the subanalyses conducted by the authors and is contradicted by other findings from the same study. Some might argue that the paradoxical finding lends credence to the perspective that the strong focus of tobacco control interventions on youth may unintentionally be glamorizing tobacco use as an adult behavior and thus may have counterproductive effects.[45] At the present time, there is little empirical evidence to substantiate this concern, and no similar concerns have been raised in the counteradvertising campaigns now underway.

Project ASSIST

Another comprehensive community intervention is the American Stop Smoking Intervention Study for Cancer Prevention, or ASSIST, an eight-year program (1991–99) funded by the NCI in collaboration with the American Cancer Society and state and local health departments.[46] The COMMIT project was the direct precursor to ASSIST and the basis for much of ASSIST's focus and content. The overall goal of ASSIST was to reduce smoking prevalence to 15 percent by the year 2000 by encouraging smokers to quit and by discouraging young people from initiating the habit. Project ASSIST was unique in that it offered the potential to reach over 90 million Americans and in that it was largely planned and implemented by coalitions organized for the sole purpose of reducing smoking rates in their own communities.

Many local ASSIST coalitions emphasized the use of public health information and advocacy to denormalize tobacco use in the community. Some strategies used by ASSIST communities to prevent and reduce youth tobacco use included youth education, encouraging enforcement of laws restricting youth access, banning tobacco advertising that is youth-oriented, environmental tobacco smoke restrictions, and increasing physicians' role in youth tobacco prevention efforts. Currently, there are few published articles evaluating the effectiveness of Project ASSIST efforts in general or relative to youth in particular.[47] One study reported that interim results regarding the impact of ASSIST suggest that this program has led to reduced tobacco consumption in ASSIST states and that this effect reflects more than increased prices from tobacco taxation. Between 1993 and 1996, ASSIST states showed a 7 percent per capita reduction in tobacco consumption as compared to non-ASSIST states.[48] Another group studied the factors related to coalition effectiveness in 10 Project ASSIST communities in North Carolina but did not evaluate individual programs for effectiveness in reducing smoking rates.[49] They found that community groups possessing an articulated plan, including specific goals and strategies for implementation, had stronger coalitions than community groups lacking these characteristics.

The efforts of several community interventions involved a particular focus on youth access to tobacco products. In some states, ASSIST funds were used to conduct checks of retailer compliance with existing laws and ordinances.[50] Numerous other examples of community intervention efforts related to youth access have been reviewed, including the development and implementation of restrictions regarding cigarette vending machines; restrictions regarding the sale of "loose," or single, cigarettes; restrictions regarding the age of people who can sell cigarettes; and requirements regarding the training of salespersons.[51] All of these are examples of attempts to alter the social environment or policy context in which tobacco products are obtained, distributed, or consumed. So far, there is little evidence as to the effectiveness of these initiatives in reducing youth tobacco consumption. As we will show shortly, however, some recent comprehensive state-based programs show promising early results.

Community-Based Prevention of Illicit Drug Use

As in the case of tobacco, many community-based interventions seek to reduce illicit substance use.[52] One such intervention is the Fighting Back program funded by the Robert Wood Johnson Foundation.[53] This ambitious effort seeks to create a multifaceted, locally directed response to harmful drug use. Drawing on previous experience in both substance abuse policy and community organization, Fighting Back has important political, educational, social service, and occupational health components. Through the creation of neighborhood management teams and other devices, the program seeks to create political networks that allow local residents to persuade politicians and public agencies to close crack houses, repair abandoned buildings, and address other social contexts conducive to drug use.

Fighting Back has a significant educational component, largely aimed at preventing adolescent initiation and use of alcohol, tobacco, or other drugs. Unlike many youth tobacco prevention programs, Fighting Back includes in its guidelines efforts to target specific individuals at greatest risk. Through early identification, assessment, and referral into treatment, the program includes an important secondary prevention component designed to prevent casual experimentation from becoming chronic harmful use.

In an effort to create a viable continuum of care, Fighting Back also maintains an outreach effort for professionals who are especially likely to encounter individuals with drug problems. Emergency rooms, correctional facilities, public housing, and other sites have been targeted as part of this effort.[54]

Important research evaluating this intervention explores both community changes in the prevalence of drug-related adverse outcomes and changes in the civic infrastructure that can be plausibly linked with the intervention.[55] Although changes in civic organization can be documented, linking changes in community-level political and social factors to changes in individual behavior and outcomes is much more difficult, reflecting many methodological problems in evaluating these approaches.[56] Despite the impressive funding and organization of Fighting Back in many locations, the efficacy and cost-effectiveness of this program is not known. However, this intervention was viewed as sufficiently promising for the Center for Substance Abuse Prevention to establish community partnership demonstrations on a similar model.[57]

Comprehensive Tobacco Control Programs

Besides the ASSIST initiative, several state health departments have developed comprehensive tobacco prevention and control programs that attempt to discourage youth tobacco use through multiple interventions. "Best practices" for this type of statewide, comprehensive tobacco control program were recently summarized by CDC,[58] which views comprehensive, statewide programs as having the potential to reduce youth tobacco use by increasing the tobacco control capacity of local programs, promoting media advocacy, implementing clean indoor air policies, and reducing minors' access to tobacco. Thus, statewide programs should (1) provide resources for organizational networking to design and evaluate coordinated interventions; (2) sponsor training sessions, conferences, and technical assistance workshops; and (3) support innovative demonstration projects and interventions at the state, regional, and local levels.

Comprehensive programs need to involve statewide organizations, as they have access to diverse communities and often have additional organizational resources to share. Organizations and individuals at the regional and local levels should also be involved.

In this section, we briefly summarize three state programs that have generated considerable national attention—from California, Massachusetts, and Florida—and their initial evaluation results. While these programs are in the early stages of development and implementation, the preliminary results suggest that these comprehensive models have significant potential for youth tobacco control.

California

In 1988, California voters passed Proposition 99, the Tobacco Tax and Health Promotion Act. It raised the tax on cigarettes from 10 to 35 cents and also increased the taxes on other tobacco products. Not only did the increase in the tobacco excise tax fund the program components, but the tax increase also serves as an important intervention component itself. Part of the tax increase was used to create the California Tobacco Control Program (CTCP), which began in 1989 and was evaluated in 1996 and 1999. California is the only state to have prohibited smoking in bars or limited it to separately ventilated areas. It has also enacted statewide laws prohibiting indoor smoking at government work sites, private work sites, and restaurants, except in designated areas.[58]

The goal of the CTCP is to reduce the prevalence of both youth and adult smoking.[59] The original components of the program were modeled after earlier community interventions and included mass media campaigns, community organization efforts, education for prevention and cessation of smoking, health care provider education, and health promotion at work sites.[60] The state's strategy focuses on specific populations, multiple interventions for multiple aspects contributing to tobacco use, and multiple channels for the interventions. An example of this is the network of local and city health departments, called Local Lead Agencies, that was developed to coordinate tobacco control programs in the community and beyond.

Funding for the CTCP has not always been consistent. In its first year, the budget was over $130 million. For several subsequent years, until 1994, the CTCP received only a portion of what the mandate proposed. Recent budgets have approached the original level, but the program was less effective when the advertising budget was reduced from $16 million in 1991 to $6.6 million in 1995. Evaluators also noted that the decline in effectiveness accompanied a shift in the advertising strategy from attacking industry practices to focusing on health hazards. [61]

More recently, the focus has shifted from components of the social learning and communications theory to changing the smoking environment in California. Recent funding has concentrated on three goals: reducing exposure to environmental tobacco smoke, reducing youth access, and countering pro-tobacco influences (i.e., reducing the social acceptability of smoking).[60]

Despite budget fluctuations, there is some evidence that the program has been effective. Several program evaluations have taken place at different stages of implementation, including surveys of adult and adolescent populations, a process evaluation that monitored CTCP program implementation, and an evaluation of the implementation and impact of school-based initiatives. Overall, the effects of the program have been positive. Although adolescent smoking increased in California in the early 1990s, it did so at a rate that was lower than in other states. Adult smoking has declined more steeply in California than in other states (from 26.7 percent in 1988 to 18.4 percent in 1998),[62] as have lung cancer rates (decreasing by 14 percent between 1988 and 1997 compared to a 2.7 percent decline in other regions).[63] Surveys indicate several important changes between 1996 and 1993: more no-smoking policies at work, less smoking in the home, majority support of policies to ban store advertisements, and a majority recollection of various media spots and antitobacco messages.[60] Overall, one study estimates that during its first nine years, California's anti-smoking program prevented 33,000 deaths from tobacco-related heart disease.[64]

Results from the CTCP's actions to influence youth behavior are similarly promising. Adults and opinion leaders overwhelmingly support tobacco vendor licensure, and law enforcement personnel believe it is an effective means to stop stores from selling to minors. Almost every school district has adopted a no-smoking policy for students and staff, and over 90 percent of students are aware of their school's policy. Adolescent smoking rates, up from 9.2 percent in 1990 and 1993 to 12 percent in 1996 (an increase of over 30 percent) and up among all subgroups, are still much lower than national rates of smoking for 12–17 year olds. More important, the rate of adolescent smoking in California has dropped by 12 percent since 1995.[62]

Massachusetts

The Massachusetts Tobacco Control Program (MTCP) is funded by the proceeds from a voter-mandated increase in cigarette taxes (from 26 to 51 cents) passed in November 1992. The goals of the MTCP are threefold: to reduce exposure to environmental tobacco smoke, to reduce youth access to cigarettes and prevent smoking uptake in adolescence, and to help adults quit smoking.[65]

The program, administered by the Massachusetts Department of Public Health, started with a statewide multimedia campaign (October 1993). Other activities at the state level include a Quit Tobacco telephone line, the Tobacco Education Clearinghouse, and projects to provide technical support and institution-building.[66] In late 1993, the media campaign was followed by funding to local health departments and school programs for reducing environmental smoke, smoking cessation activities, health education programs, assistance to primary care providers, and activities restricting youth access to cigarettes.[67]

The media campaign is the underpinning of the state-level effort to reduce smoking prevalence and change smoking norms. Television, radio, billboard, and print media were used to inform citizens of the dangers of smoking. Four themes were developed by the MTCP, each targeted at a specific population: the health consequences of smoking (adults), environmental tobacco smoke (public opinion), smoking is not the norm (African Americans), and the deglamorization of smoking (youth).

Based on a four-year longitudinal survey, a recent evaluation concluded that exposure to the television counteradvertising campaign reduced the progression toward routine smoking among youths aged 12–13 at baseline but not among those aged 14–15 at baseline. Neither radio nor outdoor (billboard) counterads influenced adolescent smoking behavior. But 12–13 year olds were more likely to have an accurate perception of adolescent smoking prevalence.

Local programming is also an important aspect of the MTCP. Community coalitions engage in community-wide education mobilization activities to raise public awareness and organize local efforts to reduce tobacco use. The activities of the local health department center around the enactment and enforcement of ordinances restricting youth access and also focus on providing smoking cessation services.[65] Local tobacco control coalitions also assist local health departments in planning and coordinating activities.[66]

The MTCP has developed several community-based smoking intervention strategies: programs designed by health workers to identify smokers in their client population; smoking cessation programs; innovative interventions for specific, at-risk populations; and programs aimed at youth with a focus on youth leadership roles in tobacco control.[65] The MTCP also functions at the regional level. All local tobacco control programs are organized into six, regional networks. The role of the networks is to facilitate communication across agencies, programs, and geographic regions; promote regional action planning and coordination of activities; disseminate information and identify best practices; and train participants.[66]

Shortly after the tax increase went into effect (January 1993), several cigarette manufactures lowered the price of their product so that in Massachusetts the price of cigarettes relative to inflation declined to the 1992 level.[67] In effect, this was a maneuver by the tobacco industry to erase the tax increase's negative consequences for consumption. Per capita consumption had, in fact, been declining in Massachusetts even before the tax increase and subsequent price decrease by some cigarette manufacturers.

Nonetheless, the MTCP appears to have precipitated a continuing decline. From 1992 to 1996, per capita consumption fell by 19.7 percent, well above the national average of 6.1 percent for the same time period.[67] An evaluation of MTCP showed an impressive 15 percent decline in adult smoking between 1993 and 1999, compared to little change in national adult smoking rates.[68]

Massachusetts has also seen a reversal of national smoking trends for youth during the MTCP. Data from the 1997 Youth Risk Behavior Surveillance Survey indicated a decrease of 2 percentage points in current youth smoking rates from 36 percent in 1995. In contrast, the national trend was an increase from 35 percent to 36 percent.[66] Further, successful purchase attempts in sting operations have dropped from 48 percent in 1992 to 10 percent in 1998.[69]

Florida

Florida is at the beginning stages of developing and implementing a comprehensive tobacco control program that includes an aggressive advertising campaign accompanied by an educational component. This is not to say that the Florida Department of Health, local health departments, and community groups have not been active in tobacco eradication activities for many years. Florida enacted youth access laws in October 1992 and again in May 1994 and has aggressively enforced these laws.[70]

What is in the planning stages in Florida closely resembles the comprehensive programs in California and Massachusetts but will be less comprehensive overall. The goals include the prevention of youth tobacco use, the promotion of youth and adult smoking cessation, a reduction in exposure to environmental tobacco smoke, and the targeting of at-risk populations.

The birth of Florida's Tobacco Pilot Program was a direct result of the settlement of the Medicaid litigation with the tobacco industry and the resulting $93 million in appropriations to begin its work. The program includes a marketing component, community partnerships, youth programs, youth access enforcement, and an evaluation component. The community partnerships were established with the intent to change social norms about smoking.

One well-known component of the program is the Truth media campaign, which seeks to counter the advertising techniques of the tobacco industry. The idea behind the Truth ads is to deglamorize smoking by attacking the integrity of the tobacco industry and by assailing the idea that smoking is cool and sexy. For example, one ad depicts an executive from the Lucky Strike tobacco brand who does not know why people are "lucky" when smoking. Adolescents from Students Working against Tobacco were actively involved in helping to design the media campaign. The Truth campaign has been hard-hitting, graphic, and sophisticated in attacking social norms and the integrity of the tobacco industry—so much so, in fact, that the Florida legislature yielded to industry lobbying by drastically reducing the advertising budget (from $24 million to $18 million), despite widespread public support for the message and the apparent success of the state's campaign.

While a full program evaluation is premature, Florida has seen substantial decreases in tobacco use among youth since the program went into effect. In fact, significant declines in youth smoking were observed almost immediately after the program was implemented. From February 1998 through February 1999, 30-day smoking prevalence rates among teens fell from 25.2 percent to 20.9 percent. For middle school students, the 30-day prevalence rate dropped from 15 percent to 8.6 percent, with declines noted for both sexes, for all ethnicities, and in cigar and smokeless tobacco use.[71]

Lessons Learned
The most important lesson from these efforts is the one drawn by a recent IOM report. When the Massachusetts and California experiences are compared to previous efforts, such as the ASSIST program, the more comprehensive, aggressive, and better-funded state programs demonstrated greater reductions in adolescent and adult tobacco use than did less intensive efforts.[72] Each of these programs targets several populations concurrently and uses multiple channels to disseminate the message. The programs are comprehensive both in using a variety

of media to reach their audiences and in incorporating multiple types of intervention (i.e., education, incentives, and regulation) at the state, regional, and local levels.

The IOM's conclusion was confirmed by a comparative analysis of these three programs plus programs in Arizona.[73] This analysis concluded that the combination of price increases and other interventions reduces both adult and teen smoking more than do price increases alone. The authors noted that both the extent of funding and efforts to protect funds from being drawn into competing uses are critical factors in whether a comprehensive program succeeds. In short, a state's commitment to the program's intensity and comprehensiveness matters.

Interventions that Focus on Adolescent Risk Taking and on
Problem Behaviors

As we noted in chapter 3, youth smoking occurs in a web of social relations that foster many types of adolescent experimentation and that also may foster problem behaviors. Because of this social context, youth smoking arises from some of the same family, peer, and community influences that are also important to sexual risk taking, participation in crime and violence, and the initiation of harmful alcohol and illicit substance use.[74] Existing prevention research regarding other adolescent problem behaviors, therefore, has potentially important implications for the design and evaluation of programs to curb youth smoking. Such interventions for older adolescents are often focused on improving academic skills. Many are also aimed at creating a sustained relationship with adult advisors or mentors who can provide social and emotional support while reinforcing appropriate social norms regarding substance abuse and other behaviors.[75] An additional approach involves family-focused interventions. There is a great deal of evidence supporting the efficacy of family-focused interventions regarding substance abuse, including interventions that address the multiple factors affecting family functioning.[76]

A small but potentially interesting literature for policymakers to consider examines the effectiveness of interventions designed to deal with behavior that indicates a propensity to use tobacco products. One such example was a randomized prevention trial to determine whether interventions targeting aggressive or disruptive classroom behavior—an early antecedent to smoking—would reduce adolescent use of tobacco.[77] Using the Good Behavior Game or the Mastery Learning Curriculum as the behavioral intervention, the authors found that tobacco use for disruptive boys who were assigned to the intervention was lower than in the control group. There were no differences for girls. These results suggest that it is beneficial to target early risk factors for tobacco use as a complement to subsequent prevention activities. This suggestion is consistent with another study finding that higher academic performance is associated with a lower probability of smoking and that policies directed toward improving academic performance may also reduce adolescent tobacco use.[78]

Two other studies examined the relationship between self-care after school and subsequent substance and tobacco use.[79] Each study concluded that unsupervised adolescents were more likely to use tobacco and other substances than were adolescents whose whereabouts were supervised by their parents or another adult. Additional research has examined the relationship between adult risk behaviors, including smoking, and adverse childhood experiences, such as child abuse and household dysfunction, concluding that an increased number of adverse events is associated with a greater risk of adolescent tobacco use.[80]

Taken together, these studies suggest that policymakers might consider a wider range of prevention efforts than traditionally associated with smoking behavior. Allocating funds to after-school and similar programs may reduce adolescent smoking by addressing some of the underlying experiences and risk factors that contribute to such use.

Summary of Prevention Activities

The results of a small number of controlled trials of community interventions and the early results from statewide, comprehensive tobacco control programs attest to their ability to affect youth smoking behavior. An important finding is that the effectiveness of school-based programs appears to be enhanced when they are included in broad-based community efforts in which parents, mass media, and community organizations are involved. These findings suggest that programs can be effective when the social policy or social environment as well as individual knowledge, attitudes, and behaviors are targeted for change. As the IOM report summarizes, studies suggest that the "combination of school and community tobacco use prevention programs can enhance the short-term impact of the school-based programs by providing a longer-term, multi-pronged approach that complements or is synergistic with school-based programs."[81]

In our view, broad-based community interventions alone are not sufficient to bring about a substantial and sustained decline in youth smoking. Community efforts, as symbolized by COMMIT, ASSIST, and other interventions, likely need to be combined into comprehensive programs with stronger advocacy, taxation, media interventions, and policy formation and implementation. As demonstrated in the more comprehensive approaches implemented by several states, comprehensive programs have the greatest chance for successfully reducing adolescent tobacco use.[82] It is also important to recognize that the limited number of evaluations with experimental or strong quasi-experimental designs seriously limits our understanding of whether community interventions are effective and, of equal importance, which of their components are most useful in reducing youth tobacco use. From a policy planning perspective, the absence of adequate evaluations makes it difficult to demonstrate which interventions provide the most benefits for the amount of resources invested.

Cessation Activities

Most adolescents are informed about the dangers of smoking[83] and the addictive nature of cigarettes, but there is evidence that they do not fully understand how difficult it will be for them to quit smoking. Adolescents make frequent quit attempts but less successful ones than adults.[84] In a twelfth-grade sample, nearly 70 percent of established smokers (those who had smoked at least 100 cigarettes in their lifetime) had tried to quit at one time, and 60 percent had tried to quit in the past year.[85] Only 3 percent achieved cessation beyond 12 months.

Adolescents may not realize the extent of their nicotine addiction and may therefore falsely expect cessation to be easily accomplished. In fact, surveys suggest that many adolescents do not expect to be smoking in five years, yet as we noted in our introduction to this book, fully 80 percent still smoke five years later.[86] Without the persistent negative health effects of smoking in evidence, adolescents may not be sufficiently motivated to complete smoking cessation, especially as cessation may involve "withdrawal symptoms such as craving, nervousness and tension, and restlessness."[87] Even though many adolescents report wanting to quit in theory, most are not taking concrete steps to that end.[83] The results from a study of a large focus group of high school smokers suggest that most adolescents are unfamiliar with the concept of a smoking cessation program or with other tools or methods that support quit attempts.[88] In attempting to quit, participants were not interested in seeking help or assistance from any professional person or service, including physicians, primarily because smoking cessation is perceived as something an individual must do alone and "cold turkey." Adolescents expressed concerns about confidentiality and parental involvement. Cessation rates in adolescent populations are also low because few medical interventions are available to them.

Smoking Cessation Interventions

The results of a number of descriptive studies and focus group studies suggest that many teen smokers are motivated to quit smoking. One study estimated that 74 percent of occasional teen smokers and 65 percent of daily teen smokers have a desire to quit, although other studies suggest that the success rate among those who do attempt to quit is low.[89] Another study found that smoking cessation rates among adolescents varied according to smoking status (46.3 percent among occasional smokers, 12.3 percent among daily smokers of 1 to 9 cigarettes, and 6.8 percent among daily smokers of more than 10 cigarettes).[90] All told, adolescent smoking cessation efforts have not been particularly successful.

Regardless of tobacco dependence, those who begin smoking at a later age are more likely to be able to quit than those who begin smoking earlier.[91] Individuals may decide to quit at different stages of tobacco use. The duration of smoking and intensity of smoking may affect quit rates of adolescents, and it would be expected that teens who have been smoking longer and/or more frequently would have a lower probability of a successful quit attempt. Differences in attitudes toward smoking, such as expectations of negative outcomes from smoking, could be expected to affect cessation success. Also, the adolescent's assessment of his or her ability to quit, called strength of self-efficacy beliefs, can influence cessation success.

The context in which smoking by adolescents occurs may be an important predictor of cessation.[83] Very few adolescent ex-smokers (less than 1 percent) had no adolescents who had never smoked cigarettes among their five closest friends.[82] Part of a successful youth cessation program should entail training adolescents to help friends quit along with them, as well as providing training to develop skills to resist peer pressure to smoke.

An important conclusion reached by several studies of adolescent smoking is the need to develop intervention strategies to keep occasional smokers from becoming daily smokers. As research has demonstrated, this would facilitate cessation interventions. Developing more effective adolescent cessation interventions should become a policy focus. Given the likelihood that even a wildly successful strategy to reduce adolescent smoking would still leave many adolescents unaffected, a successful cessation intervention could substantially reduce the morbidity and mortality costs of tobacco use.

Physician Intervention

Brief office interventions delivered by health care professionals hold great promise as a cessation strategy among smokers, especially those who are not yet addicted to nicotine. Such interventions regarding the dangers of smoking and the benefits of quitting delivered by physicians in health care delivery settings have been shown to be effective in promoting smoking cessation among adults.[92] Unfortunately, there have been very few studies of the efficacy of brief interventions for adolescent smoking cessation in health care settings.[93] These efforts must be sensitive to the specific beliefs and concerns that adolescents have about smoking cessation.

There is a clear need for training regarding smoking cessation interventions among clinicians serving adolescent patients.[94] While over 50 percent of adult smokers who had seen a physician in the past year were counseled to quit smoking, only 14 percent of smokers aged 12–17 had received cessation advice.[95] Similarly, in the 1993 Teenage Attitudes and Practices Survey, only 25 percent of 10–22 year olds reported that a health care provider had discussed cigarette smoking with them.[96] In one study, adolescents' smoking status was determined in 71 percent of visits, but physicians counseled adolescents only 17 percent of the time.[97] Research has shown that most pediatricians feel confident and prepared to address issues regarding environmental tobacco smoke with their patients but that fewer feel comfortable advising pediatric patients and their parents on how to stop smoking.[98] A number of materials (including guidelines and quick reference guides) in support of clinician-based interventions regarding smoking cessation are available from the Agency for Healthcare Research and Quality (AHRQ) or the CDC.[99]

In an attempt to encourage tobacco use prevention, the NCI recommends that pediatricians and other health professionals who care for children engage in "anticipatory guidance." This is the practice of counseling pediatric patients for potential future problems related to tobacco use.[100] For infancy and early childhood, anticipatory guidance should focus on educating parents about the relationship between environmental tobacco smoke exposure and child health problems. For young children, anticipatory guidance should involve discussing the health effects of smoking and stressing that all people are responsible for their own health. For adolescents, anticipatory guidance needs to emphasize the roles that peer pressure and peer modeling play in tobacco use, and it should include discussions of strategies for resisting or responding to this pressure.

At this point, there are no reported studies indicating the extent to which these guidelines are being implemented or are effective. Several ongoing projects involve managed care organizations, but most of these focus on adults and are too new to have reported results. Recent research suggests that adults who are counseled by physicians to quit smoking are more likely to do so than patients who are not counseled.[101] However, few primary care physicians in the COMMIT intervention used sophisticated smoking cessation interventions, such as the AHRQ clinical practice guidelines for smoking cessation, with patients.[102] Since family physicians and managed care organizations are well positioned to provide smoking cessation and counseling programs, they should be encouraged to do so. As a matter of public policy, funding should be made available to stimulate physician involvement in smoking cessation.

Although physicians can personalize powerful messages about tobacco for young patients, it is very important that youth receive anti-smoking messages from multiple sources.[103] In view of the importance of parental and familial influences on adolescent tobacco use, cessation strategies involving the entire family should be encouraged.

Youth-Oriented Smoking Cessation Programs

Almost all of the smoking cessation attention has focused on adults.[104] Our review suggests that efforts to develop and implement adolescent smoking cessation programs should be accelerated.[105] It is particularly important to target adolescents who are just at the transition point before or after habitual smoking begins. For obvious reasons, the longer the cessation interventions are delayed, the higher the probability that the smoker will become addicted to nicotine or that the addiction will become more severe. One possible approach is for states to incorporate smoking cessation programs for older adolescents as part of a broader school-based program.

By high school, prevention messages are largely irrelevant for a significant number of youth already addicted to nicotine. While there is increasing need for adolescent cessation programs, few programs have been evaluated, and there may be unexplored barriers to participation, such as fear of parents learning about their smoking behavior.

There is also a need to reconsider the use of nicotine replacement therapy for adolescents. Currently, the nicotine patch and nicotine gum are not legally available to minors. Manufacturers label their nicotine replacement therapies (NRTs) as not for sale to persons under 18, and instruct retailers about this restriction. The labeling and instructions to retailers are part of an agreement with FDA reached when the nicotine patch and gum were approved for over the counter retail sales. Physicians can prescribe NRT, but have done so only infrequently. Programs and policies dealing with nicotine replacement therapies and their use in adolescent cessation interventions should be examined for safety and efficacy. At least one study supports the safety of using nicotine patch therapy for adolescent smokers, while recognizing that more trials are needed to determine efficacy and safety.[106]

Increasing numbers of smoking cessation programs are now available for adolescents. For instance, LifeSign is a program that was first developed to aid adult smoking cessation attempts but was modified for youth smokers. LifeSign for adolescents consists of a credit card–sized computer that implements a scheduled, gradual reduction protocol. The computer first records your personal smoking pattern and then creates an individualized schedule telling you when you may smoke, at times that differ from your original pattern. Hence, on the LifeSign program, you cannot smoke when you crave cigarettes and are asked to smoke when you normally would not crave them.

Currently, the nicotine patch and nicotine gum are not legally available to minors. Manufacturers label their nicotine replacement therapies (NRTs) as not for sale to persons under 18 and instruct retailers about this restriction. The labeling and instructions to retailers are part of an agreement with the FDA reached when the nicotine patch and gum were approved for over-the-counter retail sales. Physicians can prescribe NRTs but have done so only infrequently. Programs and policies dealing with NRTs and their use in adolescent cessation interventions should be examined for safety and efficacy.

The impact of smoking cessation interventions among adolescents is not well understood.[107] Given the cost-effectiveness of smoking cessation interventions for adults, and given the large number of addicted teenagers, research on cessation programs tailored to youth is an important area and should be a high priority.[108]

Innovations

Because tobacco control is such a dynamic field, new approaches frequently emerge. While it is difficult to evaluate all of the new possibilities before they are adopted more widely, policymakers should nonetheless be aware of them. As we argue in our "Conclusion and Recommendations," a critical aspect of using the tobacco settlement funds and in developing tobacco control programs generally will be allocating sufficient resources for program evaluation. In this section, we briefly describe several promising interventions that policymakers should consider using in future program development.

Computer-Based Systems

A promising, but as yet untested, emerging innovation is the use of computer-based systems (often referred to as "expert systems" in the literature) to communicate messages about tobacco to teens.[109] Some of these innovations have been evaluated, but because most are in various stages of development and implementation, we consider them under the category of innovations. For instance, Innovative Training Systems is developing a computer game designed to educate children about the harms from tobacco products,[110] and former surgeon general C. Everett Koop is developing a similar system.[111] Two advantages of these efforts, if successful, are their low cost and adolescents' receptivity to computers. Another advantage is that the same basic systems design can appeal to both adults and children.[112]

Underlying the enthusiasm for computer-based approaches is the premise that computer programs have the potential to reach a large portion of the adolescent audience, can be adapted to individual concerns, can be implemented as designed in an infinite variety of treatment settings (or at home), and can be sustained over time at very low cost.[113] Previous research has demonstrated that tailored and individualized messages are an important factor in increasing smoking cessation rates. In a computer-based approach, each message can be specifically tailored to address the individual's particular smoking stage.[114]

The rapid development of computer technology has made tailoring messages to the individual more economical. In some studies, individuals who received tailored messages were significantly more likely to change their behavior than were individuals in a control group, at least in short-term results.[115] Tailored Internet-based interventions would differ dramatically from the prevailing socially influenced classroom interventions. These latter programs are forced to target their interventions at the entire class, with minimal latitude for tailoring, and are thus limited in efficacy. Another problem with traditional school-based interventions is that they are costly to sustain as ongoing programs.

By contrast, an effective computer-based intervention can have a much greater reach and impact than a more traditional intervention. For example, a smoking cessation intervention delivered over the Internet has the potential to reach a far larger number of people than is possible for a single health care intervention. An added attraction is that because many smokers prefer to quit on their own,[116] users can choose freely the best and most convenient times and places to participate in a smoking cessation program. The rapidly increasing reach of the Internet thus permits much greater flexibility with computer-based cessation programs than with other available programs. One potential problem with this strategy, however, is the growing economic and racial disparity in Internet access and use. Groups with high socioeconomic status (SES), those actually less likely to use tobacco, have greater access to the Internet, while those with lower SES, who actually need the intervention more, have less Internet access.

Nevertheless, a few early computer-based studies suggest that even less sophisticated computer approaches have been as effective as clinical programs among adolescent and adult smokers.[117] For adolescents, the ability of computer-based systems to provide virtually instantaneous feedback may be attractive to a population not known for a long attention span. This method of delivering smoking cessation messages to adolescents may also be attractive because it avoids the concerns about parental knowledge and so forth noted earlier.

Two new computerized self-help smoking cessation programs for adolescents provide an example of a recently evaluated program.[118] In the first intervention, the authors adapted to adolescents a computer system based on a model of changing adult smoking behavior. For the second intervention, they used a clinical teen smoking cessation program developed by the American Lung Association. The results suggest reasonable cessation attempts and initial success (14–20 percent), but cessation rates decreased 6 percent after the six-month follow-up survey. The authors note that the technology and approach are at an early stage of development but that this study nonetheless supports the feasibility of using computer-based systems in adolescent smoking cessation interventions. Their caveat is important, because another study found that the use of an expert system model did not appear to reduce adolescent smoking one year after the intervention among schoolchildren aged 13–14.[119]

Among the issues to be considered in subsequent work on computer-based intervention is how to relate the intervention message more clearly to the adolescent's current smoking status. Researchers also need to conduct experiments on whether the source of the message should be an authoritative adult or a peer. Another challenge is to learn more about how a user navigates through the computer-based system during the intervention.

Peer-Based Interventions

A major trend in school-based interventions is the use of peer-education programs like Teens Against Tobacco Use (TATU), which has had programs in many states. These programs, sponsored by the American Lung Association, train older students (usually ages 14–17) to become positive role models for middle and elementary school students (focusing on ages 9–12). TATU interventions include multiple, intensive sessions during the first phase, with boosters in subsequent years. Prevention programs often include a media literacy component (e.g., teens learn how the tobacco industry's advertising savvy has manipulated and distorted information about tobacco). A project in Kentucky and Florida focused on explaining to elementary school students the nature of tobacco's addictiveness.[120]

The concept of using teens to design antismoking programs for their peers has become an important aspect of the American Legacy

Foundation's approach to reducing adolescent smoking. Based on the assumption that teens can be more effective in addressing their peers than adults, the foundation has used adolescent focus groups to determine the shape and direction of its advertising campaign. The foundation is also organizing adolescents from around the country to take their antismoking message directly to events popular with other youth. Many states, including Florida, have been organizing similar teen events. As yet, these peer-based interventions have not been evaluated.

As a companion initiative, the foundation has established a three-year matching grant program for states to develop antitobacco youth movements. According to the foundation, youth involved in the movements "will take responsibility in the fight against tobacco use" and will work with existing state and local antismoking coalitions.[121]

Recently, researchers have also begun to recommend testing intervention models that involve youth developing their own solutions and that examine the interaction between school-based interventions and other community-based activities.[122] They also recommend that research be conducted to understand better why many youth do not smoke.

School Policies

Schools may have their own smoking policies, which can apply even to those students over 18 years old. Penalties for violations include fines, smoking education and cessation classes, informing the student's parents, and suspension and/or expulsion. In 1997, one study reported that schools were not very aggressive in enforcing no-smoking rules and considered the matter a low priority.[123] It appears, however, that schools are increasingly willing to develop, implement, and enforce no-smoking policies. Recently developed school smoking policies seem to use a combination of punishments, rather than just fining or suspending students. For example, a study of 23 schools in California found that those with smoking policies that included four components had lower rates of self-reported smoking among the students.[124] The four components were a smoking prevention education plan and three restrictions on student smoking: on school grounds, when leaving school grounds, and when near school grounds. Although the study was not controlled, these results suggest that strong school smoking policies are associated with decreased rates of youth smoking.

Although school-based smoking control and prevention programs implemented more recently have not yet been evaluated, many involve new and interesting approaches worth noting.[125] For instance, in Marysville, Washington, students who transgress the smoking rules are fined, required to attend smoking cessation classes, and ordered to complete four hours of community service. Schools in Houston, Texas, reported a reduction in smoking rates on school premises from the combination of fines and smoking education classes.

In the Schaumberg District of Chicago, in Derby, Kansas, and in Shepardsville, Kentucky, school districts have suspended or expelled students who disobeyed no-smoking policies. An official at Roosevelt High School in Casper, Wyoming, estimated that 77 violations had resulted in 367 missed days of instruction, revealing a major disadvantage of this type of policy. In lieu of suspension, the school has now started a three-hour cessation program for offenders. Indeed, school administrators must be alert to a potential backlash if parents perceive these sanctions to be too strict. In Lexington, Kentucky, parents of students at Bullitt Central High, protesting the school's expulsion-for-smoking policy, are claiming it achieves the exact opposite result by encouraging delinquent behavior in unsupervised teens. Indeed, many North Carolina high school students face suspension for a second smoking offense.[126] Instead of offering tobacco education or cessation classes as an option for those caught smoking, suspension was more likely. If implemented, this means that students could fall behind in school work, exacerbating other problem behaviors that predict tobacco use among adolescents.

Conclusion

As previously implemented, school health education, the quintessential ingredient of youth tobacco control, has contributed little toward discouraging future tobacco experimentation or addiction. Yet there is evidence that state-of-the-art education programs can reduce tobacco use. Despite the mixed results of previous school-based efforts, prevention programs based on a social influence model have been shown to have short-term effects on students of middle school age, the age when students are most likely to initiate smoking. But the reality thus far is that school systems lack both the will and the resources (including time in the curriculum) to implement state-of-the-art programs effectively and on a sustained basis. An investment in program evaluation and resource allocation is required to permit the adoption of sustained interventions.

Just as important, policymakers should identify innovative programs, some of which we identified in this chapter, and allocate funds to expand and evaluate their impact. In particular, adolescents represent a perfect audience for using the emerging computer-based antismoking strategies. The development and expansion of computer-based systems presents a unique opportunity to take advantage of technology that most adolescents are comfortable with and to adapt antismoking messages to individual needs and circumstances.

Our review suggests that policymakers should focus on taking advantage of synergies between different strategies, especially school- and community-based programs. One possibility for expanding school-based interventions is to combine them with community-based programs for families. Adolescents who have parents and siblings who smoke are more likely to have easy access to cigarettes, initiate smoking, and become regular smokers. School-based interventions can include homework assignments and other activities involving family members, to at least reinforce nonsmoking behavior among children and perhaps convince parents to consider quitting. Community-based programs can also encourage family members to quit smoking and can provide resources for cessation programs and information.

Our review also suggests that most school-based prevention programs target students in the elementary and junior high school, while high school students are often ignored. High school students may receive booster sessions, but these sessions are often unconnected to the interventions received in junior high. Adolescent smokers should be offered and encouraged to enroll in smoking cessation programs. Nonsmoking high school students are excellent candidates for participating in sting operations, lobbying for antismoking legislation, and becoming peer educators for children in their community. Interventions using peer educators should be evaluated both for their impact on the children in the program and for the effect of reinforcing nonsmoking behavior on the teens themselves.

Adult cessation programs should be emphasized, especially in connection with smoking prevention programs underway in managed care organizations. To the extent that parental smoking encourages or influences adolescent tobacco use, it is important for the health care system to involve entire families in smoking cessation programs.

REFERENCES

1. USDHHS 1994; IOM 1994.

2. Even though we do not emphasize study design and methodological issues in our comments on individual studies, we expect that this review will be useful to researchers as well.

3. A meta-analysis is a statistical technique for combining numerous small studies, where sample sizes are too small to derive meaningful results, into one larger analysis. Because the meta-analysis takes advantage of a larger sample size, statistically valid results can be derived. The methodology has been criticized for yielding artificially determined results.

4. IOM 1994.

5. Rooney and Murray 1996.

6. Tobler 1986, 1997.

7. Black, Tobler, and Sciacca 1998.

8. Bruvold 1993.

9. Murray et al. 1992.

10. Ennett, Rosenbaum, et al. 1994.

11. Ennett, Rosenbaum, et al. 1994; Lynan et al. 1999; Hansen and McNeal 1997.

12. Elder et al. 1993; Murray et al. 1989.

13. Dijkstra et al. 1999.

14. Botvin et al. 1995.

15. CDC 1999j.

16. CDC 1999j.

17. Peterson, Kealey, Mann et al. 2000.

18. Wechsler et al. 1998.

19. Rigotti, Lee, and Wechsler 2000.

20. Study finds alarming smoking rates 1999.

21. MTF 1999.

22. Naquin and Gilbert 1996.

23. Schorling et al. 1994.

24. Werch, Pappas, and Castellon-Vogel 1996.

25. Walsh et al. 1999.

26. Botvin et al. 1995; Ennett, Tobler, et al. 1994.

27. Kim et al. 1998; Petoskey, Van Stelle, and DeJong 1998.

28. CDC 1994.

29. CDC 1994; CDC 1999k.

30. Aguirre-Molina and Gorman 1996.

31. See the studies collected in IOM 1994.

32. Sowden and Arblaster 2000; Aguirre-Molina and Gorman 1996; Kaufman et al. 1994; Biglan, Ary, Yudelson, et al. 1996; Perry et al. 1992; Pentz, MacKinnon, Flay, et al. 1989.

33. Pentz, MacKinnon, Dwyer, et al. 1989.

34. Biglan, Ary, Smolkowski, et al. 1999.

35. USDHHS 1994; Manley et al. 1997; Aguirre-Molina and Gorman 1996.

36. IOM 1994; Perry et al. 1992.

37. Pentz, Dwyer, et al. 1989; Pentz, Mackinnon, Flay, et al. 1989.

38. IOM 1994; Pentz, MacKinnon, Flay, et al. 1989.

39. Tobler 1992; Aguirre-Molina and Gorman 1996; Flynn, Worden, and Secker-Walker 1994; Flynn et al. 1992; Worden et al. 1996; Sowden and Arblaster 2000.

40. USDHHS 1994.

41. COMMIT Research Group 1995a, 1995b.

42. Bowen, Kinne, and Orlandi 1995.

43. COMMIT Research Group 1995a, 1995b.

44. Lewit et al. 1997.

45. Glantz 1996.

46. Gritz 1994.

47. Based on discussions with various officials connected with Project ASSIST, we were unable to identify any additional evaluations of this program. To the best of our knowledge, no comprehensive evaluation is being planned or conducted.

48. Manley et al. 1997.

49. Kegler et al. 1998.

50. Jacobson and Wasserman 1997.

51. Forster and Wolfson 1998.

52. Hawkins, Catalano, and Miller 1992; Winick and Larson 1997.

53. Kadushin et al. 1998; Jellinek and Hearn 1991.

54. Fighting Back 2000.

55. Kadushin et al. 1998.

56. Rossi et al. 1993.

57. Winick and Larson 1997.

58. CDC 1999j.

59. Pierce, Gilpin, Emery, Farkas, et al. 1998c.

60. Independent Evaluation Consortium 1998.

61. Pierce, Gilpin, Emery, White, et al. 1998b.

62. Pierce, Gilpin, Emery, White, et al. 1998b.

63. Cimons 2000 (citing a CDC report in November 2000).

64. Fichtenberg and Glantz 2000. The authors attribute 8,300 excess heart disease deaths to budget cuts and an emphasis of youth tobacco control during the mid-1990s.

65. Connolly and Robbins 1998.

66. Hamilton and Norton 1999.

67. CDC 1996c.

68. Biener 1999; see also, Biener, Harris, and Hamilton 2000.

69. Biener, Harris, and Hamilton 2000.

70. Jacobson and Wasserman 1997.

71. CDC 1999a; Florida Department of Health, Office of Tobacco Control 2000; Bauer et al. 2000.

72. IOM 2000.

73. Wakefield and Chaloupka 2000.

74. Donovan, Jessor, and Costa 1991; Kim et al. 1998.

75. Kim et al. 1998; Petoskey, Van Stelle, and DeJong 1998.

76. Biglan and Metzler 1998.

77. Kellam and Anthony 1998.

78. Hu, Lin, and Keeler 1998.

79. Richardson et al. 1989, 1993; Mulhall, Stone, and Stone 1996.

80. Felitti et al. 1998; Anda et al. 1999.

81. IOM 2000.

82. Gritz 1994; Ross and Taylor 1998; Fortmann et al. 1995.

83. Pederson, Koval, and O'Connor 1997.

84. Engels et al. 1998.

85. Burt and Peterson 1998.

86. USDHHS 1994, 84.

87. Everett et al. 1999, 330.

88. These results echo the findings of the 1994 surgeon general's report suggesting that adolescent smokers frequently attempt to quit smoking, are typically unsuccessful, are hard to recruit and retain in formal cessation programs, and do not have positive responses to programs currently in use (USDHHS 1994).

89. Stone and Kristeller 1992; Lamkin, Davis, and Kamen 1998.

90. Sargent, Mott, and Stevens 1998.

91. Breslau and Peterson 1996.

92. Manley, Epps, and Glynn 1992.

93. Schubiner, Herrold, and Hurt 1998.

94. Perez-Stable et al. 2000.

95. Frank et al. 1991.

96. Baker, Morley, and Barker 1995.

97. Thorndike et al. 1999.

98. Frankowski and Secker-Walker 1989; Frankowski, Weaver, and Secker-Walker 1993; Zapka et al. 1999.

99. Epps, Manley, and Glynn 1995.

100. CDC 1999j; AHRQ 2000.

101. Thorndike, Rigotti, and Stafford 1998; Ockene and Zapka 1997a.

102. Ockene et al. 1997.

103. Epps, Manley, and Glynn 1995.

104. USDHHS 1994, 274–75.

105. Houston, Kolbe, and Eriksen 1998.

106. Smith et al. 1996.

107. Sussman et al. 1999.

108. Cromwell et al. 1997; Warner 1997.

109. We thank our colleague Unto Pallonen, Ph.D., for substantial assistance in thinking about and drafting this section.

110. Parent 1999.

111. Noble 1999.

112. Pallonen 1998.

113. Glasgow, Vogt, and Boles 1999.

114. Pallonenen 1998. These tailored messages are based on the transtheoretical model of behavior change, which identifies the various smoking stages that an individual encounters, from experimentation to daily use.

115. Strecher 1999; Bental, Cawsey, and Jones 1999.

116. USDHHS 1989.

117. Velicer et al. 1999; Pallonen, Velicer, et al. 1998.

118. Pallonen et al. 1998. Shiffman et al. (2000) found positive results from tailored computer programs over the other cessation methods in an adult population.

119. Aveyard et al. 1999.

120. Humana-American Lung Association Partnership Program, Teens against Tobacco Use.

121. American Legacy Foundation 2000.

122. Manske, Brown, and Cameron 1997.

123. Jacobson and Wasserman 1997.

124. Pentz, Brannon, et al. 1989.

125. These anecdotes are taken from various media reports that we monitored while preparing this book.

126. Enforcement policy guidelines for North Carolina 2000.

5

Tobacco Marketing and the Potential for Antismoking Mass Media Interventions

Given that adolescence is a time of experimentation, of emulating adults, and of challenging notions of what is acceptable or appropriate behavior, many people believe that adolescents are vulnerable to tobacco advertising and marketing strategies.[1] A prominent view is that the tobacco industry and its marketing tactics are largely responsible for the strong association between youth and smoking initiation. Although tobacco industry representatives have forcefully declared that they do not market their products to children, many people believe that there is more than sufficient evidence to suggest otherwise. In fact, one of the main criticisms of the tobacco industry during the past decade is that it has deliberately and quite effectively targeted young children and adolescents in product advertising.[2]

A wide range of countermarketing activities has been implemented in response to the perceived success of the tobacco industry. Such activities range from fairness doctrine ads in the late 1960s to statewide mass media campaigns supported by tobacco excise taxes in the 1990s. In addition, the successes of tobacco industry marketing may actually be instructive in the development of antitobacco media campaigns. As Seidel-Marks stated, "the very tools used by the tobacco industry to make cigarettes into the single most profitable legal consumer product sold can also be used to combat the smoking pandemic unleashed by tobacco products."[3]

While many tobacco control advocates may find such a perspective to be intuitively appealing, such opinions are based on a number of assumptions, including that the tobacco industry understands marketing to children in ways that other industries or sectors do not, that their marketing strategies actually influence youth smoking behavior, and that certain identifiable aspects of these tactics could be effective in countermarketing strategies. What is the evidence for any of these perspectives? Can health professionals interested in marketing tobacco prevention and control learn anything from the tobacco industry?

In this chapter, we present the results of a literature review and research synthesis to address two important questions: (1) what is the impact of tobacco industry marketing on youth smoking behavior; and (2) can countermarketing or antitobacco mass media or advertising strategies be effective in youth smoking prevention and control? In our attempt to answer these questions, we obtained information from a variety of sources: (1) tobacco industry documents, many of which have become available for public use because of the recent court battles involving the tobacco industry;[4] (2) published literature on the effects of tobacco advertising on youth; and (3) published evaluations of mass media antismoking campaigns. In addition, we reviewed books and articles on the concept of *social marketing* and its application in public health arenas.

The findings of our research synthesis suggest that although tobacco advertising is not the primary cause of adolescent smoking behavior, industry tactics do influence youth smoking. The industry's success appears due primarily to its application of sound, conventional marketing principles directed at youth rather than to any special expertise or insight regarding adolescent behavior or psychology. Applying these principles in the area of smoking prevention can be considered a type of social marketing and holds great promise for tobacco control media interventions. The unprecedented amount of resources currently available at the state and national level affords the opportunity to invest in the rigorous design, implementation, and evaluation of social marketing approaches to tobacco control.

Examples of Tobacco Industry Marketing to Youth

In 1991, a lawsuit was brought against the R. J. Reynolds Tobacco Company with the goal of ending the Joe Camel marketing campaign. The discovery process for this lawsuit, involving R. J. Reynolds and its advertising agencies, produced an enormous number of documents, interviews, and depositions. This body of information, along with additional documents that emerged from other tobacco companies as a result of the state suits against the tobacco industry, provide strong and compelling evidence that the tobacco industry has indeed developed product lines and implemented advertising campaigns that target adolescents and even younger children. Perry concluded in her recent review of industry documents emerging from the Minnesota litigation that there is ample evidence from the tobacco industry itself that (a) youth smoking has been viewed as critical to economic viability, (b) decreases in youth smoking were perceived as negative and alarming trends, and c) specific product lines and marketing strategies were successfully aimed at youth.[5]

Of the thousands of tobacco industry documents now in the public domain, relatively few refer specifically to youth under the age of 18 as a desirable market segment. Those that do so primarily address the importance of this market segment to the future economic prosperity of individual tobacco companies. For example, a 1974 R. J. Reynolds document refers to 14–24 year olds as "tomorrow's cigarette business" and suggests that the company follow the strategy of "direct advertising to the younger smokers." Other industry documents have a similar tone.

> The brands which these beginning smokers accept and use will become the dominant brands in future years. Evidence is now available to indicate that the 14–18 year old group is an increasing segment of the smoking population. RJR-T *must soon* establish a successful *new* brand in this market if our position in the industry is to be maintained over the long term. (Claude Teague, "Planning Assumptions and Forecast for the Period 1977–1986 for RJ Reynolds Tobacco Company," draft report, 1976)

Other documents provide evidence that the industry saw declines in youth smoking initiation and habitual smoking as negative and alarming and as something to which their marketing units needed to respond. As Perry documents,[5] a 1980 R. J. Reynolds Marketing Development Department memo regarding the company's decrease in the share of brands smoked by 14–17 year olds concluded:

> [The report on teenage smokers] indicates that RJR continues to gradually decline and between the spring and fall 1979 periods, RJR's total share declined from 21.3 to 19.9. Hopefully, our various

planned activities that will be implemented this fall will aid in some way in reducing or correcting these trends. (R. J. Reynolds, interoffice correspondence, July 22, 1980)

Numerous other documents provide chilling examples of industry recognition of the importance of the youth market and the need to attract young, beginning smokers for economic survival and prosperity.[6]

Industry documents also forcefully demonstrate that advertising strategies and promotional tactics were unequivocally aimed at youth markets, despite bans on such activities. A 1973 memo from an advertising agency to the marketing department of R. J. Reynolds includes the following statement:

Marlboro's share among the 14–15 segment is a phenomenal 51.0%. . . . Many manufacturers have "studied" the 14–20 market in hopes of uncovering the "secret" of the instant popularity some brands enjoy almost to the complete exclusion of others (as shown above). Creating a "fad" in this market can be a great bonanza.

A 1988 letter from the advertising agency Flanigan Enterprises establishes that R. J. Reynolds understood the effectiveness of cartoons in advertising campaigns targeting young people.

Imagine a five-year old child, who will be a future customer of your cigarettes in the next few years. How can your company begin to attract/tap into this next generation? . . . Flanigan Enterprises is proposing a children's video be made to advertise the Camel product. . . . Children love cartoons and these can be incorporated into the purchasing of cartons/packets of Camel cigarettes. ("Tapping into the Next Generation," letter from Flanigan Enterprises to Richard Kampe, president of R. J. Reynolds Tobacco Company, 1988)

This type of thinking was the foundation for R. J. Reynolds's forceful and lengthy campaign based on the now infamous Old Joe Camel cartoon character. Launched in the United States in 1988, this large-scale advertising campaign was based on a campaign in France during the 1970s that centered around a cartoon camel (referred to as the "funny camel" or "laughing camel"). R. J. Reynolds's French campaign was perceived as successful, especially because of its strong appeal among younger smokers. In the United States, the Joe Camel character displayed his "smooth moves" in print ads, on billboards, and on promotional products, such as T-shirts, caps, and jackets. Joe Camel was most often portrayed in social situations, engaged in fun and hip activities, such as playing pool, riding motorcycles, or hanging out in night clubs and bars. The Joe Camel cartoon character proved to be appealing to children of all ages, but especially among male adolescents. In an important study, a group of researchers in Massachusetts concluded, "in just three years Camel's Old Joe cartoon character had an astonishing influence on children's smoking behavior."[7] As a result of the campaign, Camel's market share among those under 18 rose from 0.5 percent to 32.8 percent.[7] Children—even very young children—were more familiar with the Old Joe cartoon character than were adults, ostensibly because this type of advertising has more appeal to children.

Along with targeted ad campaigns, tobacco companies have considered different product lines that might specifically attract teenagers, such as cigarettes flavored with honey or Coca-Cola, because "it's a well known fact that teenagers like sweet products" (1972 Brown and Williamson memo from consultants). Industry documents also show that tobacco companies perceived a need to cater products to young, novice smokers. For instance, a 1973 draft report found in the R. J. Reynolds documents stated: "[the] beginner smoker and inhaler has a low tolerance for smoke irritations; hence the smoke should be as bland as possible. . . . for the beginning smoker the cigarette smoke should have a moderate level of blended tobacco flavor, but should be as free as possible from strong, unpleasant flavors."

Additional documents demonstrate that the industry understood and appreciated the relevant psychological and behavioral traits that characterize many adolescents.

> It is important to know as much as possible about teenage smoking patterns and attitudes. Today's teenager is tomorrow's potential regular customer, and the overwhelming majority of smokers first begin to smoke while still in their teens. . . . At least a part of the success of Marlboro Red during its most rapid growth period was because it became *the* brand of choice among teenagers who smoked cigarettes. (Philip Morris, special internal report, 1981)

> Smoking a cigarette for the beginner is a symbolic act . . . "I am no longer my mother's child, I'm tough, I'm an adventurer, I'm not square . . ." As the force from the psychological symbolism sub-

sides, the pharmacological effect takes over to sustain the habit. (Draft report to the Philip Morris Board of Directors, 1969)

[Camel advertising will create] the perception that Camel smokers are non-conformist, self-confident and project a cool attitude, which is admired by their peers. . . . Aspiration to be perceived as a cool member of the in-group is one of the strongest influences affecting the behavior of younger adult smokers. (R. J. Reynolds Tobacco Company, memo, 1986)

If the desire to be daring is part of the motivation to start smoking, the alleged risk of smoking may actually make smoking attractive. Finally, if the "older" establishment is preaching against smoking, the anti-establishment sentiment . . . would cause the young to want to be defiant and smoke. Thus, a new brand aimed at the young group should not in any way be promoted as a "health" brand, and perhaps should carry some implied risk. In this sense, the warning label on the package may be a plus. (R. J. Reynolds Tobacco Company, internal draft report, 1973)

Industry documents have revealed that in internal written correspondence, R. J. Reynolds's employees used an acronym for youth, FUBYAS, which appears to stand for either "First Usual Brand Younger Adult Smokers" or "First Unbranded Young Adult Smokers." FUBYAS were broken down into several different types of youth according to their social group linkages, concepts of success, recreational interests, and attitudes toward risk-taking behavior, such as drinking, having sex, and smoking. This breakdown included the labeling of such groups as "goody-goodies," "preps," "G.Q.s," "punkers," "rockers," and "burnouts," with the last three groups viewed as the most likely to smoke. Many additional tobacco industry documents refer to "starters" or "young adult smokers" but do not explicitly state which age-group is meant; it is logical to assume that these are euphemistic references to the under-18 age-group.[6]

Youth Exposure to Tobacco Industry Marketing

Of all consumer products, cigarettes are among the most heavily advertised and marketed. Adolescence is a time of image formation, making adolescents particularly vulnerable to cigarette advertising.[7] Children of all ages shape their own self-images in multiple ways, including by what they see on television, in magazines, and through other mass media. Tobacco advertising influences children's images not only of smoking (including who smokes and the benefits of smoking) but also of the situations in which smoking takes place. When tobacco advertisements are presented in ways that resonate with children and adolescents (e.g., through the use of cartoons), and when smokers are portrayed in ways that appeal to them as well (e.g., as people who are physically attractive, socially active, popular, and cool), there is little doubt that these advertisements are finding an audience among youth.

Several studies have noted that the most popular cigarette brands among adolescents are also the most heavily advertised.[8] Research also has shown that magazine readership age is correlated with the advertising of youth brands and that the most popular youth magazines contain the most tobacco advertising.[9] One study found that 50 percent of seventh graders reported that they had seen tobacco-related magazine advertisements, 90 percent had seen tobacco billboards, and 74 percent had seen tobacco advertisements at sporting or community events.[10] In addition, more than 25 percent of these early adolescents owned a tobacco promotional item. It has also been reported that the majority of middle school students exhibited some receptivity to tobacco industry marketing strategies, which in turn was associated with susceptibility to smoking behavior.[11]

Cigarette advertisements provide adolescents with image-based information about smokers and may contribute to their attitudes regarding smoking and those who smoke. The extent to which cigarette advertising contributes to the decision to start smoking is less clear. Thus, while there is significant evidence that most youth in the United States are routinely and heavily exposed to some form of tobacco industry marketing, the impact of this exposure on smoking behavior is not as well understood.

As we noted in chapter 1, after the Master Settlement Agreement was signed, the tobacco industry shifted its advertising strategy from billboards to increased print media buying. For our purposes, the most important aspect of this shift is the increasing advertising presence in magazines aimed at the young adult readership but also read avidly by adolescents. One study found that tobacco advertising expenditures rose by 33 percent in 19 magazines (of 29 studied) with a greater than 15 percent youth audience (e.g., *Rolling Stone, Sports Illustrated, Essence,* and *Hot Rod*).[12] As of this writing, Philip Morris has voluntarily agreed to suspend such crossover advertising, but R. J. Reynolds has not.

The Impact of Tobacco Advertising on Youth Smoking

Advertising could directly influence the consumption of cigarettes in several ways: by encouraging smokers to take up the habit, by preventing current smokers from quitting, by encouraging ex-smokers to begin smoking again, and by increasing the total daily consumption of smokers.[13] Advertising can also influence broad social attitudes about smoking. Unfortunately, it is quite challenging to establish empirical links between advertising and its direct and indirect impacts on any consumer behavior, including tobacco use.

Researchers have long noted ecological associations or general correlations between tobacco industry marketing (and advertising in particular) and the consumption of cigarettes in the population. A 1942 study concluded that "without advertising, cigarette use would probably have grown; with advertising, the increase has been amazing."[14] The econometric (i.e., statistical) evidence on the effects of advertising on cigarette consumption has focused on the aggregate impact on adult smoking. With many studies finding no significant relationship and many others finding a significant but generally small relationship, the literature is indeterminate on the issue.[15] In any event, technical limitations of econometric methods, combined with a lack of studies on adolescent smoking, make this literature of little utility in trying to assess whether advertising affects smoking by children.[16] The bottom line is that there is no definitive research suggesting that tobacco industry advertising is in large part responsible for youth smoking initiation.

It is important to note that the effects of cigarette advertising bans are mixed, as different statistical analyses have come to opposite conclusions about whether bans reduce cigarette consumption in a population.[14] Some studies suggest that advertising bans could serve to reduce smoking, while other studies suggest that bans would have no significant impact. Some researchers have noted that these inconsistent findings can be explained by the fact that partial and complete bans have different effects but are not clearly distinguished from each other in studies.[17] Partial bans appear to have little effect because they afford cigarette companies the opportunity to switch advertising expenditures to other promotional media and methods. In contrast, complete bans could reduce total tobacco consumption by approximately 6 percent, an amount that may seem small but could have a large public health impact.[16]

Current evidence at hand suggests that a complete ban on tobacco advertising may have a discernable impact on youth smoking behavior but that it would likely be quite small. A significant number of youth would still be experimental and habitual (addicted) smokers. This is because, as we discussed in chapter 3, the social context is key in youth smoking behavior, with multiple factors contributing to youth smoking initiation and other forms of risk-taking behavior. However, while a complete ban on advertising might have only a limited impact on youth smoking, advertising is still an important factor in smoking behavior. Therefore, regulation of industry advertising is warranted. There is great concern that tobacco advertising and marketing—including the distribution of promotional products, such as clothing, sporting equipment, and outdoor gear—is positively associated with youth smoking.[18]

A historical review of tobacco marketing tactics and smoking rates among youth showed that smoking among females under age 18 greatly increased at the same time large-scale marketing campaigns aimed specifically at women were implemented.[19] This work demonstrates a compelling association between a major increase in smoking initiation among minor females and the introduction of gender-specific tobacco products and marketing.

Both adolescents' ability to recognize cigarette advertisements and their reporting that an ad was likeable or appealing have been linked to higher levels of smoking and intentions to smoke in the future.[20] Youth awareness of tobacco marketing campaigns, receipt of free tobacco samples, and receipt of direct mail promotional paraphernalia were found to be associated with susceptibility to tobacco use in cross-sectional studies.[21] However, because these promotional items are not randomly distributed, selection bias could partially explain this finding. In other words, we cannot say that being aware of marketing campaigns and receiving promotional items lead or cause youth to smoke, because these youth may be predisposed, for reasons not observable by researchers, both to notice and participate in marketing tactics and to smoke.

Stronger evidence for an association between exposure to tobacco industry advertising and smoking comes from longitudinal analyses. One such study in California reported that adolescents who had received a tobacco promotional item and/or had an interest in tobacco advertising (i.e., had a favorite advertisement) were significantly more likely to initiate smoking in the following three years.[22] This study also found that approximately one-third of smoking experimentation in California between 1993 and 1996 could be attributed to promotional activities of the tobacco industry. Similarly, a longitudinal study of Massachusetts youth found that exposure to brand-specific magazine advertising at baseline in 1993 was significantly related to brand-specific smoking initiation four years later.[23]

Several additional studies have found potential links between advertising and increased susceptibility to smoking among adolescents.[24] An examination of trends in smoking initiation rates among adolescents and marketing expenditures by the tobacco industry concluded, "although other influences cannot be ruled out, we suspect that the expanded tobacco marketing budget, with its increased emphasis on tactics that may be particularly pertinent to young people, affected adolescent initiation rates."[25]

The public stance of the tobacco industry has been that their marketing of products is not geared toward encouraging nonsmokers—especially adolescents—to initiate smoking. The industry argues that advertisements and other promotional activities are meant to encourage current smokers to maintain brand loyalty or to switch brands to that being advertised. A number of experts, however, have challenged this claim, as the evidence shows that most smokers—including youth smokers—are strongly brand loyal.[26] Brand loyalty is solidified as adolescents move toward smoking more than half a pack per day. By twelfth grade, less than 2 percent of daily smokers and less than 1 percent of smokers smoking half a pack or more per day had no brand preference, a "striking fact" that "helps to show why tobacco companies might have a strong motivation to induce young people to establish a preference for their brands at an early age."[27] Given the amount of resources the industry invests in marketing/advertising and given the low rate at which smokers switch brands, it has been argued that it is beyond reason to believe that the purpose of advertising is solely to encourage brand switching among current smokers.[28] The industry's own behavior argues against this position.

Public Health Mass Media Campaigns

Mass media strategies have been used for broad-based public education regarding a variety of public health issues, including tobacco use, prevention and control. Mass media efforts are viewed as particularly appropriate for reaching youth, who are often heavily exposed to and greatly interested in media messages.[29] Further, as others have suggested, media-based health promotion efforts have the potential to reach large segments of the population (especially those who are less educated) and to lower barriers to participation in health-related programs.[30]

Adolescents have been targeted by antitobacco media campaigns in several communities and in several states, but research results regarding the campaigns' development and impact are sparse.[31] Researchers at the University of Vermont demonstrated that combining traditional school-based prevention efforts with a mass media campaign increased intervention effectiveness.[32] In a study of two communities, the one that received a mass media intervention along with an educational program for four years had an almost 40 percent lower rate of smoking than the one receiving the educational program alone. The researchers also found that the media intervention was particularly effective among high-risk youth, defined as students who reported ever smoking at baseline (grades 4–6) and had two or more smokers in their immediate social or family environment. A subsequent cost analysis of the media intervention estimated (in 1996 dollars) that the cost per exposed student was $41, the cost per averted smoker was $754, and the cost per life year gained was $696.[33] If the campaign were to be implemented nationwide, economies of scale were viewed as producing significant decreases in these costs, which are already impressively low compared not only to media interventions but to other public health interventions as well.

Goldman and Glantz recently reviewed research on the effectiveness of various antismoking advertising strategies and conducted a qualitative study using 180 focus groups involving more than 1,500 adults and youth.[34] They concluded that "aggressive" public education campaigns that focus on "industry manipulation" (i.e., the goal of the tobacco industry to recruit young smokers and the tactics used to achieve this goal) and the negative effects of secondhand smoke are likely to reduce cigarette consumption and denormalize smoking. According to these researchers, incorporating messages of industry manipulation into antismoking campaigns resonates with youth because such messages emphasize that people are not acting independently in their decision to smoke. Advertising strategies that focus on youth access, the short- and long-term health effects of smoking, and romantic rejection were found to have less potential for effectiveness.[32]

Several states have received attention for multimillion-dollar statewide mass media campaigns that included a focus on youth. These include California and Massachusetts, with funds from tobacco excise tax increases, and Florida, with funds from its settlement with the tobacco industry. As we described in chapter 4, Massachusetts and California both experienced a decrease in overall smoking rates that researchers have partially attributed to the media campaigns, although neither state witnessed a decline in adolescent smoking.[35]

The Florida Department of Health used money from its separate settlement with the tobacco industry to implement a hard-hitting media campaign aimed specifically at youth, starting in 1998. Between 1998 and early 2000, current cigarette use declined by 54 percent among middle school students and 24 percent among high school students.[36] More detailed data from Florida suggest that in 1998, 18.5 percent of middle schoolers reported smoking at least one cigarette in the past month. By 1999, this rate had dropped to 15 percent, and in early 2000, it was lower still, at 8.6 percent. Smoking in the past month declined among high school students as well, dropping from 27.4 percent in 1998 to 20.9 percent in early 2000. Florida's decline in youth smoking has been observed for both males and females and across racial and ethnic groups and is larger than any other decline witnessed in the United States since 1980. While it is difficult to scientifically attribute all or a certain proportion of the decline in youth smoking to Florida's countermarketing and communications activities, evidence from trend analyses strongly suggest that these efforts—many of which were designed with significant input from youth—are having a significant impact on youth smoking behavior. Process evaluation data suggest that 95 percent of Florida teens recognize the ads, which to date primarily have focused on the manipulative and deceptive practices of the tobacco industry.[36]

Interestingly, all three states—California, Florida, and Massachusetts—experienced the diversion of funds away from tobacco education and control by the state legislature during their media campaigns.[37] The tobacco industry itself played a major role in criticisms of and the diversion of funds from the efforts in California and Florida, where the media campaign focused heavily on industry manipulation and deception. In California, the industry worked by lobbying and influencing both legislators and Department of Health Services administrators in an attempt to "limit the scope and aggressiveness of the media campaign."[38] In their article on the history of the California media campaign, Balbach and Glantz further write that the dramatic response of the industry to this well-funded and professionally designed campaign is evidence of a belief that such campaigns can indeed have an impact on smoking behavior.[37]

The Meaning and Importance of a Social Marketing Approach

Although there have been numerous attempts to communicate prevention messages about tobacco and other substances through advertising or mass media campaigns, the use of true marketing strategies in these efforts is rare. In fact, the majority of the "marketing" that has been conducted in regard to substance abuse prevention in general should more accurately be called "social advertising." There are important differences between mass media or social advertising strategies and the alternative concept of social marketing. Social marketing is defined as the "design, implementation, and control of programs calculated to influence the acceptability of social ideas, involving considerations of product, planning, pricing, communication, distribution and marketing research."[39] In short, social marketing applies techniques and strategies from the business sector—specifically from commercial marketing—in the planning and implementation of social improvement or change.

Several essential elements of the social marketing process have been defined, including (1) the use of a consumer orientation in the development of intervention techniques, (2) the use of exchange theory (which posits that marketing involves a type of persuasion that attempts to facilitate the voluntary exchange of resources—e.g., money, time, freedom, happiness, health—between a consumer and a producer), (3) audience segmentation and analysis strategies, (4) an emphasis on pretesting in market segments and formative research in intervention development, (5) the use of an information system to track the process by which the campaign was implemented, and (6) a strong management process that includes feedback and control processes.[40]

The differences between a traditional mass media approach and social marketing are further outlined in table 3. In summary, social marketing differs from mass media or social advertising in that the target audience is divided into clear segments and in that different messages or ideas are developed, pretested, and reformulated for these segments. In addition, in social marketing, the entire intervention strategy is managed and analyzed with a strong focus on the process by which the campaign is designed and implemented. Social marketing has been described as a disciplined approach that uses conventional market research and management techniques for rigorous planning and decision-making processes.[41] A social marketing approach has a strong formative component, meaning that the interpretations, reach, and impact of a social marketing campaign are analyzed on a continual basis as the campaign is developed and implemented, with the results fed back to campaign designers and implementers. This is in contrast to most public health marketing campaigns, which typically are implemented in a one-shot fashion, without much market segmentation and without collecting information along the way to feed back to the campaign designers and implementers.

Several examples of successful social marketing campaigns for public health have been described in the literature.[42] These include attempts to market products (e.g., condoms or oral rehydration therapy), services (e.g., childhood vaccinations), and even behaviors or health practices (e.g., breast-feeding). There are obvious differences between marketing campaigns that attempt to sell products or tangible "things" and those that attempt to convince people not to engage in a certain type of behavior (e.g., tobacco use). As a developmental psychologist involved in commercial marketing argued, it is far easier to sell new products than to create new behaviors; and it is especially difficult to use advertising to promote the avoidance of a familiar product (e.g., cigarettes).[43] However, "demarketing," or "deselling," is viewed as an important way to reduce demand for certain products or behaviors that threaten health.[44]

We should, however, recognize the limitations of and barriers to the social marketing of public health ideals and goals. Most health professionals are not trained in market research or in the management processes involved in social marketing. Thus, attempts to implement social marketing campaigns could fall short of meeting the prerequisites of a successful marketing intervention. Well-executed social marketing campaigns require human resources, a long-term commitment, and significant financial resources. Barriers to the social marketing of public health include difficulties in identifying and classifying narrow audience segments, obtaining appropriate "consumer" or behavioral data on the targets of the intervention, developing strong yet simple product concepts in reaching vulnerable populations (including those

TABLE 3. Mass Media vs. Social Marketing Approaches to Public Health

Technique	Mass Marketing	Social Marketing
Use of techniques from commercial marketing in the planning and implementation of social improvement or change (i.e., encouraging people to stop smoking)		√
Target audience defined	√	√
Target audience defined in terms of its needs and the perceived costs and benefits involved in meeting those needs		√
Audience segmentation by sociodemographics, such as age, geographic region, or race	√	√
Audience segmentation by core values, behavioral characteristics, lifestyle, class, etc.		√
Consumer orientation in development of intervention: "addresses the client's needs and interests in the development and promotion of products and services" (L&F)		√
Use of exchange theory: "marketing's orientation towards satisfying consumer interests through the utilization of techniques that facilitate *voluntary* exchanges between the consumer and the producer" (L&F)		√
Pretesting in market segments before intervention is widely disseminated		√
Use of pretesting to refine intervention before it is widely disseminated (formative research)		√
Use of channel analysis in distribution and promotion (a channel is a medium through which targeted segments can be reached with information, products, or services) to:		√
Determine which channel is most effective given limited resources (usually ends up being a public service announcement or posters/fliers/brochures)	√	
Determine which channel is most effective at reaching the target population		√
Marketing mix concept: the four P's of marketing plans (product, price, place, and promotion)		√
Process tracking system to evaluate program delivery and utilization trends over time		√
Management process		√
Consumer orientation in evaluation: looking at results of intervention with the question "how well did we understand our target poulations' needs and wants, and how well did we meet those needs?		√

most negatively oriented to the marketing message), and implementing and maintaining long-term strategies.[45]

There are many reasons to believe that a more disciplined and consumer-oriented approach to health communications and mass media interventions could be more effective. Social marketing requires empirically based audience segmentation and a consumer- and process-oriented approach to message tailoring, packaging, and dissemination. Thus, social marketing requires a different way of thinking about interventions and target audiences, which potentially could lead to significant improvements in traditional public health activities. Importantly, social marketing challenges the view that when a health promotion campaign fails, the defect resides in the people targeted by the campaign rather than in the campaign itself.[46] Often in public health, when a mass media campaign fails to produce the desired change in knowledge, attitudes, or behaviors, the assumption is that these desired outcomes are essentially intractable or that people are just not ready to change. A social marketing approach, however, is designed around the premise that most marketing campaigns fail because they do not reach the right people with the right message at the right time. Maibach and Holtgrave link the growing acceptance of social marketing in public health with its "progress toward replacing traditional, paternalistic approaches to public health with consumer-driven approaches."[47] Rather than deciding that the public should want a reduced risk of a certain disease or condition as a result of a change in behavior, "public health practitioners must learn to package, position and frame their programs to appeal to more salient, powerful, and influential core values: freedom, independence, autonomy, control, fairness, democracy, and free enterprise."[48]

Siegel and Doner emphasize that it is especially important for public health advocates to emphasize core values rather than offer simplistic health messages when attempting to confront "opposition framing" (i.e., the ways in which opponents will frame or define an issue). For example, in opposing municipal smoking bans in restaurants, the tobacco industry used a frame based on the notion of a "level playing field" for its core position: that restricting smoking in one city places its businesses at an "unfair advantage" compared to competitors in nearby cities without such regulation. Siegel and Doner write that the core values stirred up by this opposition framing included fairness, equality, justice, and economic opportunity. In response to this opposition, Siegel and Doner further suggest that public health messages need to be situated in or framed to include appeals to the same set or an equally appealing set of core values. Thus, public health responses can also target the notion of a level playing field, by emphasizing that "singling out restaurant workers as the one occupational group not deserving of basic health protection afforded to nearly all other workers creates an unlevel playing field for these workers" or that "failing to protect citizens in this city from secondhand smoke when more than 200 cities nationwide have already afforded these protections to their workers creates an unlevel playing field for our residents."[46] Both of these framings appeal not only to the core value of health but also to the same set of values targeted by industry opposition: fairness, equality, justice, and economic opportunity.

In deciding what types of core values are important to target, the designers of media campaigns would be well served in taking a community-based approach.[49] Such an approach would include community (or target audience) members as key participants in the conceptualization and development of the campaign. Those targeted to receive the campaign are likely the best source of information about which core values are salient or are going to resonate in the community. A community-based approach also would involve community members in planning, data collection, analysis, and interpretation. Any antitobacco campaign that does not emphasize community participation will be more likely to neglect local beliefs, values, and behaviors and thus will be less likely to produce campaigns that will be effective in changing smoking behavior.

Three Examples of a Social Marketing Approach

The media campaign implemented in California during the 1990s is a good example of social marketing in practice. From its very beginning, the campaign was designed to address core values rather than convey the traditional public health message "Don't smoke because it is bad for your health." The initial fifteen months of the campaign—as explained in a print ad marking the advent of the campaign—intended to go "right at the tobacco companies' predatory marketing—the selective exploitation of minorities, the seduction of youth, the selling of suicide."[50] The campaign promised to "talk about a shared community opportunity and a shared community menace." This campaign was aimed at a number of identified core values, including the values of truth in advertising, fairness in presenting information to the public, protection of groups perceived as somehow vulnerable, and community health. Intense premarket focus group studies and other research were conducted to identify these core values and messages that would resonate with different audiences, including youth. Subsequently, tailored messages and campaign products were developed and rigorously tested before being marketed. In addition, the entire campaign was professionally overseen with a strong and formative management process. Evaluation data suggest that the campaign has been successful in reducing overall tobacco consumption in the state, although the specific impact on youth is less clear.

The University of Vermont media intervention for elementary school students described earlier is a good example of the use of social marketing principles in public health practice.[51] The important features of this intervention have been described as including (1) a clearly identified target group whose perceptions and interests in smoking were determined before the mass media intervention was fully developed, (2) adherence to a set of strategic principles derived from previous research (e.g., the use of variety and formats that appealed to the target group and the avoidance of commands to not smoke), (3) pretesting in the target group, (4) identification and use of the most effective media channels for the target population, and (5) implementation of several concepts to ensure audience attention (including the repetition of messages using multiple channels over a long period of time, where the messages were novel, targeted at very specific issues, and provided attitudinal alternatives).[52]

As a third example, McKenna and Williams's description of a tobacco counteradvertisement campaign aimed at teenagers illustrates how this effort may have benefited from a more rigorous social marketing approach.[53] This campaign employed some of the techniques of good social marketing. Research from focus groups that included many different segments of the target audience was used to design the campaign. In addition, consumer response to the materials was tested after the campaign was implemented. Unfortunately, however, this market testing came too late, as it revealed that the central campaign message (about the "predatory marketing techniques" of the tobacco industry) was not being communicated clearly to the intended teenage audience. In fact, the message was so confusing to the target audience that the campaign was halted. In their discussion of this failed campaign,

McKenna and Williams espoused some of the fundamental principles of social marketing: "These negative test findings underscore the critical need for ongoing audience research throughout the creative process to ensure that campaign planners stay 'in tune' with their consumers."[53]

Tobacco Marketing vs. Public Health Social Marketing: Similarities and Differences

It is imperative that health practitioners involved with attempts to improve social conditions, to change behaviors, and to promote public health policy employ the concepts and principles of effective social marketing. For those working in the area of youth tobacco control, an important educational resource is the tobacco industry itself.

From our review of tobacco industry documents and other literature on tobacco marketing strategies, several key lessons can be articulated. First, it is important to recognize that the marketing strategies of the tobacco industry have tended to meet the requirements for effective marketing in general: the process was disciplined and well managed, the consumer was "heard" through formative research, and the product was responsive to consumer wants and needs.[54] The tobacco industry has long used these basic marketing tools in strategies that go far beyond simple advertising campaigns. Cigarette audiences of all ages are clearly segmented by gender, social class, recreational interests, and values; and there is pretesting and significant formative research before promotional campaigns are broadly implemented. The cases of Dakota and Uptown cigarettes forcefully illustrate the targeting tactics of the tobacco industry. These two brands were intended to be marketed to clear, narrow audience segments. Dakota cigarettes were to be marketed to young, working-class "virile" females who enjoy such recreational events as tractor pulls and do not have professional career aspirations. In contrast, the Uptown brand of menthol cigarettes was being targeted toward urban African Americans who enjoy big-city night life. Both of these brands underwent test marketing before being dropped, although negative publicity after exposure of the industry's targeting tactics may have played a larger role in the decision to drop the brands than did lethargic sales in test markets. In cities where Uptown was being test-marketed, there was a well-coordinated and well-publicized protest among African Americans. They objected to a large corporation targeting a product known to have negative health effects in their communities, which already were facing serious public health challenges and discrimination.

Regarding youth, information from R. J. Reynolds industry documents regarding FUBYAS and segmentation of adolescents into groups based on behaviors, attitudes, recreational interests, and propensity to smoke (as described earlier in this chapter) is another case in point. Although one might not condone the industry's effort to segment the youth market, the creation of clear and numerous audience segments— and the development of products and campaigns specific to those market niches—is important for any marketing effort. In fact, R. J. Reynolds's own internal documents suggest that the company learned from the Uptown experience that not enough market research was conducted before the new brand was introduced. Had advertising executives asked African Americans across a number of social strata for their opinions regarding a menthol cigarette targeted specifically at blacks, they would have been able to predict the fate of this brand before its introduction. Thus, the perceived failure here was not the targeting of a brand to a specific market niche but failing to do the appropriate pre-market testing and research before introducing the brand.

A second lesson to be learned from the tobacco industry is that the exchange that tobacco advertisers are trying to promote is not as simple as "cigarettes for money." What is being promoted are core values or attributes desirable to youth—for example, a cool demeanor in social situations, a rugged sort of individualism, athletic ability, sex appeal, and romantic attractiveness. Promotional gimmicks based on proof of purchase (e.g., as sports-related clothing or paraphernalia or admittance to a music concert) promote exchanges that involve the acquisition of desired objects or a fun, exciting experience. The exchanges being promoted are also reinforced by associating them with recognizable characters or symbols (e.g., Joe Camel or the Marlboro Man) or events (e.g., extreme sports competitions) that appeal to youth, which in turn serve to embody and further promote the desired exchange. Once the link between product and symbol is established, these appealing images of smoking are efficiently transmitted and reinforced.

A third lesson is that even though the tobacco industry has engaged in savvy and high-quality marketing tactics, we should not give the industry or its advertising firms credit for having some secret knowledge or magical marketing strategies for enticing youth to smoke.

Industry documents reveal that the industry heavily invested in understanding youth market segments and tailoring products and ad campaigns to those identified segments. These documents, however, do not reveal that the industry has any type of special insight into, or understanding of, youth attitudes and behaviors. Thus, the most important thing to understand about tobacco industry tactics and youth is that the principles of sound marketing have been implemented effectively and that significant financial and human resources have been devoted to this endeavor. In addition, of course, the product being promoted is highly addictive. This combination of knowing how to market, having the resources to do it right, and the addictive nature of the product likely explains the bulk of the industry's marketing success.

Given what we understand about social marketing and some key aspects of successful marketing campaigns, efforts to market smoking prevention to youth need to include elements standard to any marketing plan. These include (a) the use of market research for audience segmentation, (b) the use of adolescent psychology and exchange theory for creating campaign messages and strategies, (c) evaluative and formative research in message development, and (d) a well-formulated dissemination strategy that is managed and processed as it is implemented. Market segmentation leads to the development of different messages for different types of youth, based on sociodemographic characteristics (e.g., age, gender, and ethnicity) and core values, rather than negative health messages. For example, focusing on tobacco industry deception in antismoking campaigns was identified as an important core message in California's and subsequently in other states' mass media campaigns.[55] Other campaigns have focused on the core value of romantic or physical attractiveness, focusing on the negative effects of smoking on teeth, breath, and overall body scent. Members of the communities or subpopulations targeted by a campaign need to help identify the core values or message content that form the heart of the campaign.

Market segmentation also needs to be thought of in broader terms. Social marketing can reach beyond adolescents to influence parents, teachers, clinicians, community organizations and institutions, people who make movies, television shows and music videos, and policymakers at the local, state, and federal levels. Dissemination strategies also require keen vision regarding message placement, including where and at what times. Reliance on public service announcements on the radio and television is not an ideal message placement strategy for most audience segments, because many of these announcements air at undesirable hours.

Although there are many similarities between marketing tobacco products and the social marketing of smoking prevention, there also are some important differences between the two endeavors. This includes the fact that the tobacco industry is now forbidden to market its products to children and maintains that it has refrained from doing so in the past. While one might argue that the industry has been quite shrewd in getting around the social (and now legal) sanctions against marketing to children, it also might be the case that industry tactics would be even more effective if tobacco advertising could be explicitly directed toward children or youth. Public health campaigns aimed at smoking prevention face no such age restrictions and thus may have a competitive edge over the industry in this regard.

On the other hand, tobacco industry has the significant advantage that the successful marketing of its products will generate revenue that can be reinvested in marketing. Successful social marketing campaigns may lead to great social achievements, but they will not generate money. Thus, these campaigns will always expend a great deal of money without generating any new resources. Also, the tobacco industry will no doubt continue to invest resources and exert political influence in an attempt to remove anti-industry messages from media campaigns.[56] This means that as "more states embark on anti-tobacco advertising campaigns . . . public health advocates need to understand the importance of helping to establish the rules by which this money will be spent and monitoring the process of spending it."[54]

The apparent success of antismoking media campaigns—both nationally and, more recently, at the state level—convinced the American Legacy Foundation to devote a substantial proportion of its nearly $200 million in annual expenditures to a professionally designed media campaign. Many of the ads in this campaign have emphasized the health consequences of smoking, presented in a novel, graphic manner. Others have focused on the deceptive practices of the tobacco industry, including both denial of the addictiveness of nicotine and intentional (yet again denied) targeting of children. The ad campaign was inaugurated in early 2000. Two of the ads were immediately attacked by the tobacco industry as vilifying the industry and thereby violating the multistate settlement's prohibition on industry vilification. Initially, major television networks refused to air these and other foundation ads, and the foundation withdrew the two ads challenged by the industry. Subsequently, the foundation reintroduced one of these ads, as well as others in the same series. Foundation ads are played on the Web site <www.thetruth.com>, as well as on television. Given the novelty of this campaign, the determination of its impact and the ultimate resolution of any industry objections must await the passage of time.

Conclusion

Sophisticated mass media campaigns have the potential to have a positive effect on the attitudes and behaviors of youth regarding tobacco use, although the impact of such campaigns is challenging to evaluate and has not yet been fully demonstrated. The literature suggests that mass media interventions increase their chance of having an impact if the following conditions are met: (1) the campaign strategies are based on sound social marketing principles, (2) the effort is large and intense enough, (3) target groups are carefully differentiated, (4) messages for specific target groups are based on empirical findings regarding the needs and interests of the group, and (5) the campaign is of sufficient duration.

There is ample evidence that the tobacco industry has engaged in marketing tobacco products to youth and that this marketing has had some impact on youth smoking behavior. Some of the tactics used by the tobacco industry (and other industries that market products to youth) can also be used by public health advocates in marketing smoking prevention. Some may find this notion of social marketing, which takes its cues from the business sector, ironic at best and inappropriate or even offensive at worst. Some people may not want to emulate the tools and strategies of those who promote consumption and strive to manipulate behavior. Social marketing also has been criticized as too often focusing on individuals and their behaviors, rather than "upstream causes," which are typically socioeconomic, ecological, or political in nature.[57] Yet social marketing principles have been described as being well suited for and effective at translating educational and behavioral-change messages into concepts and products that will be accepted and responded to by target populations in an attempt to produce social goods. The bottom line is that social marketing has the potential to improve public health.

There are, however, two caveats we would like to issue. First, some tobacco control advocates are concerned that the psychology of some antismoking messages aimed at youth may unintentionally be enticing adolescents to smoke. This counterproductive effect may be occurring when smoking is portrayed as an adult behavior that is off-limits to youth—a "forbidden fruit" that becomes more alluring when it is deemed inappropriate for youth.[58] Advertising can prompt behavior, even negative behavior. A developmental psychologist with experience in advertising wrote: "This is behind the 'don't put peas up your nose' phenomenon in child rearing. I do not recommend giving this command to a preschooler. And while you are at it, maybe you shouldn't tell your teenager not to smoke."[59] The messages and values being communicated in antitobacco marketing campaigns aimed at youth cannot be based solely on the concept that adolescents should not smoke because they are too young and that smoking is an adult behavior choice. If this is the fundamental message being imparted, it is possible that counterproductive effects may ensue. Interestingly, the tobacco industry recently launched its own media campaign against youth smoking. The television and print ads in this campaign take a variety of forms, with the majority emphasizing in some fashion that smoking is an adult behavior that is not appropriate for adolescents. Some have argued that such tactics are not likely to be effective, since defining smoking as an adult behavior makes it more alluring and interesting to youth. A cynic might even suggest that the tobacco industry and its marketing gurus know that this approach is at best benign and are thus implementing it precisely because of its potential for counterproductive effects.

Second, we need to be careful not to overestimate either the effects of tobacco advertising on smoking or the potential gains of even well-crafted social marketing approaches to mass media interventions. Social marketing, like any other tobacco control policy or strategy, is not a magic bullet that will work on its own. Interventions in this area need to be implemented in conjunction with other tobacco use prevention and control efforts, such as youth access interventions, multiple-component community interventions, and tobacco excise tax increases.

In summary, there is much that health practitioners and policy-makers can learn from those who market tobacco products. Just as tobacco marketing can influence smoking behavior, social marketing is a promising approach to smoking prevention, although it does require significant resources and skillful execution. The resources available from the recent settlement between the tobacco industry and state attorneys general provide an unprecedented opportunity to engage in an intensive, high-quality social marketing campaign to test and evaluate the premise that tobacco marketing tactics can be met head-on and countered. Indeed, as we described earlier, a significant portion of the settlement resources being overseen by the American Legacy Foundation is specifically designated for this purpose. Thus, the time is right to design, implement, and rigorously evaluate social marketing strategies in youth tobacco control.

REFERENCES

1. Giovino 1999.
2. Richards, Tye, and Fischer 1996; Perry 1999.
3. Seidel-Marks 1998.
4. Joe Camel Campaign: Mangini v. R. J. Reynolds Tobacco Company Collection <galen.library.ucsf.edu/tobacco/mangini/>; Brown and Williamson Collection CD-ROM <galen.library.ucsf.edu/tobacco/bw.html> .
5. Perry 1999.
6. See Perry 1999 and Hastings and MacFadyen 2000 for additional examples of industry documents regarding youth tobacco marketing.
7. Botvin et al. 1993.
8. DiFranza et al. 1991; Arnett and Terhanian 1998; Cummings et al. 1997; Pierce et al. 1991.
9. DiFranza et al. 1991; King et al. 1998.
10. Schooler, Feighery, and Flora 1996.
11. Feighery et al. 1998.
12. Turner-Bowker and Hamilton 2000. See also Sanchez and Goldberg 2000.
13. Warner 1986.
14. Borden 1942.
15. Chaloupka and Warner 2000.
16. Warner et al. 1986.
17. Saffer and Chaloupka 1999.
18. Altman et al. 1996; Gilpin and Pierce 1997; Pierce and Gilpin 1994; Gilpin, Pierce, and Rosbrook 1997.
19. Pierce and Gilpin 1994.
20. DiFranza et al. 1991; Unger, Johnson, and Rohrbach 1995.
21. Evans et al. 1995.
22. Pierce, Choi, et al. 1998.
23. Pucci and Siegel 1999.
24. Aitken and Eadie 1990; Aitken et al. 1991; Biener and Siegel 2000; Sargent et al. 2000.
25. Gilpin and Pierce 1997.
26. Cummings et al. 1997; Tye, Warner, and Glantz 1987.
27. Johnston, O'Malley, and Bachman 1999a.

28. Tye, Warner, and Glantz 1987.

29. Giovino 1999; Jernigan and Wright 1996.

30. Jason 1998; Macaskill et al. 1992.

31. Siegel 1998.

32. Worden 1999; Flynn, Worden, and Secker-Walker 1994.

33. Secker-Walker et al. 1997.

34. Goldman and Glantz 1998.

35. Heiser and Begay 1997; Traynor and Glantz 1996; Popham et al. 1994.

36. Florida Department of Health, Office of Tobacco Control 2000.

37. Balbach and Glantz 1998; Siegel et al. 1997; Givel and Glantz 2000.

38. Balbach and Glantz 1998.

39. Lefebvre and Flora 1988.

40. Lefebvre and Flora 1988; Chapman et al. 1993; Ling et al. 1992.

41. Chapman et al. 1993.

42. Ling et al. 1992; Maibach and Holtgrave 1995.

43. Rust 1999.

44. Lefebvre and Flora 1988; Chapman et al. 1993; Ling et al. 1992; Maibach and Holtgrave 1995; Rust 1999.

45. Bloom and Novelli 1981.

46. Chapman et al. 1993.

47. Maibach and Holtgrave 1995.

48. Siegel and Doner 1998.

49. Israel et al. 1998.

50. Balbach and Glantz 1998.

51. Worden 1999; Flynn, Worden, and Secker-Walker 1994; Worden et al. 1996; Secker-Walker et al. 1997.

52. Worden 1999; Pechmann and Reibling 2000.

53. McKenna and Williams 1993.

54. Chapman et al. 1993.

55. Balbach and Glantz 1998.

56. Siegel 1998; Balbach and Glantz 1998.

57. Maibach and Holtgrave 1995; Walack et al. 1993.

58. Rust 1999; Glantz 1996.

59. Rust 1999.

6

Teenage Smoking Behavior and the Cost of Cigarettes

The effects of cigarette price increases on discouraging youth smoking is clearly one of the best-documented and most encouraging stories in all of tobacco control. Although the evidence is not unequivocal, there is a consensus among economists who have studied the relationship between price increases and cigarette consumption that higher prices do indeed decrease smoking by young people.

In this chapter, we examine the impact of raising the cost of cigarettes as a means for controlling teenage tobacco use. This chapter is considerably more technical than the rest of the book. To the extent possible, we have attempted to frame the discussion in lay terms so that readers can reasonably follow the economic analyses. But because the issue is largely described in complex econometric studies, it is inherently more difficult to explain than the other material we cover.

Overview

Most studies have found that raising the price of cigarettes reduces cigarette consumption for both adults and youths. While there is, as we show shortly, no unanimity among economists as to the specific amount of reductions in the quantities of cigarettes demanded resulting from increasing prices, there is a great deal of agreement about the general direction of the relationship between price and demand. In contrast with most of the literature, a few studies by economists have not found greater price responsiveness among children than among adults.[1] A recent debate, inaugurated by conflicting interpretations of the same empirical data set, has broken out among health economists as to whether higher prices discourage youth smoking initiation per se.[2] Despite these uncertainties, the overall strength of the evidence supporting the proposition that higher prices reduce youth smoking led a group of economists who had substantial experience working on tobacco economic issues to call for increased cigarette taxation, primarily to reduce youth smoking.[3]

The cost of cigarettes faced by teenagers can be raised through both price and nonprice measures. Policymakers at the federal, state, and local levels can increase the price of cigarettes by raising cigarette excise taxes—perhaps the most direct route of action. A wide variety of other measures will also lead to cigarette price increases. For example, the recent $206 billion settlement between 46 states and the tobacco industry increased the wholesale price of cigarettes by approximately 50 cents per pack.[4] Similarly, the governmental system of tobacco price supports and supply controls that has been in place since the late 1930s has acted to raise cigarette prices, albeit to a very modest degree.[5]

It is also possible that the tobacco industry itself might decide to raise prices, independent of any government-imposed tax increases or costs related to lawsuits. The industry could decide to shift its current strategy of maximizing long-run profits in favor of a strategy that focuses on short-run profit maximization. Industry executives might reason that smoking is on the decline in the United States and that it may be to their financial advantage to exploit current smokers' addiction to cigarettes at the expense of reducing the number of future smokers. While this is certainly an interesting possibility, no empirical evidence exists to support this potential strategy shift.

While each of the possibilities just outlined may raise the price of cigarettes, each also has very different distributional consequences (i.e., affecting different population groups in differing ways). In the case of excise tax increases, income is transferred from smokers to the government. In contrast, the tobacco quota and price support program transfers income from smokers to tobacco farmers (producers). For reasons described shortly, our guess is that the settlement will transfer income from smokers to state governments and producers.

In addition to increasing the cost of cigarettes via the price mechanism, policymakers have at their disposal a variety of nonprice measures that have the potential for imposing significant "costs" on teenagers. For instance, clean indoor air laws may act to reduce opportunities for teenagers to smoke by forcing them to limit their smoking to relatively few and perhaps inconvenient settings. Moreover, teen access laws—such as those that ban vending machine sales, impose harsh penalties on individuals who sell cigarettes to minors, and prohibit minors from possessing cigarettes—make it more difficult and costly for minors to obtain and smoke cigarettes.

Organization of the Chapter

In the sections that follow, we explore in somewhat greater detail the potential for various price and nonprice measures to raise the cost of cigarettes to teenagers. First, however, we examine the evidence from studies related to the impact of price changes on adult smoking behavior. There is considerable evidence that adult smoking behavior has a significant impact on teenage smoking behavior and that price increases appear to reduce smoking on the part of adults. Thus, if price increases are effective in getting adults to quit smoking, we can expect fewer teenagers to smoke. After presenting a brief overview of the adult cigarette demand literature, we turn to the comparatively few studies that have focused on the impact of cigarette price changes on teenagers. Many of the issues, and much of the evidence, discussed here are covered in greater detail in Chaloupka and Warner's study of the economics of smoking.[6]

Excise Taxes and the Demand for Cigarettes

A variety of rationales have been offered by legislators, policymakers, smoking control advocates, and others for increasing federal, state, and local cigarette excise taxes. Such rationales include covering the costs that smokers impose on others; generating revenue for government coffers; providing an economic incentive for smokers to reduce, if not eliminate, the amount they smoke; and preventing teenagers and young adults from starting to smoke. These rationales have come under increasing attack from the tobacco industry and its supporters, who have in part argued that cigarettes are already fully taxed and that smokers already pay for any harms caused by smoking.

Cigarette prices vary considerably from state to state. Most of this price variation is due to differences in state excise taxes on cigarettes. As is shown in table 4, 1999 tax rates varied from a low of 2.5 cents per pack in Virginia to a high of $1 per pack in Alaska and Hawaii, with an

TABLE 4.   Cigarette Excise Taxes, July 31, 1999

State	Cents per Pack
Alabama	16.5
Alaska	100.0
Arizona	58.0
Arkansas	31.5
California	87.0
Colorado	20.0
Connecticut	50.0
Delaware	24.0
District of Columbia	65.0
Florida	33.9
Georgia	12.0
Hawaii	100.0
Idaho	28.0
Illinois	58.0
Indiana	15.5
Iowa	36.0
Kansas	24.0
Kentucky	3.0
Louisiana	20.0
Maine	74.0
Maryland	66.0
Massachusetts	76.0
Michigan	75.0
Minnesota	48.0
Mississippi	18.0
Missouri	17.0
Montana	18.0
Nebraska	34.0
Nevada	35.0
New Hampshire	37.0
New Jersey	80.0
New Mexico	21.0
New York	56.0
North Carolina	5.0
North Dakota	44.0
Ohio	24.0
Oklahoma	23.0
Oregon	68.0
Pennsylvania	31.0
Rhode Island	71.0
South Carolina	7.0
South Dakota	33.0
Tennessee	13.0
Texas	41.0
Utah	51.5
Vermont	44.0
Virginia	2.5
Washington	82.5
West Virginia	17.0
Wisconsin	59.0
Wyoming	12.0

Source: National Cancer Institute: State Cancer Legislative Database Program, 1999; Office on Smoking and Health, Centers for Disease Control and Prevention, State Tobacco Activities Tracking and Evaluation System, 1999.

average tax rate of 40.5 cents per pack. Currently, 13 states require that at least a portion of the revenue generated from cigarette excise taxes be devoted to tobacco control programs.

The extent to which higher cigarette taxes will reduce smoking prevalence rates and the quantity of cigarettes smoked by smokers depends on the degree to which cigarette tax increases are passed on to smokers and how responsive smokers and prospective smokers are to price increases. Or, as economists would say, it depends on the price elasticity of demand for cigarettes (more commonly referred to in economics as just the price elasticity of cigarettes). In arithmetic terms, the price elasticity of demand is simply the percentage change in the quantity demanded divided by the percentage change in price. In other words, the price elasticity provides a summary measure of how much we can expect the demand for cigarettes to decline if the price of cigarettes is increased by a certain amount. For example, if a 10 percent increase in the price of cigarettes yields a 4 percent reduction in the amount of cigarettes smoked, then the elasticity of demand is 0.4 (i.e., 4 divided by 10). The price increase can result from higher taxes, increased production and marketing costs, or industry attempts to maximize profits.

A number of studies have examined the degree to which excise tax increases are passed on to consumers in the form of higher cigarette prices. The consensus view is that prices tend to rise by at least as much as the value of the tax. Two of the early studies of this issue, for example, found that for each 1-cent increase in the tax, the retail price of cigarettes rose by 1.065 and 1.101 cents, respectively.[7] A more recent study found that a 1-cent rise in a state's excise tax would translate into a 1.11-cent increase in the price of cigarettes.[8]

Determining the extent to which teenagers are responsive to cigarette price increases has proven to be a somewhat more difficult proposition, one that has produced inconsistent results. From a purely theoretical standpoint, economists argue that teenagers can be expected to be more responsive than adults to price increases, for several reasons.[9] First, because teenagers have lower disposable incomes than do adults, cigarette purchases represent a higher fraction of their total income. Second, because teenagers are particularly susceptible to peer pressure, cigarette price increases may cause a ripple effect in that fewer teens may take up smoking if the price increases cause existing teen smokers to either reduce the quantity of cigarettes smoked or give up smoking entirely. Third, the addictive nature of cigarettes suggests that teenagers could indeed be more responsive than adults to changes in cigarette prices, as it is easier to start smoking than to quit. In fact, one could argue that teenagers will be more responsive to price changes than are adults as smokers make the transition from one stage of smoking (i.e., never-smoker, experimenter, regular user, and quitter) to another. Thus, in principle, any factor that can deter or reduce consumption, especially in adults (who are established smokers), is likely to have a larger effect on teenagers who are initiating smoking.

Studies of Adult Cigarette Demand

Empirical studies of the elasticity of demand for cigarettes have followed a long tradition, dating back more than half a century.[10] The bulk of these studies have focused on the adult or overall demand for cigarettes, with comparatively few focused on teenage cigarette demand.

An early review of cigarette demand studies that were completed between 1970 and 1982 and used data from the United States reported that estimates ranged between −0.40 to −1.30 (meaning we would observe anywhere from a 4 percent to a 13 percent reduction in cigarette demand for every 10 percent increase in price).[11] The range of price elasticity estimates found in these studies appears to be attributable to differences in data and statistical techniques.

In an effort to summarize and synthesize the studies on the adult elasticity of demand, a 1993 National Cancer Institute (NCI) expert panel reviewed the relevant literature and concluded that most estimates of the adult elasticity of demand have clustered around −0.40.[12] As described earlier, this implies that a 10 percent increase in the price of cigarettes will reduce consumption by 4 percent. More recent studies of the elasticity of demand have also produced estimates that tend to cluster around −0.40.[13]

Many studies used aggregate time series data to construct statistical models of the demand for cigarettes, with the unit of analysis being either the nation or the state rather than the individual. In this type of analysis, an attempt is made to explain per capita cigarette consumption as a function of price, per capita income, and various measures of aggregate demographic characteristics. One study, for example, analyzed data from 46 states between 1963 and 1980 to develop their cigarette demand model.[14] The results of their model indicated a price elasticity of −0.22. Another researcher also used time series data to construct demand equations for cigarettes and generated a price elasticity estimate just under –0.5.[15] A third researcher used aggregate time series data from 1947 to 1978 to examine the determinants of cigarette demand.[16] At the average price and consumption level for the data included in the model, this study estimated price elasticity of demand at –0.37.

Only a few studies have used micro-level data, where the unit of analysis is the individual rather than the state or nation, to construct cigarette demand models. The main advantage of using microdata is that it allows one to look at the impact of prices and other policy variables on the various transition stages of smoking. It also permits researchers to assess the effects of policy variables on population subgroups and to avoid some of the biases that may creep into aggregate data analyses. For example, Lewit and Coate[17] used data on respondents to the 1976 Health Interview Survey to estimate price and income elasticities of adult cigarette demand. The authors noted that using data on individuals is preferable to using states as the units of observation because the latter approach produces biases in elasticity estimates. This bias results from the fact that sales figures based on taxes paid fail to reflect adequately actual consumption, as there may be smuggling or bootlegging of cigarettes from low-tax to high-tax states. To eliminate the potential for producing biased estimates, Lewit and Coate's analysis excluded individuals who lived in communities where the price of cigarettes exceeded another price found within a 20-mile-wide band around their place of residence. The estimates obtained from this "restricted sample" indicated an overall price elasticity of –0.42.

Not all studies found such responses. Using seven years of National Health Interview Survey data covering the period 1970 through 1985, one group of researchers constructed several models of adult cigarette demand.[18] Their results indicated that the adult price elasticity of demand was unstable over time, ranging from 0.06 in 1970 to –0.23 in 1985. These figures, however, demonstrated that adults might be somewhat less responsive to cigarette price changes than previously thought.

In an effort to analyze the impact of a price increase of 25 cents per pack of cigarettes in California, Keeler et al.[19] used aggregate monthly time series data for the period 1980 through 1990.[20] They found that the overall short-run elasticity of demand was between –0.3 and –0.5, and the long-run elasticity fell in the 0.5 to –0.6 range. Moreover, their study presented some evidence that antismoking regulations reduced the quantity of cigarettes smoked during the 1980s. Their conclusion about the strength of this relationship, however, was tempered by the fact that the regulation index and time trend variables were correlated, making it difficult to tease out the independent effect of the regulation variable.

Finally, several studies have applied a *rational addiction model* to cigarette demand. In a rational addiction model, the individual's prior cigarette use predicts future consumption because it is rational for one who is addicted to nicotine to continue smoking regardless of the price increase. Thus, an addicted smoker will be less likely to quit if the price is increased. This modeling approach maintains that there are important linkages between past, current, and future cigarette consumption that should be accounted for in demand estimation efforts. For example, Becker, Grossman, and Murphy[21] used a rational addiction framework and cigarette sales data from 1955 through 1985 to estimate cigarette demand. Their results indicated that a 10 percent permanent increase in the price of cigarettes reduced cigarette consumption by 4 percent in the short run and 7.5 percent in the long run. Using a similar analytic framework, Chaloupka[22] found that men had a long-run price elasticity of –0.60, while women were unresponsive to price changes. Earlier, Mullahy[23] estimated several cigarette demand models accounting for past consumption and found that the average price elasticity obtained was –0.47.

Studies of Teenage Cigarette Demand

The NCI expert panel noted earlier concluded that prices influence teenage cigarette consumption "at least as much as adult consumption." Yet the relative dearth of studies devoted to calculating teenage cigarette price elasticities prevented the panel from arriving at a more precise estimate. Several influential studies of teenage cigarette demand are discussed in this section.[24]

Given our concern with the effects of cigarette prices, regulation of public smoking, and other influences on the smoking behavior of teenagers, the underlying conceptual model of teenage cigarette demand must address the external influences on teenage smoking choices. These include (1) the budgetary constraints imposed by cigarette prices, family income, and the teenagers' own disposable income; (2) public influences (laws on smoking) that alter the smoking opportunities available to teenagers and signal the social acceptability of smoking; and (3) opportunities for learned or acquired behavior from parents, siblings, peers, or adult celebrities (e.g., sports figures).

As the first of these three influences indicates, part of the underlying conceptual framework is a standard microeconomic model of choice. Teenagers make consumption choices about cigarettes and other goods based on the resources available to them (family income and their own disposable income) and the costs of other goods and services. This conceptual model typically leads to statistical models that portray cigarette demand as a function of cigarette prices, the prices of other goods and services, the family's or the adolescent's own income, and the presence of nonprice restrictions that may raise the effective price of smoking.[25]

In addition to microeconomic theory, social psychology has contributed to the development of conceptual models of teenage smoking behavior. In particular, several empirical studies of teenage smoking have relied, to one extent or another, on social learning theory, as developed by Bandura.[26] Social learning theory has generated considerable insight into the motivations for smoking and has in fact served as the basis for much of the empirical work conducted by noneconomists on smoking initiation and maintenance. According to Bandura, social learning is achieved through the following processes: attention, retention, motor reproduction, and motivation or incentive. For instance, a teenager may try a cigarette (motor reproduction) after observing a parent smoking (attention) and may continue smoking in response to peer pressure (motivation or incentive). With these processes in mind, it is easy to see how a teenager's peers and family members could play an important role in the decisions to initiate and continue smoking. The application of social learning theory to smoking behavior has been strongly supported in a large number of studies that have attested to the influence played by peers and family members on an individual's smoking behavior.[27]

The influences of parental and sibling smoking can also be imbedded in an economic model. Initiation, for instance, may be facilitated by easy access to cigarettes through peers who smoke, and there may be relatively little parental pressure to not smoke. These factors can be viewed as reducing the total "cost" to teenagers of smoking, as alluded to in chapter 3.

One of the early empirical studies of teenage smoking behavior found rather large price elasticities of demand.[28] The researchers used data from the Health Examination Survey to estimate cigarette demand functions for teenagers.[29] Specifically, they examined two measures of smoking behavior: whether the teenager smoked (i.e., "participation") and, if so, the quantity smoked per day. The estimated elasticities for both smoking participation and quantity smoked were large (i.e., −1.19 and −1.44, respectively) in relation to those found in other studies. An important contribution of this study was that it stimulated subsequent studies in this area to assess the impact of price changes on the various stages of smoking behavior. For the most part, researchers have looked at the impact of prices on initiation and on the quantity of cigarettes smoked by smokers, with relatively little attention being devoted to how price increases may influence teenage smokers' decisions to quit.

The conclusion that youth cigarette demand is more price elastic than is adult demand was widely accepted until a study published in 1991 indicated that prices did not have a statistically significant impact on youth smoking.[30] The authors attributed this result to the inclusion in their models of an index of restrictions on smoking in public. These restrictions, which had an important impact on the price variable, had not been included in most previous studies of cigarette demand. Moreover, an analysis of NHANES II (a national household survey of health attitudes and behaviors) survey data found that the price elasticity of demand for young adults (defined as individuals between 17 and 24 years of age) was also insignificant.[31]

A recent study of the impact of cigarette price increases on young adults (i.e., college-age students) analyzed survey data from the 1993 Harvard College Alcohol Study.[32] Based on the results from the model constructed for the survey, the overall estimated price elasticities range from −0.906 to −1.309, with approximately half of the response due to the impact of price on smoking participation and the remaining half due to the impact of price on the number of cigarettes smoked by smokers. Noting that their sample was not a random sample of all young adults, the authors suggested that the price elasticity of cigarette demand by young adults who have not completed their education and have relatively little income may be even higher, given the evidence that cigarette demand is relatively less elastic for individuals with more education or higher income.[33]

Another study found similar evidence, based on 13 waves of the National Health Interview Survey conducted between 1976 and 1992.[34] The researchers estimated that demand was more than twice as elastic for their sample of young adults, ages 18 to 24 years (total elasticity of −0.58), as for their full sample (total elasticity of −0.25). Other recent studies provide additional support for the proposition that young people are more sensitive to cigarette price increases than are adults.[35]

In general, researchers examining the effects of price on smoking participation using individual-level data from cross-sectional surveys have assumed that much of the price effect estimated for youths reflects the impact of price on smoking initiation, while the estimate for adults is largely capturing the effects of price on smoking cessation. A few recent studies have attempted to examine directly the impact of cigarette prices on smoking initiation. With retrospective data from the 1978 and 1979 smoking supplements to the National Health Interview Survey, one study examined the ages at which survey respondents reported that they began smoking.[36] While the authors found that a number of socioeconomic and demographic factors had a significant effect on smoking initiation, their estimates for cigarette prices were insignificant.

These results were supported by another study's finding that the estimates for the effect of cigarette taxes on the probability of starting to smoke on a daily basis between the eighth and twelfth grade were not statistically significantly.[37] Taken together, these studies raised doubts about the hypothesis that higher cigarette prices lead to significant reductions in youth smoking.

Yet a debate between two of the research teams involved has served only to obfuscate the conclusions. For example, Dee and Evans[38] reexamined the longitudinal data used by DeCicca et al., arguing that DeCicca et al.'s finding that price has no impact on smoking initiation was largely the result of the way in which their sample was constructed; they found a negative and significant impact of cigarette taxes on smoking initiation. Specifically, Dee and Evans obtained an estimated price elasticity of smoking onset of –0.63, which is consistent with several other recent studies of youth smoking employing cross-sectional data. This exchange illustrates the sensitivity of elasticity estimates to the particular data and methods used by researchers.

An important issue that had not been previously examined, whether and how smokers compensate for higher prices, recently received some research attention. Using data from the 1979 smoking supplement and the 1987 cancer control supplement to the National Health Interview Survey, Evans and Farrelly investigated the compensating behavior by smokers in response to tax and price changes. Specifically, they found consistent evidence that although smokers reduced daily cigarette consumption in response to higher taxes, they also compensated for the reduction in several ways. In particular, smokers in high-tax states consumed longer cigarettes and those that are higher in tar and nicotine, with young adult smokers most likely to engage in this compensating behavior.[39] As a result, the authors argued that the perceived health benefits associated with higher cigarette taxes are likely to be somewhat overstated. Given this compensating behavior, they suggest that if cigarette taxes are to be used to reduce the negative health consequences of smoking, taxes based on tar and nicotine content would be appropriate.[40]

The Evans and Farrelly study in a sense serves as a reminder of the dynamic nature of the teen smoking problem. We cannot take for granted that, say, a single tax increase will elicit the desired effect once and for all. As these researchers illustrate, there may be some unexpected (and undesirable) side effects. Moreover, it is also important for policymakers to ensure that cigarette taxes are periodically adjusted upward to account for inflation. Otherwise, the "real" value of the tax and its ability to reduce cigarette consumption will simply erode over time. Along these lines, it is interesting to note recent research indicating that teenagers who move from high-tax to low-tax states may take up smoking at a later age.[41] This finding is important for policy formulation because it supports the need for interventions targeted at young adults and provides further justification for a comprehensive tobacco control strategy.

Although appreciable numbers of teenagers and young adults manage to quit smoking,[42] until recently researchers have neglected to study the impact of cigarette prices, clean indoor air laws, and other public policy measures on smoking cessation by young people. Rather, the focus of the econometric analyses of prices and regulations on both adult and teenage smoking behavior have tended to assess the impact of alternative public policies (e.g., clean indoor air ordinances) on smoking initiation and on the number of cigarettes smoked by smokers. However, researchers using longitudinal data from Monitoring the Future surveys found that a 10 percent increase in the real price of cigarettes will increase the probability of smoking cessation by, on average, 12 percent for young males and 19 percent for young females.[43]

Summary

In conclusion, the evidence on the degree to which teenagers are responsive to changes in cigarette prices is decidedly mixed. On the one hand, from a theoretical perspective, there are compelling reasons to believe that teenagers will be at least as responsive to price changes as are adults, whose elasticity of demand appears to be in the –0.40 range. A number of studies provide empirical support for this assertion. On the other hand, several published studies indicate that price does not have a statistically significant influence on teenagers' smoking behavior. Perhaps the best interpretation of the collective evidence remains that of the 1993 NCI expert panel: youth are likely to be as responsive to cigarette price increases as are adults and possibly more so.

Because cigarette price increases have been relatively small (i.e., under a dollar and in many cases just a few cents), it is difficult to predict with confidence the impact that a large price change—say, on the order of a dollar or two per pack—would have on teenage cigarette consumption. In principle, however, large tax increases could generate proportionately larger demand responses, as cigarette purchases start to impinge more significantly on teenagers' incomes. In any event, if large-scale price changes materialize, their impact on consumption should be carefully monitored.

Finally, two important caveats should be borne in mind when drawing conclusions about the likely impact of excise tax increases on teenage smoking. The first is that some of the previous studies in this area may have failed to control adequately for the effects of clean indoor air ordinances and teen access laws. From a statistical point of view, this may have led the authors of these studies to overestimate the impact of prices. If states and locales with high cigarette prices are also inclined to pass stringent antismoking laws, and if only a price variable is included in a given statistical model, then the price variable will also pick up the effects of the antismoking laws.[44]

The second caveat is that price increases may not affect all teenage subpopulations equally. A study showed, for example, that young men are much more responsive to cigarette price changes than are young women and that young black men are more responsive than young white men.[45] As a result of these and other findings on the differential impact of prices, the study's authors conclude, "There is clearly not a 'one size fits all' strategy for discouraging young people's smoking." The need to provide different messages for different population groups is one we have already encountered in this book—for example, with media strategies.

Policy Implications

From a policy perspective, the literature on the impact of cigarette price increases on cigarette demand is somewhat difficult to decipher. While it is reasonably clear that adults are responsive to price increases—and that, in fact, there is an emerging consensus among economists on the magnitude of the effect—the impact of higher prices on teenage smoking behavior remains uncertain.

Apart from the conflicting empirical results found in the literature, there are several reasons to believe that prices can be expected to have a relatively minor direct impact on teenagers' cigarette consumption. Given that all states currently prohibit the sale of cigarettes to minors, increasing the price of cigarettes should, in principle, have little or no impact on teenagers, because if laws were rigorously enforced, teenagers would be unable to purchase cigarettes anywhere. Obviously, state and local enforcement efforts are imperfect, and in reality teenagers are often able to buy cigarettes through vending machines, convenience stores, and other outlets as well as to obtain them from family members, friends, and even strangers. Nevertheless, as efforts to enforce teen access laws (including bans on vending machine sales, sales of cigarettes to minors, possession, etc.) increase, the actual price paid for cigarettes will represent a smaller and smaller fraction of the total costs of acquiring and smoking cigarettes. In other words, in areas with strict enforcement, teenagers will have to go to greater and greater lengths to get cigarettes, such as traveling long distances, arranging for older friends and perhaps strangers to purchase cigarettes for them, and stealing from adults.

This reasoning, if correct, has several important implications. To begin with, recent studies of the impact of price increases on teenagers' smoking behavior may have produced misleading results. Specifically, if higher prices are correlated with greater degrees of regulation and enforcement efforts, and if these phenomena are not adequately accounted for, then the demand models will generate biased estimates of the impact of prices on cigarette consumption. From a theoretical point of view, it seems likely that such a strong correlation exists. In areas of the country where antismoking sentiment is high (e.g., California), state legislatures will be inclined to pass a wider range of antismoking measures, including tax increases and clean indoor air laws, relative to areas of the country that are more sympathetic to the tobacco industry's concerns (e.g., North Carolina).

There are a number of reasons why models of teenage cigarette demand have typically failed to account sufficiently for both antismoking regulations faced by teenagers and accompanying enforcement efforts. First, most of the regulations aimed specifically at reducing youth smoking, such as removal of vending machines and restrictions on vendor sales to minors resulting from the Federal Synar Act, have only recently been implemented. The full effects of both state and local regulations are likely to influence smoking behavior over time. Second, as is discussed in chapter 7, a comprehensive database of local anti-smoking ordinances simply does not exist. Finally, more work needs to be done to develop more refined measures of smoking restrictions and the degree to which these measures are enforced. In sum, the failure to account for the impact of regulations means that estimates of the impact of prices on consumption may be overstated.

Interestingly, this argument may not apply to demand models that rely on data that are 20 or more years old. As recently as the mid-1970s, many states still did not prohibit the sale of cigarettes to minors, and enforcement efforts in states and locales that had laws on the books were virtually nonexistent. As a result, the price paid for cigarettes accounted for a large proportion of the total cost of smoking faced by minors.

Another implication of the argument that price may be declining in importance vis-à-vis regulations is that stepping up teen access law enforcement efforts may produce significant benefits, in terms of reduced teenage smoking, as such efforts will drive up the cost of smoking faced by minors. Moreover, even though the direct impact of price increases on teenagers is unclear, they may have a substantial indirect effect. More precisely, as we have seen in our review of adult cigarette demand studies, higher prices appear to reduce consumption to a moderate degree, with a 10 percent increase in price generating a 4 percent reduction in consumption. As a number of studies have found, children and teenagers appear to be influenced by the smoking behavior of their older siblings and parents. Indeed, a study found that by age 18, the smoking rate for teenagers who live in a household with a smoker (either a parent or an older sibling) is twice as high as the rate for teens living in a nonsmoking household.[46] Thus, to the extent that higher excise taxes reduce smoking by an adult or older sibling in a household, these studies suggest that a further positive effect will be to reduce teen smoking. More generally, in light of the strong influence that parental smoking behavior has on teenage smoking patterns, smoking control initiatives that primarily target adults, such as workplace smoking bans and bans on smoking in other public places, will also act to reduce teen smoking rates.

Policymakers should therefore adopt a broad-based smoking control program, not just one that is targeted at teenagers. An increase in the federal cigarette excise tax is an obvious component of a comprehensive tobacco control program. Another important component would be to strengthen tobacco control laws and their enforcement to discourage parents from smoking. A third generic policy intervention would be to encourage physicians and other health care providers to counsel families with adult smokers that they should stop smoking to discourage their children from initiating cigarette consumption.

Along these lines, another finding from the Wasserman et al.[47] study regarding the influence of adult behavior on teen smoking is the increased probability of teen smoking in single-parent homes. To be sure, the societal problems facing single parenthood are not easily susceptible to policy interventions. Nevertheless, other research suggests that providing appropriate after-school activities may reduce teen smoking.[48] Additional research to determine the extent to which such activities may be useful in reducing a range of problem behaviors, including smoking, should be encouraged.

NOTES

1. Chaloupka 1991; Wasserman et al. 1991.
2. DeCicca et al. 1998; Dee and Evans 1998.
3. Warner et al. 1995; see also Gruber and Zinman 2000 for a similar recommendation.
4. Cigarette makers lift wholesale prices 1999.
5. Sumner and Alston 1984; Zhang and Husten 1998.
6. Chaloupka and Warner 2000.
7. Barzel 1976; Johnson 1978.
8. Keeler et al. 1996.
9. Chaloupka 1998.
10. Wasserman 1988.
11. Lewit and Coate 1982.
12. National Cancer Institute 1993.
13. See, e.g., Keeler et al. 1996; Barnett et al. 1995; Harris 1994.
14. Baltagi and Levin 1986.
15. Fujii 1980.
16. Warner 1981.
17. Lewit and Coate 1982.
18. Wasserman et al. 1991.
19. Keeler et al. 1993.
20. This period includes an increase of 25 cents per pack in the state excise tax on cigarettes, which occurred on January 1, 1989.

21. Becker, Grossman, and Murphy 1990.

22. Chaloupka 1990.

23. Mullahy 1985.

24. Some of the material presented in this subsection was taken, with permission, from previous work of Chaloupka and Warner (2000).

25. This can be viewed either in a one-period framework or as a multiple-period dynamic choice. The qualitative impact is similar in each view, but there are important differences in the details of short- and long-run responses (See Mullahy 1985; Becker and Murphy 1988).

26. Bandura 1977.

27. See, e.g., Syme and Alcalay 1982; Hirschman, Leventhal, and Glynn 1984; Conrad, Flay, and Hill 1992; Biglan et al. 1995; Distefan et al. 1998.

28. Lewit, Coate, and Grossman 1981.

29. Much of what we report here was taken, with permission, from previous work of Chaloupka and Warner (2000).

30. Wasserman et al. 1991.

31. Chaloupka 1991.

32. Chaloupka and Wechsler 1997.

33. Townsend 1987; Chaloupka 1991; Townsend, Roderick, and Cooper 1994; Farrelly and Bray 1998.

34. Farrelly and Bray 1998.

35. Lewit et al. 1997; Evans and Huang 1998; Chaloupka 1998.

36. Douglas and Hariharan 1994; Douglas 1998.

37. DeCicca, Kenkel, and Mathios 1998.

38. Dee and Evans 1998.

39. Evans and Farrelly 1998.

40. This idea was first suggested by Harris 1980.

41. Gruber and Zinman 2000.

42. See, e.g., Rowe et al. 1996; Chen and Kandel 1995.

43. Tauras and Chaloupka 1999. The average ages of the males and females included in the sample were 23.01 and 23.25, respectively.

44. Wasserman et al. 1991.

45. Chaloupka and Pacula 1999.

46. Wasserman et al. 1998.

47. Wasserman et al. 1998.

48. Richardson et al. 1989, 1993.

Regulating Youth Smoking Behavior

Various forms of regulation offer potentially important mechanisms for reducing adolescent smoking. Regulation can restrict youth access to tobacco products, determine product content, restrict advertising, raise the price of tobacco products through taxes, and penalize adolescent use of tobacco products. Regulatory activity can have both direct and indirect effects. Such actions can directly restrict adolescent opportunities to use tobacco and indirectly affect behavior by raising the cost of obtaining tobacco products, as discussed in chapter 6.

Just as important, regulation sends a set of signals from the community to adolescents about what conduct is acceptable. By restricting where adolescents can purchase tobacco products and by restricting the time and place where people can smoke in public, the community sends a signal that smoking is to be discouraged. As we discussed in chapter 1, legislators are more responsive to laws regulating youth access to tobacco products than they are to regulating adult access. Since sales of tobacco products are prohibited to minors in all states, laws designed to restrict youth access are less controversial than laws regulating clean indoor air. Nonetheless, there is considerable opposition among libertarians and business groups to stringent youth access restrictions.[1]

Serious attempts to regulate youth access date from the late 1980s. At this point, it is not clear how effective these laws are in reducing adolescent smoking prevalence. We know that aggressively enforced youth access restrictions can substantially reduce illegal sales to minors, but we do not yet know whether and how that translates into reduced adolescent tobacco consumption. There are reasons to believe that, short of dramatic reductions in youth sales, substantial declines in youth smoking as a result of stopping illegal sales to minors may not be feasible.[2]

Advertising restrictions and taxes, arguably the two most important regulatory strategies, have been covered in chapters 5 and 6. In this

chapter, we discuss other restrictions on youth access to tobacco products and examine the literature on their effectiveness. We start with an
analysis of trends in state and local laws restricting youth access to
tobacco products and then examine how effective these laws have been.
Next, we discuss various proposals for regulating tobacco products
and how such regulations might influence adolescent tobacco use.
Then we consider some innovations in regulatory policy.

Youth Access Restrictions

In the past decade, the issue of regulating youth access to tobacco products has received considerable policy attention. Prior to this time, most
intervention activities regarding adolescent tobacco use were focused
on discouraging individual adolescents from smoking. Starting in the
late 1980s, when the evidence that adolescents have easy access to
tobacco products was mounting, concern and action proliferated
regarding broader environmental factors affecting the ability of youths
to purchase or otherwise obtain cigarettes. In response, many policies
have been implemented at the local, state, and federal levels regarding
the distribution and sale of tobacco products.[3] These policies include
regulation of sellers, regulation of buyers, restrictions on the distribution of free products or samples (including coupons), and regulation of
the means of tobacco sale (where and how it can be sold). The latter policy includes state and local efforts to restrict or totally ban vending
machine sales of tobacco.

At the present time, all states prohibit the sale and distribution of
tobacco products to minors through a variety of youth access laws, or
policies that involve age restrictions for selling tobacco. All 50 states
and the District of Columbia prohibit the sale of tobacco products to
people under the age of 18. In contrast, laws banning adolescent purchase or possession of cigarettes vary by jurisdiction. Some tobacco
control advocates have argued that purchase and possession laws are
more difficult to enforce than restrictions on the seller and are part of an
effort to shift responsibility for tobacco sales from retailers to minors.[3]

Trends in State and Local Tobacco Control Laws
Affecting Adolescents

In this section, we describe trends in state and local laws and ordinances specifically aimed at adolescent tobacco use. Most of these laws

attempt to restrict youth access to tobacco products. Our source for the state law information is the Centers for Disease Control and Prevention's State Tobacco Activities Tracking and Evaluation (STATE) system.[4] Our information about local ordinances restricting youth access comes from a data set compiled by the Americans for Nonsmokers' Rights Foundation (ANRF).

Youth access restrictions are one class of policies aimed at reducing smoking initiation by children and adolescents. Such restrictions include a ban on single-cigarette sales or the provision of tobacco samples, as well as bans on youth purchase, possession, or use of tobacco products. Restrictions on purchases from vending machines and self-service displays are also intended to restrict youth access by forestalling opportunities for illegal purchases and shoplifting by underage smokers.

In what follows, we first describe state policies regarding youth access restrictions. State legislation can alter the policy environment in a state, in part by limiting policy options at the local level. Second, we analyze a useful—albeit limited—data set that illuminates important trends in youth access policies at the local level. Later in the chapter, we discuss the effects of clean indoor air ordinances.

State Laws

Most tobacco control laws and ordinances are enacted at the state and local levels. There is some interplay and conflict between the two. One of the most important developments has been enactment of preemption legislation in many states that limits local regulation of tobacco use. State preemption usually prohibits a locality from either acting at all or enacting an ordinance that is stronger than the state law.

The number of preemption laws increased during the 1980s and rapidly increased during the mid-1990s. Twenty-one states have enacted preemption laws addressing at least one youth access issue (sales to minors, vending machines, or distribution), with 10 preempting all aspects of youth access. Of these preemption measures, 76 percent were enacted between 1993 and 1996. Since 1996, no state has enacted a law preempting stronger local ordinances.[5] Laws in fourteen states now preempt local regulation of tobacco displays, promotion of tobacco products, and sampling of tobacco products.

Increased state preemption may be a perverse result of the 1992 federal Synar Amendment, which required states to enforce existing laws that restrict sales to minors. As part of the political bargaining to secure state compliance with Synar requirements, tobacco industry lobbyists convinced many legislatures to include language preempting stronger local ordinances. Most state preemption laws were passed after adolescent prevalence trends had reversed from declines or stable smoking figures in the 1980s to significant increases in the early 1990s. While there may be no direct connection, it may be that the tobacco industry determined that local ordinances were having an effect on smoking rates and hence pushed aggressively to block them through preemption.

Aside from preemption laws, state governments pursue many policies to regulate youth smoking. In all likelihood, the extensiveness of a state's tobacco control policies will affect youth tobacco use.[6] As of December 31, 1998, all 50 states except Arizona and Kansas had enacted laws prohibiting sales of all tobacco products to minors.[7] Thirty-four states (of 35 requiring licenses for sale of tobacco products) had enacted laws with provisions for licensure suspension or revocation for tobacco sales to minors. All states plus Washington, D.C., had laws carrying some penalty for a first violation of laws prohibiting the sale of tobacco to minors. By December 31, 1998, 42 states had enacted laws prohibiting the purchase, possession, and/or use of tobacco products by minors, thus penalizing adolescent smokers. Forty-one states and Washington, D.C., had also passed vending machine access restrictions (either limited placements, locking devices, supervision, or bans in areas accessible to youths) by 1998, but only 34 of those states had articulated penalties to businesses for violations of the law.[8]

Local Ordinances

Many tobacco control advocates favor local ordinances over state laws. This preference reflects a strategic calculation that the tobacco industry is politically effective at the state level but may be less able to block strong local ordinances.[9] As we have noted, however, the tobacco industry has been effective in limiting the power of local ordinances through state preemption laws. Given the sheer number and variety of regulatory efforts, it is difficult to generalize reliably about local policies. Perhaps due to these difficulties, the existing scholarly literature is especially sparse in describing patterns of such regulations or their impact on youth.

To provide some context to the policy debate, we analyze a new and useful data set regarding local ordinances that is maintained by ANRF. At our request, ANRF provided data from local ordinances pertaining only to adolescent tobacco use. We obtained two ANRF data sets, from June 1998 and June 1999, to explore local policies during recent years. These data included detailed information on local policies dating back to the 1970s. Because most youth access laws and regulations were enacted during the 1990s, we confined our attention to local ordinances passed over the past decade. (For purposes of presentation, the small number of ordinances passed in the decades prior to 1990 were combined in a "pre-90" category.) To examine geographic variation in local policy and to facilitate comparison with other data sources, we divided the ANRF data into the four major census regions of the United States.[10]

This data set has some limitations. Most important, it relies on self-reporting from local jurisdictions and therefore is likely to understate the number, variety, and extent of local antismoking ordinances. Also, ANRF has necessarily altered some aspects of the data set over time to improve data quality and usability, complicating efforts to construct reliable measures of important regulatory trends.[11] Despite these limitations, ANRF data are the best available to document the great regional variation in tobacco regulation. These data also illuminate some important trends in local regulation of youth tobacco use.

ANRF collects data regarding local ordinances regulating vending machines, tobacco sampling, self-service displays, single-cigarette sales, licensing, and restrictions on the use or purchase of tobacco products. ANRF also explores ordinances containing provisions either totally or partially limiting access to vending machines, such as supervision, locking devices or tokens, and exemptions for adult-only areas. The data on tobacco sampling restrictions include bans on the distribution of tobacco samples to anyone, regardless of age. Since the distribution of tobacco samples to minors is already prohibited in all 50 states, separate local ordinances restricting tobacco sampling to minors only were not included in the data set.

The data set contains ordinances passed to restrict self-service displays. This means that all tobacco products must be kept behind or above the counter, so that they are not accessible to the general public. Ordinances passed that only limit the distance that tobacco may be displayed from the store clerk are not included in the data set. Ordinances that require tobacco retailers to obtain licenses and that contain provisions for the suspension or revocation of the license for failure to comply are included. The data presented here do not include licensure ordinances that only provide fines, not suspension/revocation. This omission will understate the actual level of activity regarding illegal sales to minors.

The data set contains information on ordinances banning the sale of single or multiple cigarettes from a pack, originally sealed by the manufacturer. Ordinances that ban possession or use of tobacco products by minors are included in the data set but have only been included since June 1998.[12]

Figures 8 through 13, at the end of the chapter, indicate the most important patterns in the ANRF data. Perhaps the most important feature of the available data is the stark difference across both regions and states in regulatory activity. In every category examined, localities in the southern states passed substantially fewer regulations than were observed in other census regions. Most prominently, 20 southern localities enacted some restrictions on vending machine sales. In contrast, 171 northeastern localities, 157 north-central localities, and 187 localities in western states enacted similar measures.

States also differ sharply in their regulatory action. Certain states appear to pursue more aggressively youth access restrictions at the local level while others do not, with little consistency between adjacent states. Of the localities passing ordinances in the western region, 75 percent were in California. New Jersey and Massachusetts were equally dominant in the northeastern region, with approximately 80 percent of the localities in those two states. Within the north-central region, licensure was widely enacted, with legislative measures spread over several states in roughly equal number.[13] Yet in the northeast, 75 percent of the licensure ordinances were enacted by Massachusetts localities.

Figure 14, also at the end of the chapter, displays the number of localities in each state that passed youth smoking ordinances captured within the ANRF data. For presentation purposes, only the top 12 states are shown. The top 5 states—California, New Jersey, Massachusetts, Minnesota, and Illinois—account for 80 percent of all known regulations in the ANRF database.

Local regulation appears to have peaked during the mid-1990s. Although different types of regulations were passed in different regions at different times, 1994 and 1995 were the years of most intense regulatory activity at the local level. The small number of enacted regulations during the late 1990s is especially puzzling given escalating public attention to tobacco issues.

States and regions also appear to differ in the type of regulation enacted by local governments. A commonly enacted ordinance is to require tobacco product sellers to be licensed. Together, Illinois and

Massachusetts localities enacted 114 such measures (37 and 77, respectively), whereas only one southern locality did so. Perhaps more surprising, only one California locality (and only 11 other localities in western states) enacted similar measures.

The next most frequently passed type of ordinance is to ban self-service displays. An overwhelming majority of the localities that passed self-service display restrictions were in Massachusetts, New Jersey, and California (with 64, 55, and 55 restrictions, respectively).

Tobacco activist states also differ in their approaches to solving the problem of youth access to tobacco. Northeastern localities appear to focus on youths' ability to buy or to steal tobacco without the knowledge or the approval of tobacco sellers. These localities were the most likely to limit use of self-service displays, vending machines, and free samples. Compared with other regulatory strategies, such access restrictions require limited oversight of the tobacco marketplace and require limited monitoring resources to ensure seller compliance with legal norms. In contrast, Illinois and Minnesota have chosen relatively more intense monitoring and law enforcement approaches. Illinois and Minnesota localities enacted 47 and 20 youth possession/use ordinances, respectively—the majority of all such ordinances enacted across the country as captured by the ARNF data.[14] These states were also leaders in requiring merchants to purchase licenses before they can sell tobacco products and in threatening suspension and/or revocation of that license.

Youth Access Laws and Tobacco Sales

The Synar Amendment

One objective in the Public Health Services' Healthy People 2010 Objectives is to increase to 100 percent the number of states with retail licensure systems that include license suspension or revocation for violations of state laws restricting tobacco sales to minors (youth access restrictions).[15] The primary vehicle to obtain that objective is the Synar Amendment, described in chapter 1, which requires states to enact and enforce laws restricting the sale and distribution of tobacco products to minors or risk losing substance abuse block grant funding. The Synar Amendment has led to a number of developments in state-level youth tobacco control activities, including passage of legislation on minimum age for purchase, increased enforcement efforts, and the increased use of undercover, or "sting," operations.[16] But the Synar Amendment may

be fueling the growth in laws penalizing youth purchasing or possession of tobacco products. When states moved to enact laws to implement Synar, the tobacco industry was often successful in attaching provisions to preempt stronger local action or to penalize youth tobacco
possession and use.

So far, Synar has not been a very effective mechanism, as the early
evidence suggests that compliance has been disappointing. Even with
the leverage from the Synar Amendment, few jurisdictions seriously
enforce laws regarding the sale of tobacco to minors.[17] In what amounts
to a devastating indictment of governmental failure to enforce the
Synar Amendment, one study recently analyzed 1997 substance abuse
block grant applications from 59 states and territories.[18] Of these, 19
applicants failed to meet statutory requirements but were not sanc-
tioned, 15 failed to conduct any enforcement inspections, and 18 found
no violations at all. While data from subsequent years may show some
improvement, only a few states are aggressively enforcing youth access
restrictions. The U.S. Department of Health and Human Services has
demonstrated no inclination to sanction states for failing to comply
with the Synar Amendment.[19] As we discuss shortly, this presents a
potentially significant problem for the FDA's strategy of relying on
states to enforce FDA regulations. An important aspect is that even
those states enforcing Synar vigorously (e.g., Florida) are unable to
determine the effect on adolescent tobacco consumption rates.[20]

Enforcement
What seems to make a difference regarding illegal tobacco sales to
minors is whether or not the laws are enforced. Aggressive and ongoing enforcement is the key to reducing illegal sales to minors. Numerous sting operation studies show that absent enforcement, illegal
tobacco sales to minors are common, with older minors more able to
purchase cigarettes than younger minors.[21] Local licensure and license
removal for vendors who sell tobacco products to minors, combined
with ongoing enforcement efforts, could influence vendors' willingness
to sell cigarettes to minors.

A study of what is likely the gold standard of enforcement, in
Woodridge, Illinois, produced very encouraging results: illegal merchant sales to minors fell from 70 percent to 5 percent over one and a
half years of compliance checks following implementation of a youth
access ordinance; experimentation with and regular use of cigarettes by

adolescents fell by more than 50 percent.[22] In another study, enforcement contributed to retail outlets reducing their cigarette sales to minors significantly (compliance with the law in three intervention communities rose to 82 percent, compared to 45 percent in three control communities), but analysts found no evidence of a decline in smoking by youth.[23] In this study, three communities in an intervention group enforced tobacco sales laws, while three matched communities in the control group did not. The findings suggested that increased enforcement enhanced vendors' compliance with Massachusetts' tobacco sales laws, thus reducing illegal sales to minors.

Subsequent studies found that the passage and sustained enforcement of legislation have proven to be an effective means of reducing illegal sales to minors.[24] For example, researchers have found that frequent enforcement schedules (every two months) could result in a four-fold reduction of illegal sales to minors. Two-month enforcement intervals were more effective at reducing illegal sales than were either 4- or 6-month intervals, which were more effective than no enforcement. Similarly, a randomized trial of an intervention to reduce tobacco sales to minors in some California communities found that "tobacco sales to minors can be reduced through a broad-based intervention."[25] In another study, illegal sales rates dropped from 75 percent prior to the intervention to zero after the intervention.[26]

An evaluation of the impact of an intervention to increase compliance with tobacco purchasing laws monitored 319 outlets in six community pairs, where one of the communities in the pair was randomly assigned to an active enforcement program.[27] The results showed a dramatic increase in compliance with the law in both the intervention and control communities. The authors stated that their finding of no intervention effect, which contradicts the studies just described, may be explained by "contamination" from publicity about the enforcement intervention and hence almost universal awareness of the project sting operations among retailers in both the intervention and the control communities.

In response to public pressure, the tobacco industry has embarked on a highly publicized and controversial campaign to encourage merchant compliance with youth access restrictions and to reduce teen smoking behavior. This campaign has been strongly opposed by tobacco control advocates, who argue that it is just an attempt to put a kinder, gentler face on pernicious attempts to obscure the industry's continued attempts to market their products to adolescents. Advocates have thus publicly opposed state or local group willingness to cooperate with the industry's efforts.

The effects of the Tobacco Institute's "It's the Law" campaign—which was a public relations effort purportedly designed to eliminate the sale of tobacco products to minors—appear to have been minimal. A survey of tobacco retailers revealed that less than 5 percent of retail respondents were participating in the program and that there was no significant difference between participating and nonparticipating retailers in terms of their willingness to sell cigarettes to minors (86 percent vs. 88 percent).[28] Another study found that vendors participating in the "It's the Law" program were just as likely to make sales to minors as were nonparticipating vendors.[29]

The Effectiveness of Youth Access Restrictions

Even if the enforcement of youth access laws reduces illegal sales to minors, the evidence that this actually translates into reduced tobacco consumption is limited. Most early studies only looked at whether restrictions on sales to minors reduced the rate of such illegal sales; they failed to examine the impact of enforcement interventions on smoking behavior. In studies that have looked at both sales and behavior, the two did not always go hand in hand. For example, an important study found that reduced sales to minors were not accompanied by changes in adolescents' perceptions of their access to cigarettes or in their smoking behavior.[30] Similarly, other researchers have concluded that, while interventions to reduce tobacco sales to minors can be effective, multiple supply- and demand-focused strategies are needed actually to reduce tobacco use.[31] And some studies reported either insignificant changes in adolescents' perceptions of the ease of purchasing tobacco products[32] or insignificant differences in tobacco purchase success.[33] A recent study that confirmed these results still found that adopting local youth access laws reduced the propensity of 12–15 year olds to progress to more routine smoking over a four-year period as compared to jurisdictions without such laws.[34] Even though access to cigarettes was not reduced, the authors speculate that the laws served to change community norms and standards regarding smoking initiation.

In contrast, an observational study of the impact of antismoking legislation in one suburban community that mounted the nation's most aggressive youth access program found that both merchant sales and adolescent smoking behavior were reduced after the law was passed.[35] Data from student surveys suggested that both experimentation and habitual use of cigarettes decreased by over 50 percent between the pretest and posttest observations. Further inquiry suggested that a reduction in use was still apparent after seven years, largely because of rigorous and ongoing enforcement activities.[36] Similar results were observed in a follow-up study to an experiment with differential enforcement arrangements. There were significantly fewer smokers in communities with regular enforcement under licensure laws than in communities that did not regularly enforce the laws.[37]

The Effectiveness of Youth Access Restrictions Combined with Other Interventions

Some researchers have evaluated the impact of youth access strategies when combined with other interventions. For example, one study investigated the effects of a community education and law enforcement intervention in a two-year controlled trial.[38] The primary conclusion was that an educational intervention alone (directed at merchants, law enforcement agencies, and the community at large) had a limited effect on reducing illegal sales to minors but that education plus enforcement significantly reduced illegal over-the-counter sales. Another study assessed the impact of an intervention involving community mobilization, merchant education, changing consequences for clerks, publicity about clerks refusing to sell, and feedback to store owners and managers about sales to youth in rural Oregon.[39] The analyses suggested that the intervention led to a significant (62 percent) reduction in sales in the intervention communities.

Similar results were observed in a randomized community trial in 14 Minnesota communities. The goal of the intervention was to make youth access a community-wide issue. Intervention communities organized to enact local ordinances, change retail merchants' behavior, and promote enforcement to halt illegal sales to minors. Although youth smoking rose in both intervention and control communities, the rate of increase was much smaller in intervention communities. The authors concluded, "this study provides evidence that a community mobilization intervention resulting in policy adoption and enforcement to reduce youth access to tobacco can affect adolescent smoking rates," yet they also were careful to note that the results reflect only short-term effects.[40]

We add a note of caution: In the 14 communities in the intervention trial, youth who reported ever smoking were very likely to cite social sources for cigarettes, although older youth and those reporting weekly smoking also reported purchasing their own tobacco.[41] Despite a reduction in purchase attempts, adolescents' perceptions of availability of cigarettes from friends or family members showed increases in intervention communities.[42]

A recent longitudinal study supporting the more positive results found that "12–15-year old Massachusetts youths living in towns that had a local tobacco sales ordinance in 1993 were significantly less likely to become established smokers over the next 4 years than were youths living in towns without an ordinance."[43] Of equal interest, the adoption of local ordinances prohibiting sales to minors reduced the progression to routine smoking among the adolescents surveyed. Because of a small survey sample size, it is not possible to draw broad conclusions from this study. In conjunction with other recent research, however, it indicates that youth access restrictions may help change adolescent attitudes and general social norms. As the authors also note, the attendant media attention to enacting such an ordinance may mobilize and educate the entire community.

Taken together, these studies show why a comprehensive tobacco control strategy is needed. Both a perception of the threat of enforcement[44] and education about the laws and fines associated with selling to minors[45] may reduce the number of stores willing to sell to minors. By contrast, earlier research demonstrated that merchant education regarding youth tobacco access laws failed to produce sustained refusal to sell cigarettes to minors.[37]

Limitations to Youth Access Restrictions

The preceding discussion points to a limitation of youth access laws. Aside from commercial sources, they do not restrict access to cigarettes from other sources, such as friends, siblings, and parents. If the only or primary way in which youth gained access to cigarettes were through illegal sales, we might expect the enforcement of youth access laws to have a powerful effect on smoking behavior. However, youth cite a number of "social sources" (e.g., family, friends, or even strangers), as well as stealing cigarettes, as substitutes for commercial tobacco purchases.[46]

If stringent enforcement encourages adolescents to procure cigarettes from social sources, a side effect of these laws may be the strengthening of smoking bonds, the inflating of perceptions of smoking prevalence, and a bolstering of the social normalcy of smoking. Still, strict compliance by merchants would make it harder for teens to obtain cigarettes. As a result, adolescents might be less likely to smoke at all, to offer cigarettes to others, and to be exposed to smoking by others.

Another limitation of youth access laws is that high rates of merchant compliance with restrictions on cigarette sales to minors are needed before such laws will reduce adolescent cigarette use.[47] Several studies have shown that just reducing illegal sales is problematic. If, for example, only one out of four stores will sell tobacco to minors, adolescents can direct their purchases to that one store. Young people will learn where cigarettes can be purchased.[48] More important, the studies evaluating compliance with laws prohibiting tobacco sales to minors suggest that programs lacking in repeated compliance monitoring and substantial penalties for illegal sales will have only short-term effects. To be effective, a compliance program must encompass repeated monitoring, merchant education, community involvement, and fines. Unless retail compliance with illegal sales laws is substantial, perhaps as high as 90 percent,[49] the effects of these laws will be limited.[50] States and localities must be prepared to make considerable investments for enforcement to be successful.

Developing an effective compliance program faces political and resource barriers that require community support to overcome. Without such support, youth access restrictions will not achieve their desired effectiveness. Well-implemented and enforced laws may have the ability to contribute to reduced adolescent tobacco use, even though such effects have not yet been clearly demonstrated. Thus, ordinances limiting youth access to tobacco may reduce smoking prevalence and change perceptions about the availability of cigarettes.[51] At a minimum, these laws also express important social norms, which may indirectly discourage adolescent use.[52]

Several additional studies are now under way to assess the effectiveness of youth access restrictions, but the results are not yet available. Even if these studies are unable to determine that youth access restrictions actually reduce youth cigarette consumption or to replicate previous successes,[53] this does not mean that such strategies should be abandoned. Public policy should not facilitate youth access to tobacco products. Reducing illegal sales to minors will, at a minimum, make it more difficult for teens to obtain tobacco products.[54]

Clean Indoor Air Laws: Indirect Effects

Policy efforts to restrict smoking in public places proliferated during the late 1980s and early 1990s.[55] Such efforts have included state and local restrictions on smoking in public facilities, outdoor spaces, work sites, hospitals, restaurants and bars, and hotels and motels, as well as on airline flights.[56] While the intent of most of these efforts is to reduce exposure to environmental tobacco smoke, it is also believed that such restrictions can have a positive impact on current smokers by reducing daily cigarette consumption or by promoting total cessation.[57] Restrictions on smoking in public places are designed to create an environment where nonsmoking is the cultural norm. An equally important indirect effect on adolescent tobacco use would be the extent to which these laws encourage parents to quit smoking, given the importance of parental tobacco use as a factor in adolescent use.

The published research regarding the effects of policies directly restricting public smoking on adolescents is limited. Some econometric studies of teenage and young adult smoking behavior found evidence that clean indoor air laws may reduce teenage cigarette consumption. For example, restricting smoking in public places can be an effective smoking control measure for both teenagers and adults, with reductions in cigarettes consumed of up to 6 percent for adults and 40 percent for teenagers.[58] Restricting smoking in schools, in particular, reduces the average number of cigarettes smoked by young smokers.[59] For young adults, laws restricting smoking in restaurants and schools significantly lowered college students' smoking prevalence rates.[60] Policies restricting smoking in private workplaces have had a positive impact on the probability that young female workers will quit smoking, but there is no indication that such policies lead males toward smoking cessation.[61]

Although no one knows for certain precisely why clean indoor air laws, especially those covering the workplace, may be effective in reducing teenage smoking, one can speculate that they simply reduce the opportunities available for youths to smoke. Alternatively, or perhaps in conjunction with these reduced opportunities, at a social psychological level, clean indoor air laws may be a useful vehicle for sending a message to teenagers that smoking is socially unacceptable.

Summary

It is undeniable that the current state of regulatory, judicial, and legislative pressure on the tobacco industry and tobacco retailers represents an unprecedented and concentrated regulatory assault on youth access to tobacco products. As one study noted, although "it seems reasonable to assume that reducing the number of retailers that sell tobacco to minors illegally will reduce minors' access to tobacco, which will in turn reduce youth smoking rates, it is surprising how little evidence is available to support those assumptions."[3] More evidence, in the form of controlled trials of interventions, is needed to support the intense growth of activity in the area of youth access restrictions. Furthermore, it is clear that in the face of increased enforcement of youth access laws, tobacco remains an alluring and addictive substance of great appeal to youth. What can be said with the evidence at hand is that youth access interventions can lead to a general reduction in illegal sales of cigarettes to minors. Whether this will translate into actual and sustained reductions in youth tobacco use remains to be seen.

Product Regulation

One of the most interesting and challenging contemporary concerns in the field of tobacco control relates to the issue of product regulation. In 1996, the FDA claimed jurisdiction to regulate cigarettes and smokeless tobacco products, with the intent of protecting children.[62] Following a lengthy investigation, the agency concluded that nicotine is a drug and that cigarettes and smokeless tobacco products are drug delivery systems. Motivated by the fact that the vast majority of smokers begin smoking prior to adulthood (former FDA commissioner David Kessler called smoking "a pediatric disease"), the agency targeted its regulatory efforts at reducing children's access to tobacco products and the industry's ability to promote smoking among children.

As we noted in chapter 1, on June 20, 1997, representatives of the state attorneys general and lawyers for the tobacco industry, embroiled in a number of tobacco-related lawsuits, announced a proposed "global settlement" that included a number of public health measures. Prominent among these was granting FDA regulatory authority over tobacco products. Although the proposal had a number of important strings attached, it explicitly accorded FDA the authority gradually to require the removal of nicotine from tobacco products, a concept that had been suggested three years earlier by two prominent nicotine addiction researchers.[63]

Because it included a number of policy measures and legal protections for the tobacco industry, implementation of the "global settlement" required congressional legislation embodying many of its provisions. Congress struggled with the issue, with the Senate eventually producing a bill with more substantial public health provisions than those written into the settlement proposal. The legislation died on the floor, however, and the FDA's claim of regulatory authority (discussed shortly) was taken to the federal courts by the tobacco industry. The tobacco industry challenged these regulations as being beyond the FDA's scope of authority. In *FDA v Brown & Williamson Tobacco Corp.* (529 US [2000]), the U.S. Supreme Court agreed with the industry and ruled that the FDA could not promulgate most of the regulations.

Throughout this period, and quite independent of the political machinations, tobacco control scholars have been debating what form, if any, nicotine product regulation ought to take.[64] At present, all nicotine-containing pharmaceuticals must go through the conventional FDA regulatory review and approval procedures, a process that typically takes years and costs millions of dollars. In contrast, cigarette manufacturers introduce novel nicotine delivery systems, designed to look like cigarettes,[65] with no governmental regulatory review of any kind. One result is a very unbalanced regulatory playing field, in which the safest nicotine-bearing products ever developed—the nicotine pharmaceuticals—must meet high and expensive regulatory standards, while the most dangerous nicotine-bearing products ever marketed—cigarettes and related products—are introduced by the cigarette companies at no regulatory cost or effort.

With scores of patents outstanding on innovative nicotine delivery devices, many held by the tobacco companies, it has become clear to many tobacco control professionals that rational and rationalized regulation of all nicotine-containing products is necessary. Precisely what form that regulation will take is not known. The complexities in answering this question are truly profound.[66] A committee of the Institute of Medicine of the National Academy of Sciences has been examining the scientific basis for evaluating the safety and efficacy of novel nicotine delivery products. And medical and scientific bodies in other countries, as well as the United States, are addressing similar questions as well.[67]

The principal issue relating to product regulation is how to ensure that the health risks associated with smoking cigarettes are effectively reduced. Although not the focal point of attention, a clear concern is to design regulation in such a manner that children will not be enticed into using either tobacco products or their less harmful (but still risky) substitutes. One fear associated with introducing ostensibly less haz-ardous nicotine-bearing products is that children will experiment with them, with a subset finding themselves addicted and conceivably even-tually "graduating" to the more dangerous forms of nicotine delivery, including smoking cigarettes. For children who would have experi-mented with and become addicted to cigarettes anyway, no additional disease exposure would be experienced. However, if ostensibly less hazardous products attract kids who eschew tobacco per se, a net addi-tion to health risk could be experienced.

The development and regulatory review of nicotine replacement pharmaceuticals demonstrates attention to this concern. The original version of nicotine gum, for example, was designed to taste bad, in part so that children would not find it a viable alternative to regular gum. All nicotine replacement products are evaluated with regard to their potential to addict. Still, as more products come onto the market and as pharmaceutical company products are positioned to compete more directly and aggressively with tobacco products, the risk of appealing to children cannot be discounted. Thus, while product regulation may hold the key to reducing harms to addicted adult smokers, as some sci-entists believe, it may also wave a red flag before the eyes of those con-cerned with saving youth from addiction and disease.

FDA Restrictions

In 1997, the FDA implemented a number of regulations regarding youth access to tobacco. These regulations made it a violation of federal law to sell tobacco products to anyone under the age of 18 and to fail to request an identification card for anyone appearing to be under 27. In addition, the regulations established a minimum cigarette pack size of 20 cigarettes, banned free samples of cigarettes and smokeless tobacco, prohibited cigarette sales through vending machines (with some excep-tions), and banned self-service displays of tobacco products. As we noted earlier, the regulations were struck down by the U.S. Supreme Court. FDA's tobacco regulatory apparatus has been dismantled and can only be revived if Congress grants explicit regulatory authority.

To implement the regulations, the FDA signed agreements with states to delegate enforcement responsibility to the states. Without FDA support, financial and enforcement responsibility rests exclu-sively with the states. But the record so far indicates that few states actively and aggressively enforce their own laws, and states' compliance with the Synar Amendment, as we noted earlier, has been minimal.

To a certain extent, the Master Settlement Agreement (MSA) settling the litigation between the tobacco industry and the state attorneys general over reimbursement for Medicaid costs of treating tobacco-produced diseases imposes restrictions that the FDA (or other federal regulatory agencies) would have otherwise considered. For instance, the MSA imposes restrictions on tobacco marketing and advertising to youths. Because the MSA does not address the FDA's authority to take other steps to regulate tobacco products, further FDA regulatory action is needed to reduce the associated harms from the product itself.

Regulatory Innovations

As with the prevention strategies discussed in chapter 3, there are several ongoing experiments with different regulatory approaches. Although these strategies have not yet been evaluated, and although several are highly contentious among tobacco control advocates, they represent developments that state policymakers should watch closely.

Penalties for Possession and Use

A controversial initiative that has emerged recently is the increasing willingness of policymakers to fine underage youth for using tobacco products. Until recently, policymakers focused on penalizing the vendor for an illegal sale to minors, as opposed to penalizing the user.[68] Under pressure from retail merchants' associations, and perhaps out of frustration that "supply-side" policies have not adequately discouraged youth tobacco consumption, policymakers have begun to enact laws that fine minors for smoking in public or possessing tobacco products. Tobacco control advocates have vociferously protested this approach as an attempt to shift attention away from vendors who sell tobacco products to minors. Regardless, this shift appears to be gaining momentum, as more jurisdictions have been enacting such laws. At this point, however, we have no information on whether user fines will be effective in discouraging youth from smoking.

Minors caught smoking or in possession of cigarettes can face a variety of penalties, ranging from a ticket or fine to an appearance in smoking courts, suspension from school, denial of a driver's license, or any combination of these. Fines differ widely in severity—some starting as low as $25—and increase with repeat violations. Fines can also be combined with tobacco education or cessation classes. In Naperville, Illinois, a suburb of Chicago, adolescents caught smoking may choose between a $100 fine or a one-week tobacco education program. In Clayton, Missouri, a suburb of St. Louis, minors are fined and required to attend smoking education classes run by the county.

Some areas allow for the removal or denial of the offender's driver's license. For example, minors in Florida may lose their license or be legally prohibited from attaining one if found in violation of the state's 1997 possession law. Driver's license suspension or denial appears to be reserved for repeat offenders; licenses are usually reinstated within a period of three to six months.

According to the National Youth Court Center, there are more than 620 peer courts nationally, with 41 in Oregon alone. In Oregon, the punishment for underage tobacco use is determined by other teenagers. An attorney acts as the judge, but teen volunteers defend and prosecute teens between the ages of 12 and 17 for minor offenses, including smoking.[69] As yet, there is no systematic evaluation of whether the teen courts are effective in reducing underage tobacco use. An important aspect of such an evaluation would be to determine whether teens respond more favorably to decisions by their peers than to punishments decided by adults.

The phenomenon of teen smoking courts merits close watching. Florida, Indiana, Utah, and various counties in other states are experimenting with such smoking courts, where teens must appear with their parents. The experience is more like participating in a prevention program than attending a traditional court. For example, in Plantain, Florida, a trip to the teen smoking court includes a lecture by a throat cancer survivor, an antismoking video, and an appearance in front of the judge. Violators under age 16 see an additional video, while older teens attend a four-hour class at the local chapter of the American Lung Association. Florida also offers eight hours of community service as a substitute for paying fines and court costs, totaling $53.[70] The smoking court in Linn County, Oregon, "tries" first time offenders using teen prosecutors and teen juries in an attempt to stop tobacco use before the transition to routine or addicted smoker status.

Two impediments could limit the effectiveness of laws penalizing adolescent tobacco use. First, enforcement may raise the unwanted specter of the dreaded "smoking police." Sting operations are costly and time-consuming, and police are hesitant to become "smoking cops,"[71] arguing that they have more pressing duties. Enforcing laws penalizing underage tobacco use is likely to be a particular problem. Nevertheless, in Naples, Florida, police go undercover to enforce the law and reported that in a little over two months in 1998, they had issued 157 $25 fines. In Wichita, police are used in schools to enforce the law. Indeed, the fines can be used to fund the enforcement program, including further sting operations against merchants selling tobacco products to underage youth.

Second, there is a potential backlash from youth who are fined or forced to attend tobacco court or antitobacco programs. Reports in the media suggest that these youth will defiantly smoke as a result of the fine. We do not suggest that these experiments should not continue, but these potential concerns should be monitored.

Vendor Penalties

There do not appear to be any significant innovations regarding actions against retail vendors who sell tobacco products to minors, but there are some nascent trends to watch. One trend is local licensure of tobacco vendors and increasing penalties for illegal sales to minors. Fines in Utah start at $250 and go up to $10,000. Despite the potential financial penalty for noncompliance, the volume of violations in that state was so great that a tobacco court was instituted in 1998. Local licensure is important because municipalities are more likely to monitor compliance and threaten licensure removal than are state agencies.[59]

Restrictions on Self-Service Displays

One means of restricting youth access to tobacco products is to remove these products from areas where youth can go. For example, restrictions on vending machines have been effective in eliminating them as a source of cigarettes for minors. An emerging trend is to restrict self-service displays of cigarettes. Vendors oppose such restrictions because self-service displays enhance sales. (Not coincidentally, tobacco companies pay large "slotting fees" to vendors as an incentive to display their brands.) Stores in Yolo County and Coeur d'Alene, Idaho, are required to remove cigarette displays to locked cabinets behind the counters; this not only limits the amount of stolen cigarettes but may reduce the number of underage attempts to buy cigarettes. In Mesa, Arizona, teen activists were successful in getting the city council to ban self-displays from area stores.

Restrictions on Billboard Advertising

The fight to limit billboard advertising by the tobacco industry reached its high point with the tobacco settlement agreement (MSA), which stipulated a ban on all outdoor advertisements by April 23, 1999, and also banned tobacco advertising on transit systems. Even before the settlement, several communities had banned or restricted the use of billboard advertising. Most restrictions concerned the area in which the ads were located. "Youth zones" were designated as areas where there are schools, parks, religious sites, libraries, and residential neighborhoods, and cigarette ads could not appear within 1,000 feet or more of these areas. Billboard ad content was restricted to black-and-white print of the product and the price in Snohomish County, Washington. As part of independently reached settlements with the tobacco industry, Florida, Texas, Mississippi, and Minnesota removed all billboard ads before the remaining states did so.[72]

Lessons and Parallels from Alcohol and Illicit Drug Use

Adolescent tobacco use is just one form of substance use that has attracted sustained attention from policymakers, clinicians, and the general public. Substance abuse policies vary greatly depending on whether the substance is legal (tobacco and alcohol) or illegal (marijuana, cocaine, etc.). This varied policy history provides some useful insights for tobacco regulation, even as it also highlights several unique features that distinguish tobacco from other substances.

Public Policies toward Substance Use

Public policies differ depending on the substance being used. Each substance has a different set of effects on the user, resulting in differing legal sanctions. Unlike the case of smoking, heavy use of alcohol and illegal drugs can visibly impair an individual's ability to function. Thus, the use of illegal substances may involve the law enforcement and social service systems, as might the excessive use of alcohol. For example, drunk drivers may be subject to criminal penalties or sent for treatment.

Another striking contrast between tobacco and other substances is the sharp difference in mortality and morbidity associated with these substances. Tobacco regulatory policies are therefore likely to have a greater public health impact than could be expected from other substance abuse interventions. Illicit substances appear to pose relatively small health risks to the majority of adolescents who consume these substances. Most adolescents who use illicit substances consume small amounts during short drug-using careers.[73] Much of the mortality and morbidity associated with illicit substances is therefore concentrated in the small minority of adolescents who make the transition from experimental to routine use as adults.

Because the social and health problems of nontobacco substances are concentrated in a small minority of actual users, public policies include intensive interventions for the small population of individuals experiencing the greatest risk. In response to the resulting social harm, many public health commentators advocate harm reduction as the appropriate strategy to regulate intoxicant use.[74]

Teen smoking presents a very different set of social concerns and a very different natural history that alters public regulatory strategies. Unlike most adolescents who use illicit substances, most teen smokers will eventually consume large amounts of tobacco, over long smoking careers. Adolescent smokers are far more likely than illicit drug users to become chronic users and subsequently to experience specific adult illness related to tobacco use.[73] Because the volume and duration of smoking are central to the subsequent public health consequences of teen smoking, use reduction has been the focus of tobacco regulatory policy. Efforts to reduce adolescent smoking are usually implemented in less coercive fashion than is common for alcohol and illicit drugs.

An additional contrast between tobacco and other substances arises in the targeting of substance abuse policy. Alcohol and tobacco are largely regulated through age-specific policies. Use of these substances is tolerated (and commercially promoted) as legitimate adult behavior, even as adolescents are forbidden to engage in such behavior. Such regulations communicate an inherently ambiguous message to adolescents, whose development typically includes experimentation with adult behaviors and roles.

In contrast to both alcohol and tobacco, illicit substances are subject to stringent regulation and social stigma that applies across all age-groups. Existing data suggest that uniform, strongly enforced social norms have an especially pronounced impact on preventing both illicit substance use and its subsequent trajectory. Adolescents are sensitive to the perceived risks and social stigma in their decisions about marijuana and cocaine use.[75] Prevalence rates of self-reported substance use decline as teens report that marijuana and cocaine bring health and other risks. Use of illicit substances also declines if larger numbers of adolescents report that they would disapprove of regular users.

The volume of news coverage of drug issues and the volume of antidrug advertisements declined during the early 1990s, contributing to increased adolescent consumption of illegal drugs.[74] This account is similar to that presented in Michael Massing's drug policy analysis *The Fix*.[76] Massing recounts how government antidrug efforts strongly emphasized adolescent marijuana use during the early-1980s. Ten years later, policymakers placed less emphasis on this issue, given the rise to public prominence of other social problems, such as adult crack addiction and HIV infection among injection drug users. At a minimum, such shifts influenced subsequent changes in adolescent substance use.

Tobacco Regulation and the Creation of Black Markets

A parallel between tobacco and other substances arises in the potential creation of illegal markets (so-called black markets) in response to changes in public policy. Many policymakers and commentators express concern that higher taxes and more stringent regulation will encourage the growth of a black market in tobacco. The fear of black markets played an important role during the 1998 congressional consideration of the McCain legislation's provision to impose higher cigarette taxes. Opponents of higher taxes claimed that an increase would create an illegal black market, citing what happened in Canada when taxes were raised substantially (although, as we now know, tobacco companies fueled the black market activities there).[77]

Illegal sales play an important role in many markets in which taxes or public regulation drive a large wedge between mandated prices and actual costs of producing and distributing a product.[78] For instance, a significant black market exists in untaxed and unregulated alcoholic beverages and illicit substances. Such activities can be reduced, but rarely eliminated, through aggressive law enforcement.

Because they are easily concealed and transported across state lines and have a long shelf life, cigarettes are conducive to illegal sales. There is also evidence that subsidiaries of U.S. firms participate in such activities.[79] A recent newspaper account documents that black market sales in Canada were at least tolerated by tobacco producers, some of whom allegedly signed contracts to serve black market suppliers.[80] Within days of this report, the Canadian government sued several tobacco companies to recoup the lost tax revenues resulting from their allegedly fraudulent conduct of smuggling cigarettes to evade Canadian taxes.

Economic theory suggests that the social costs of a tobacco black market are likely to be smaller than those associated with current markets for marijuana or illicit drugs. Much of the violence in illicit drug markets arises from organized rivals who seek to dominate a local market.[81] Given the continued existence of legal tobacco markets, and given the relative ease with which individuals could divert legal tobacco products into illegal uses, the profit margins available to tax-evading cigarette smugglers are likely to be smaller than those available for cocaine and other intoxicating substances.

Policymakers also have ample tools to scrutinize whether the tobacco black market is growing. If the volume of taxed tobacco sales begins to decline as a proportion of self-reported smoking in survey data, policymakers have the option to reduce existing taxes or to make other policy changes that minimize black market sales. (National policy changes are likely to create fewer opportunities for criminal intervention.) Age-specific regulations are especially unlikely to spawn a large and organized illicit market. Adolescent smokers are a small extension of a large legal market and often obtain cigarettes from relatives and friends or from legitimate merchants who fail to comply with existing age-based regulations.

Conclusion

Regulation has considerable potential for discouraging adolescent tobacco use. But for all of the attention to regulatory strategies during the 1990s, surprisingly limited data are available to determine how effective regulation might be. Several reasons account for this. First, entrenched and well-financed opposition to federal and state regulation has resulted in diluted regulatory policies, state preemption of

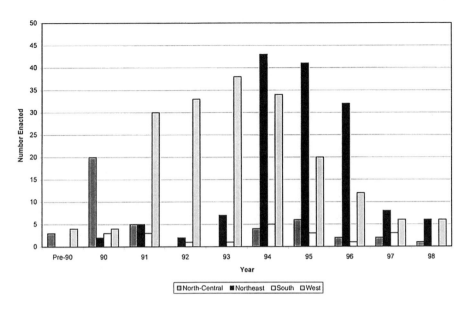

Fig. 8. Vending machine (total) ordinances. (Data from ANRF 1998.)

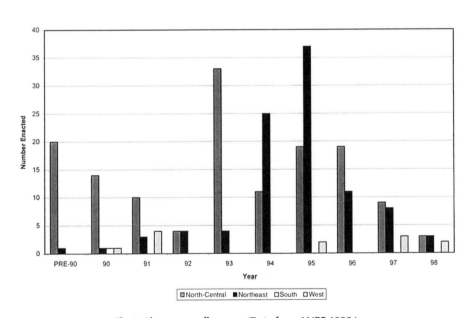

Fig. 9. Licensure ordinances. (Data from ANRF 1998.)

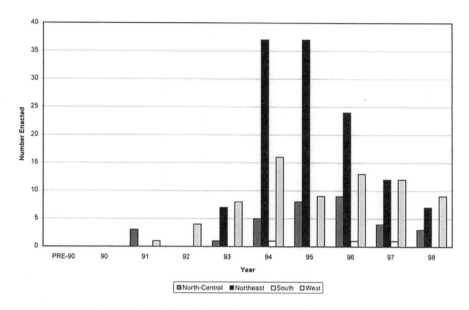

Fig. 10. Self-service displays ordinances. (Data from ANRF 1998.)

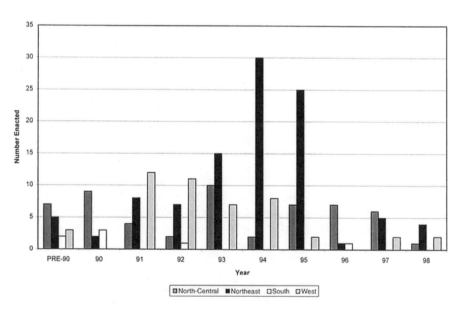

Fig. 11. Sampling ordinances. (Data from ANRF 1998.)

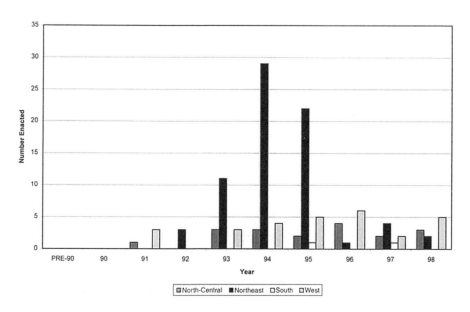

Fig. 12. Single-cigarette ordinances. (Data from ANRF 1998.)

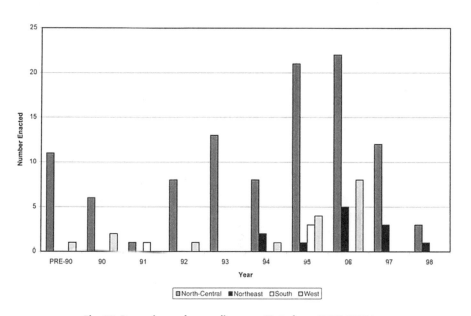

Fig. 13. Possession and use ordinances. (Data from ANRF 1998.)

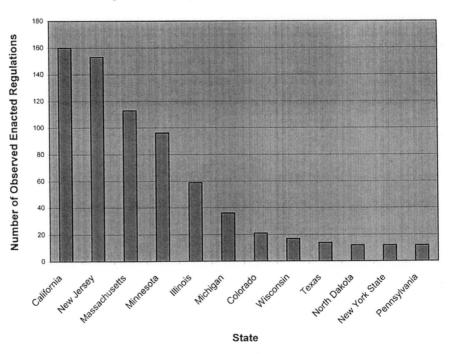

Fig. 14. Observed regulations as compiled by the American Nonsmokers' Rights Foundation

stronger local ordinances, or limits on the FDA's ability to regulate tobacco products. Second, the laws that have been enacted have suffered from a lack of enforcement. This is particularly evident at the state level, calling into question federal strategies to partner with state agencies. Third, researchers are now conducting studies to determine whether youth access restrictions do more than just reduce the level of illegal sales to minors. If subsequent research indicates that regulations also reduce adolescent smoking behavior, this will provide a strong justification for more stringent restrictions.

In part because of restrictions on FDA jurisdiction, especially on product regulation, we have not yet found the optimal mix of policy strategies for regulating adolescent smoking behavior. For the time being, state and local regulation of adolescent tobacco use will remain the focal point of these regulatory efforts. We return to the question of what regulatory policy to pursue in our "Conclusion and Recommendations."

REFERENCES

1. See, e.g., Sullum 1998.

2. Levy and Friend 2000, Jason et al. 1996a.

3. Forster and Wolfson 1998.

4. The STATE system was developed by the Centers for Disease Control and Prevention in the Office on Smoking and Health, National Center for Chronic Disease Prevention and Health Promotion. More information on the STATE system is available at <http://www2.cdc.gov/nccdphp/osh/state>.

5. CDC 1999g—as of publication date, January 8, 1999.

6. Luke, Stamatakis, and Brownson 2000.

7. Arizona and Kansas have enacted laws prohibiting the sale of chewing tobacco only. In Alabama, Alaska, and Utah, it is illegal to sell tobacco products to anyone under the age of 19.

8. CDC 1999g.

9. Samuels and Glantz 1991; Jacobson, Wasserman, and Raube 1993.

10. U.S. Bureau of the Census 1994.

11. In addition, the ANRF has been revising its data system. Up to June 1998, the ANRF did not differentiate between restrictions on use and purchase and did not include ordinances banning possession of tobacco products. Inclusion of possession ordinances and the distinction between purchase and use ordinances in later versions of the data set make it difficult to construct accurate trend information.

12. Our discussion henceforth refers only to ordinances restricting either use or purchase.

13. The states referred to are Illinois, Michigan, and Minnesota. These are also the most active states in any type of ordinance in this region.

14. From our monitoring of tobacco list servers, we know that this is a substantially underreported category in the ANRF data.

15. USDHHS 1999.

16. Jacobson and Wasserman 1997.

17. Jacobson and Wasserman 1997; Forster and Wolfson 1998; DiFranza 1999.

18. DiFranza 1999.

19. DiFranza 1999.

20. Jacobson and Wasserman 1997.

21. Jacobson and Wasserman 1999. See also Jason et al. 1991, 1996b; Feighery, Altman, and Shaffer 1991.

22. Jason et al. 1991.

23. Rigotti et al. 1997.

24. Jason et al. 1996a.

25. Altman et al. 1996.

26. Altman et al. 1999.

27. Cummings et al. 1998.

28. DiFranza, Savageau, and Aisquit 1996.

29. DiFranza and Brown 1992.

30. Rigotti et al. 1997.

31. Altman et al. 1996; Stead and Lancaster 2000.

32. Pierce, Gilpin, Emery, Farkas, et al. 1998; Rigotti et al. 1997.

33. Forster et al. 1998.

34. Siegel, Biener, and Rigotti 1999.

35. Jason et al. 1991.

36. Jason et al. 1991, 1996b.

37. Jason et al. 1999. In this study, the researchers merged experimental, social, and regular smokers into one group for comparison against nonsmokers in the two types of communities.

38. Feighery, Altman, and Shaffer 1991.

39. Biglan et al. 1999.

40. Forster et al. 1998.

41. Forster et al. 1997.

42. Forster et al. 1998; Altman et al. 1999.

43. Siegel, Biener, and Rigotti 1999.

44. Cummings et al. 1998.

45. Gemson et al. 1998.

46. CDC 1996a, 1996b; Levy and Friend 1999.

47. DiFranza and Rigotti 1999.

48. Levy and Friend 1999.

49. Rigotti et al. 1997.

50. Levy and Friend 1999 (citing Feighery, Altman, and Shaffer 1991, 2000); Jason et al. 1996a; Rigotti et al. 1997; and Forster et al. 1998. As Levy and Friend (1999) note, even a 75 percent compliance rate means that an adolescent can purchase tobacco, on average, every fourth try. They add, "Since news about sellers travels quickly among smoking youth, those continuing to sell to minors are likely to increase their sales" (13–14).

51. Hinds 1992; Forster et al. 1998.

52. However, the possibility that these laws would encourage adolescent rebelliousness cannot be ruled out.

53. Forster et al. 1998.

54. Jacobson and Wasserman 1999.

55. Rigotti and Pashos 1991; Jacobson and Wu 2000; Brownson et al. 1997.

56. Jacobson and Wu 2000. There has also been a strong voluntary movement among large businesses to limit smoking at the work site, forcing the now familiar sight of smoking breaks in building vestibules.

57. Brownson et al. 1997; Farkas et al. 1999; Farrelly, Evans, and Sfekas 1999.

58. Wasserman et al. 1991.

59. Chaloupka and Grossman 1996.

60. Chaloupka and Wechsler 1997.

61. Tauras and Chaloupka 1999. Moreover, the remaining restrictions Tauras and Chaloupka considered (i.e., a restaurant restriction, an "other indoor" restriction, and an overall restriction index) did not have a positive impact on smoking cessation in any of the models tested.

62. Wines 1996.

63. Benowitz and Henningfield 1994.

64. Warner, Slade, and Sweanor 1997.

65. R. J. Reynolds 1988.

66. These issues are explored in detail in Tobacco dependence 1998.

67. Henningfield et al. 1998; R. J. Reynolds 1988.

68. Jacobson and Wasserman 1999.

69. Teen courts connect 2000.

70. These details are taken from Navarro 1998.

71. Jacobson and Wasserman 1999.

72. Under current constitutional law, narrowly tailored advertising restrictions based on a sound public health rationale are permitted. The government cannot restrict the content of any truthful ads but can limit the timing and location of the ads.

73. Kleiman 1993.

74. Des Jarlais 1995.

75. Bachman, Johnston, and O'Malley 1990.

76. Massing 1998.

77. Gleckman 1998.

78. Reuter 1985; Rose-Ackerman 1978.

79. Drew 1998.

80. Marsden 1999.

81. Kleiman 1993.

Conclusion and Recommendations

Just since the publication of the Institute of Medicine's and surgeon general's reports in 1994, there has been a vast upsurge of tobacco control research and policy, much of it aimed at reducing adolescent tobacco use. As significant as this activity has been, we can take little comfort given stubbornly high rates of adolescent tobacco use. Yet the data showing declines in adolescent smoking since 1996 may indicate that youth prevention policies are beginning to take effect. It also takes time to absorb the vast amount of research now available and translate it into effective policy.

Smoking remains deeply rooted in American culture despite several decades of public health policy and public health advocacy designed to reduce tobacco use. Adolescents are no more immune (and perhaps less immune) than others to the attractions that smoking provides. No single policy or clinical intervention can dramatically reduce adolescent smoking, but a comprehensive strategy can address many of the influences contributing to youth smoking behavior. By comprehensive strategy, we mean a combination of multiple intervention strategies, such as governmental policy at the federal, state, and local levels; program interventions aimed at individuals, families, schools, and communities; and research, including policy and program evaluation. A comprehensive program includes multiple targets, short- and long-term components, a focus on both adult and adolescent tobacco use, and community involvement in developing and implementing the approach. Our recommendations are grounded in the belief that a policy and research strategy must be comprehensive rather than specifically targeted at either children or adults.

We believe that states have an obligation to use their resources and public health powers to discourage smoking in general and adolescent tobacco use in particular. As one of this book's authors wrote many years ago, "society has an obligation to its members to create an environment supportive of smokers' desire to quit and free of seductive enticements to children to start."[1] Thus, we strongly advocate that the states devote significant resources to expanding, improving, and evaluating comprehensive tobacco prevention and control activities. Any sense that the negotiated settlement between the states and the tobacco industry has "solved" the health-related problems associated with tobacco seems premature at best and illusory at worst.

Even before the Master Settlement Agreement (MSA), there was a wide and exciting variety of policy experimentation. The funding that will flow to the states through the MSA offers policymakers and tobacco control advocates an unprecedented opportunity to design, conduct, and evaluate numerous interventions. With the American Legacy Foundation's ability to fund a critical mass of antitobacco advertisements and messages, along with the states' ability to fund antismoking programs, the opportunities for changing the dynamics of adolescent smoking are limited only by our imagination and willingness to invest adequate resources. There is considerable public support for well-designed and effective programs.

One of the exciting aspects of working in tobacco control is the constantly changing research and policy environment. New studies are being published every day, expanding our understanding of the problem and how to attack it. New approaches are constantly being developed and tested. For policymakers confronted with the task of responding to the volume of research and the number of new programs, this moving target presents a daunting task. We hope that this book and the suggestions that follow will make that task somewhat easier.

Organization of the Chapter

We first offer recommendations for a comprehensive tobacco control program. Most of our recommendations are for interventions that can be undertaken by state and local officials or by other tobacco control advocates right away. Then we discuss longer-term changes that must be implemented to address the social context of adolescent smoking. Next we offer a research agenda that builds on existing knowledge regarding adolescent tobacco use. After reviewing our reasons for favoring a comprehensive approach to tobacco control, we add a few concluding remarks.

Recommendations for Policy and Program Interventions

The following recommendations are designed to be implemented in the short run, but should also be viewed as the foundation of a longer-term strategy to reduce adolescent tobacco use. Rather than a hierarchy, readers should view the following recommendations as a menu of choices for creating a comprehensive program. One point we want to stress is the need for policymakers and tobacco control advocates to experiment with different combinations and strategies. No one strategy is likely to be "right" for every state or community. Also, it is unlikely that every state enjoys sufficient political support to implement every element of a comprehensive program or has the resources to implement them thoroughly.

Another important point is to view reducing adolescent tobacco use as a long-term endeavor. We expect that this problem will be solved, if at all, only with a long-term commitment of resources that take advantage of potential synergies across interventions. Over time, the mix of strategies that succeed across states will become known and strategies can be adapted to reflect expanding knowledge.

Equally important, there is great potential for these interventions to be cost-effective. Even modest gains from prevention and cessation efforts could lead to substantial reductions in the morbidity and mortality costs of smoking. State officials should build on previous work to create more effective prevention programs with a high payoff potential.

Invest in Antismoking Media Campaigns Aimed at Adolescents

As we discussed in chapter 5, tobacco marketing efforts appear to be an important influence on adolescent smoking behavior. In response, social marketing can effectively convey a counteradvertising strategy designed to prevent adolescent tobacco use. To increase effectiveness, a tobacco control program should include a mass media or social marketing component to counter the allure of industry marketing tactics.

Antitobacco media strategies directed at adolescent smoking can consist of multiple approaches. One strategy is to put restrictions on the tobacco industry's marketing (advertising) to children; another is to provide antismoking advertisements and mass media messages. Ideally, both aspects should be in place. Tobacco advertising restrictions alone are unlikely to change adolescent smoking behavior unless combined with a strong and consistent antismoking counteradvertising message. For one thing, a complete ban on tobacco advertising would not result in the cessation of youth smoking. Restricting tobacco advertising (as the MSA does) is a sound policy strategy, but advertising is merely one influence on adolescent tobacco use and is not likely the dominant factor. For another thing, advertising restrictions will make it harder, but not impossible, to market tobacco products to adolescents.

Antismoking ads must be placed in time periods and on media to which adolescents are regularly exposed. Until recently, counterads have been beset by a lack of exposure. Free public service announcements often occupy less desirable airtime (e.g., late at night). With the settlement allocations to the American Legacy Foundation and to the states, more resources are now available to purchase airtime during more desirable time periods. Some states, including California and Massachusetts, have already begun purchasing time to air antismoking ads.

A subject of ongoing debate is how to structure the antismoking ads. Among the issues is whether to create an educational or "just say no" approach or to attack the tobacco industry directly and thereby attempt to turn adolescents' natural rebelliousness into anger against the industry. Another approach is appealing to teen vanity, with ads focusing on the fact that smoking makes their clothes smell and their breath stink.

In what amounts to a natural experiment, several states are trying different strategies. We will have a better understanding of which strategy or combination of approaches is more effective once the ad campaigns are evaluated. At this point, we are not prepared to recommend a particular media strategy among those now being tried. In the end, we expect states to adopt a mix of countermarketing strategies that invoke graphic descriptions of tobacco's health hazards and remind adolescents of what information the tobacco industry has been hiding from them. In all media interventions, it is important that the message resonate with some "core values," or issues that are important to the intended audience segments.

The evidence of a decline in adolescent smoking rates in California, Massachusetts, and Florida following hard-hitting state sponsored antitobacco campaigns suggests that a sustained media campaign against smoking can be a successful strategy. One thing seems clear. According to the available evidence, one-shot or short-lived campaigns are not likely to change behavior. Even though the Florida campaign has done well in a short period of time, its results might not be sustained if the campaign ends prematurely. Rather, a plan for a multiyear campaign that utilizes a strong social marketing approach with an anti-smoking message is needed to sustain any effects.[2] Initial reports from the American Legacy Foundation indicate that this is the strategy it plans to pursue.

Antitobacco messages should also be aimed at young, middle-aged, and older adults, as well as children. As we have argued, there are likely to be indirect effects if adults quit smoking, and media strategies designed to encourage adult cessation should be pursued.

Since the American Legacy Foundation has dedicated a significant sum to counteradvertising strategies, states should attempt to coordinate their countermarketing strategies with the foundation's efforts. To be sure, coordination in a rapidly changing environment is not easy, but it would maximize resource use and help avoid wasteful duplication. Since the foundation's approach will be national in scope,[3] states may want to design specific and complementary countermarketing strategies to reach well-defined audience segments in the state with culturally appropriate and resonating messages. Careful audience segmenting and targeting is especially important, given the immense diversity in the adolescent population in general. General messages aimed at all adolescents—or even at large subgroups based on gender or ethnicity—appear less effective than more specific messages that are tailored to more narrowly defined audience subgroups. Such market segmentation has long been recognized by the tobacco industry, which has developed different products to reach specific groups based not only on gender but also on values, recreational interests, other behaviors, and social class.

Design and Implement Teen Cessation Programs

Almost all of the smoking cessation attention has focused on adults. Our review of the literature suggests that efforts to develop and implement adolescent smoking cessation programs should be accelerated to determine whether adolescent cessation rates can be increased. It is particularly important to target adolescents who are just at the transition point before or after habitual smoking begins. The evidence at hand suggests that, although the processes by which nicotine dependence develops in adolescence are not well understood, teenagers certainly can and do become addicted to nicotine. For obvious reasons, the longer cessation interventions are delayed, the higher the probability that the adolescent smoker will become addicted to tobacco or that the addiction will become more severe. By high school, prevention messages may have limited value for a significant number of adolescents already addicted to nicotine, beyond reinforcing the importance of quitting.

Until now, certain cessation therapies, nicotine replacement therapy (NRT) in particular, have been unavailable to persons under 18 absent a physician's prescription, and very few studies have assessed NRT's efficacy and safety in adolescents. NRT may also be an important addition to existing cessation strategies tailored to adolescents' unique developmental and psychosocial needs.[4] Given many adolescents' expressed desire to quit smoking, policymakers should reconsider the use of NRT for adolescents. This area presents a significant opportunity for changing adolescent tobacco use patterns. Physician involvement in using NRT is essential.

Adolescent cessation efforts may have other potentially positive effects. As younger adolescents see successful cessation efforts, they may be encouraged to forgo smoking altogether or to enroll in cessation programs earlier in their smoking histories.[5] With fewer role models using tobacco, this might induce significant change in the adolescent culture of tobacco use. To achieve this result, it may be necessary to provide adolescent smokers with either free cessation therapies or subsidies to pay for them. If expensive pharmaceutical products become legally available for teens, many adolescent smokers may not be able to take advantage of them absent some financial support.[6] Even among teens whose families are able to finance their cessation therapy, many teens report that—for myriad reasons—they do not want parental involvement in their cessation attempts.

Develop and Evaluate School- and Community-
Based Interventions

We would like to be able to recommend specific school- and community-based programs that have proven to be effective in reducing adolescent tobacco use. Regrettably, the existing evidence will not support such recommendations. CDC has suggested using two programs, Life Skills Training and Toward No Tobacco Use (discussed in chap. 4), which provide good starting points for developing and implementing effective school- and community-based efforts. However, two studies suggest that few schools are implementing smoking programs that adhere to most of the CDC's guidelines.[7] Prevention programs based on a social influence model have been shown to have positive short-term effects on middle school students, who are most likely to initiate smoking. These programs play an important subsidiary role in articulating a consistent antismoking message.

The obvious problem is that states will not easily be able to take programs off the shelf and implement them. In turn, this forces state officials to review more closely the literature we discussed in chapter 4. To be sure, this also presents an opportunity for states to develop and evaluate innovative programs, but at a higher cost. We suggest that policymakers focus on taking advantage of synergies between different strategies, especially school- and community-based programs. To do so effectively, it is important to establish partnerships with teachers, school administrators, and other people who work with adolescents and preadolescents on a regular basis.[8]

School- and community-based efforts are predominantly delivered at the local level, although a state-local collaboration makes sense. States can provide adequate funding, but actual implementation should be at the local level. We also suggest that states cooperate with community groups, local businesses, and antismoking coalitions to develop and evaluate more effective school- and community-based programs. Tobacco control advocates and coalitions can play a significant role in working with school officials, other community leaders, and public health professionals to develop and implement broader interventions.

Our review suggests that most school-based prevention programs target students in the elementary and junior high schools, while high school students are often ignored. High school students may receive booster sessions on prevention, but these sessions are often unconnected to the interventions received in junior high. As we suggested earlier, the high school population might be the primary target for smoking cessation programs, but booster sessions should be provided, especially in light of increasing smoking initiation among young adults. High school students are also excellent candidates for participating in sting operations, lobbying for antismoking legislation, and becoming peer educators for children in their community.

Computer-Based Interventions

School and community-based interventions should also explore the use of computers in their programs. Because of the enormous potential of computer technology to bring individualized antismoking messages and programs to adolescents, we recommend that states invest in computer technology and Internet-based antismoking programs. Adolescents represent a perfect audience for using emerging computer-based antismoking strategies. The development and expansion of computer-based systems presents a unique opportunity to take advantage of technology that most adolescents are comfortable with and to adapt antismoking messages to individual needs and circumstances. As we discussed in chapter 4, an important reason for recommending this strategy is its ability to reach numerous adolescents at much less cost than through school-based interventions. We do not, however, recommend abandoning school-based efforts, because social interaction is an important component of the intervention. But a complementary computer-based strategy can reinforce messages delivered in school.

Involving Peer Groups
Many states, including Florida, are relying heavily on peers to design and convey antismoking messages. Most important, young people may have a much better idea of what kinds of messages and strategies will resonate with their peers than do adults. That is a major reason why the American Legacy Foundation's 11-member board includes one youth member and why the foundation is involving numerous young people in developing its media counteradvertising campaign.

Younger adolescents may be more responsive to antismoking messages when they are delivered by older adolescents rather than by adults. Older adolescent nonsmokers or former smokers may become role models over time. Interventions using peer educators, such as the Teens against Tobacco Use program described in chapter 4, should be evaluated both for their impact on the children receiving the program and for the effect of reinforcing nonsmoking behavior on the teens themselves.

One aspect that peer intervention might reiterate is the health risk of tobacco use. Despite the ubiquity of antismoking messages, some evidence suggests that adolescents underestimate the risks of smoking and overestimate their peers' approval of smoking. Reminding adolescents of true risks, actual smoking prevalence, and the difficulty of quitting would at least provide them with adequate information. Another aspect would be to develop interventions focusing on social interaction skills between peers, to reduce social pressure to use tobacco.

Involving Parents

Convincing parents to adopt voluntary no-smoking (or at least partial no-smoking rules in the home can be an important strategy in changing the social context of tobacco use. Aside from reducing exposure to ETS, making the home smoke-free actively discourages adolescent experimentation with tobacco. The home environment is an area where significant efforts regarding education and risk reduction can be effective. Even though fundamental privacy protections limit the reach of public policy in this area,[9] parents (even those who currently smoke) can be encouraged to make their homes smoke-free. There are many interventions that could result in less smoking in the home without infringing on privacy.[10] These include educating parents about the value of voluntarily instituting no-smoking rules at home, smoking cessation programs for adolescents and adults, community-based interventions to educate parents about the dangers of ETS to children, and physician-based counseling.[11]

Involving the Community

An important justification for continuing community-based efforts is to engage the entire community, especially parents, in antitobacco activities. The state can continue to educate merchants about the consequences of illegal tobacco sales to minors and provide a broad-based antismoking message to the public. States can also use the settlement funds to support community attempts to develop neighborhood- and community-based approaches. Community organizations could be provided with grant funds to design and evaluate promising community-based strategies. One potential model is the SmokeLess State National Tobacco Prevention and Control Program funded by the Robert Wood Johnson Foundation and administered by the American Medical Association. This program funds the development of statewide antismoking coalitions to engage in media education, policy development, and tobacco prevention efforts. These coalitions are designed to include adolescents in planning various activities.

As detailed in Michael Massing's book *The Fix*,[12] community involvement heightened public awareness about adolescent drug use. Efforts by voluntary parent groups played a significant role in changing public attitudes and public policy toward adolescent drug use. These groups provided important political support for substance abuse policies and helped change adolescent attitudes, including a rise in the perceived risk and a decline in social acceptability of marijuana use. Sustainable antismoking interventions also require the mobilization of constituencies that can provide long-term political support. One challenge facing school- and community-based interventions is to address adolescent smoking in the context of broader developmental issues and to recognize that for some youth, smoking serves as a marker for other adverse circumstances or problem behaviors.

Community organizations play an especially important role in mobilizing and sustaining public support for antismoking efforts. They can also play a significant monitoring role to ensure proper implementation of antismoking measures. Such groups can continue to support restrictive no-smoking laws and to oppose statewide preemption laws. Antismoking coalitions can support voluntary restrictions by publicly rewarding private businesses that do not sell tobacco products to minors or that impose smoking restrictions.

Increase Cigarette Prices

There is no question that increasing the cigarette tax is an important step governments can take to reduce adolescent smoking, especially as a complement to the other strategies we recommend that state officials adopt. Raising excise taxes and thereby increasing the price of cigarettes is likely to have an observable impact on youth smoking. Adolescents are price-sensitive. Even if they still have access to cigarettes through friends and family, higher prices are likely to result in fewer routine adolescent smokers and perhaps fewer cigarettes consumed by occasional adolescent smokers. What remains uncertain is how teens would respond to a truly substantial price increase. At this point, the evidence does not support a specific percentage tax increase that we could recommend. However, economic theory suggests that a substantial price rise may have a proportionately larger impact on teen smoking than have smaller tax-induced price increases.

Rising prices may also have an indirect effect by reducing adult smoking behavior. To the extent that higher taxes discourage adult smoking, they are likely indirectly to reduce adolescent smoking. At a minimum, adolescents will have a harder time obtaining free cigarettes. When coupled with stringent enforcement of illegal sales to minors, this makes it more difficult and costly for adolescents to obtain tobacco products. It also becomes less likely that parents will encourage or tolerate adolescent tobacco use and more likely that they will become role models for not smoking.

Therefore, efforts to increase state and federal tobacco excise taxes are justified and should continue. A higher federal tax would be particularly appropriate because it would uniformly raise the cost of smoking cigarettes and avoid cross-border or bootlegging problems. These problems arise when the price of cigarettes is much lower in one state than another; residents cross the border to purchase cigarettes, or the products are smuggled across the border by bootleggers who do not pay the state's tax. Another important reason for supporting a federal tax strategy is the burgeoning phenomenon of Internet tobacco sales, which are free of state taxes. If these sales boom,[13] states will lose anticipated revenue, and tobacco manufacturers will be under less pressure to raise prices. Independently of whether the federal government acts to regulate or tax Internet tobacco sales, states should include tax increases as part of a comprehensive strategy to reduce adolescent tobacco use.

As a longer-term strategy, one of our interview respondents proposed an addictions tax in the form of excess profits.[14] This would essentially work along the lines of the "look-back provision" from the proposed McCain legislation, where tobacco manufacturers would be penalized if the rate of youth smoking does not decline by a specified percentage over a certain number of years. The higher the sales to minors, the greater the tax on the industry.

Implement Policies That Further Regulate Tobacco

Youth Access Restrictions

Even though we lack evidence linking youth access restrictions to reductions in overall smoking rates, there is good reason to support and expand these laws, subject to certain conditions. First, rigorous enforcement of the prohibition against tobacco sales to minors (including stings, large fines, and licensure removal) is needed. As we have already argued, eliminating illegal sales to minors would almost certainly result in lower adolescent smoking rates, by making cigarette acquisition more expensive. Just as important, a clear message would be sent about society's commitment to antismoking policies. If states are unwilling to enforce the laws aggressively, responsibility should be delegated to local governments. At the very least, advocates should continue working to remove laws preempting local governments from aggressive antismoking regulation and enforcement. Second, states should require tobacco vendors to obtain licenses to sell tobacco and should permit removal of a vendor's license for illegal tobacco sales to minors, rather than just maintaining an escalating fine structure. Licensure removal is a much greater enforcement threat than are just fines, and it matches law enforcement sanctions imposed for other serious offenses, particularly alcohol sales to minors. Third, whatever fines are imposed should be sufficient to make enforcement programs self-financing. Since restricting illegal sales to minors retains widespread public support, operating the enforcement program without using general tax revenue would further insulate the program from attack.

Although most of the enforcement of youth access restrictions will occur at the state and local levels, the federal government plays an important role through the Synar Amendment. So far, the federal government has been lax in overseeing state-level enforcement. Absent pressure from the federal government, states are not likely to be aggressive enforcers.

In general, youth access restrictions are best enforced at the local level. Local governments are more likely to remove vendor licenses and to collect fines than are state agencies. Where that is not feasible, as with Synar authority, it will be up to the federal government to withhold substance abuse block grant funds if states ignore their enforcement responsibilities. One role that antitobacco advocates and coalitions might play is to bring pressure on the federal government to enforce the Synar provisions.

Penalizing Tobacco Possession and Use

The effectiveness of such interventions as fines and penalties for adolescent possession and use of tobacco products is unknown at this point. But if such programs as tobacco courts, suspension of drivers' licenses, or fines for tobacco use actually reduce adolescent tobacco use, tobacco control advocates should reconsider their opposition. If we are serious about inhibiting teen smoking, we should encourage programs that do so. As long as these programs do not substitute for enforcing laws against illegal sales to minors, we see nothing inappropriate about penalizing adolescent tobacco use and possession.[15] After all, we have had such a system in place for many years to penalize underage alcohol use. Why should tobacco be treated differently? In principle, these laws can encourage participation in smoking cessation interventions, as is routinely done for alcohol and illicit substances. Such initiatives can be managed effectively through a state-local governmental partnership.

If these programs are to be effective, they will need to be enforced. Most importantly, merchant enforcement policies need to be in place and vigorously implemented. The scope of the law should be determined in the state legislature, but enforcement should remain at the local level. The obvious problem will be to convince public officials that enforcement is worthwhile. As we discuss shortly, research determining whether laws penalizing youths actually reduce teen smoking behavior will be instrumental in generating public support for an active program.

Product Regulation

Because of disputes regarding FDA jurisdiction over tobacco products, product regulation has languished. This is unfortunate, as serious product regulation has great long-term potential for reducing adolescent use of tobacco products. Because the Supreme Court refused to uphold FDA authority to regulate tobacco products, advocates will need to develop a strategy for direct congressional enactment of such authority. Once authority is granted, the FDA will still need congressional support for adequate funding and political muscle.

Product regulation, such as changing the composition of cigarettes to reduce the nicotine content or provide a less hazardous cigarette, rests primarily with the federal government. States can theoretically put pressure on the federal government to be more aggressive, but they have no independent authority in this area, because the federal government preempts the field.

Advocates should also be preparing the foundation for product regulation. For example, is gradually reducing the nicotine content of tobacco a feasible approach? If feasible, is this strategy desirable? Should the FDA, once given authority, demand that the tobacco industry manufacture a less hazardous cigarette? The issues in this area are enormously complex and currently the subject of a study by the Institute of Medicine and various groups of tobacco control experts worldwide. The widely held belief, however, is that regulatory resolution of the issues will prove enormously important to the future of tobacco-produced disease.[16]

Advertising and Marketing Restrictions

The settlement with the tobacco industry includes a number of restrictions on advertising and marketing aimed at youth. This is a positive development that states should expand by enacting laws banning self-service displays. With some exceptions, courts have generally upheld similar restrictions if they are adequately limited to protecting children.

Invest in Program Evaluation

One possible explanation for the mixed results of smoking prevention and control programs for youth is inadequate program evaluation. One of the most significant barriers to implementing effective prevention programs is the failure to evaluate a successful small-scale and tightly controlled intervention and then translate the findings into a broad intervention involving the entire community.[17] Once an intervention has reached the community, it is often assumed to be effective without any further evaluation. The failure to evaluate youth prevention programs is a serious deficiency in being able to defend additional investments in youth tobacco control efforts. It is especially important to assess the long-term outcomes of behavioral interventions.

We therefore recommend that tobacco control interventions (especially those with innovative programs) should generally include an evaluation component. In our experience, one reason for the lack of program evaluation is that many promising programs are developed and implemented by groups lacking knowledge of how to construct an appropriate evaluation. States do not often make evaluations a condition of receiving funding. As a model, states might look to such organizations as the Robert Wood Johnson Foundation. Each of its grant programs routinely requires any demonstration program to include an independent evaluation component. States should make available training on how small grantees and local community organizations can conduct an evaluation. Transferring technology, skills, and knowledge to community groups is an important way to encourage community involvement and to help them assess the results of their efforts.[18] States should also continue surveillance and monitoring of tobacco use trends as part of their overall evaluation responsibilities.

Invest in an Information Clearinghouse and
Dissemination Strategy

Dissemination of information about effective strategies is important. It is already difficult for state policymakers to wade through the vast tobacco control literature to identify intervention strategies and to separate what works from what has not been successful. With the continuing growth in tobacco control research and with the expected program innovations likely to emerge based on that research, it will be important to devise a mechanism for coordinating and sharing that information.

We propose that a consortium of state and federal officials establish an information clearinghouse that would collect, analyze, and share information. To a certain extent, the American Legacy Foundation may end up playing that role. We recommend that the foundation and the federal government establish an independent center along the lines of the Center for Substance Abuse Prevention (CSAP), which is funded by the government to act as a clearinghouse for information on substance abuse research, programs, and policies. CSAP provides up-to-date information about substance abuse programs and research results. Without such an equivalent center for tobacco control, a great amount of useful information will remain inaccessible to state policymakers. As we noted earlier, many community organizations could also benefit from such a transfer of knowledge.

For those involved in day-to-day work on tobacco control, there are several useful sources of information, many available for free on the Internet, from such organizations as the Advocacy Institute and the Campaign for Tobacco-Free Kids. Either of these organizations could perform a broader clearinghouse function aimed at policymakers who are not likely to follow events on a day-to-day basis. Another option for dissemination would be to work through such national organizations as the National Governors Association or the National Conference of State Legislatures. Provided with direct access to research results and program innovations, policymakers can make optimal use of the settlement funds.

Even for those working full-time on tobacco control, it remains a daunting task to keep up with the flow of information. Thus, a CSAP equivalent for tobacco control must also be provided with resources to synthesize and analyze the volume of research and program evaluations policymakers need to understand.

Data Collection

Our analysis of existing data on local ordinances indicates a gap that needs to be corrected. Right now, there is no accurate and comprehensive data collection system available to report on trends in local laws regarding tobacco restrictions. The Americans for Nonsmokers' Rights Foundation is attempting to fill that void, but its current data capabilities do not provide sufficient comprehensiveness to permit adequate analysis. Advocates need to think about ways to provide more accurate and complete data on local laws.

Definitions

As we noted in our introduction to this book, there is little agreement on how to define important and commonly used terms in tobacco control. It would be helpful if advocates could develop a standard nomenclature and definition for tracking and monitoring smoking data trends. Doing so would facilitate data analysis and avoid problems in comparing survey data. This would also make it easier to provide accurate reports on trends to the public. Perhaps a conference among tobacco researchers and advocates exclusively devoted to resolving definitional disparities could generate a consensus.

Changing the Social Context

Beyond program interventions designed to change an individual adolescent's smoking behavior, policymakers need to think about how to alter the social context in which smoking takes place. As difficult as it may be to alter individual adolescent behavior, it may be that much more challenging—and potentially more important—to change the social environment influencing that behavior. Many of the issues affecting tobacco use, such as adverse childhood events, stress, poor academic performance, and school dropout rates, are not issues that tobacco control policy can fix. We recognize that changing the social context is a long-term strategy that requires much broader social policy and program interventions. Without diminishing the importance of these concerns, we believe that the expertise and resources of the tobacco control community are best targeted to those interventions most closely connected to tobacco use.

We nonetheless believe that state policymakers should begin to explore ways to create a broader social context to discourage tobacco use. Some approaches, such as laws limiting or eliminating smoking in public places, can be pursued easily by states or local governments. Other related policy concerns, such as dealing with family structure and adverse childhood events, are much more difficult for policymakers to attack.

Prevention efforts in other areas, including adolescent mental health, HIV prevention, and school failure, have yielded favorable evaluation results.[19] Such interventions as teen mentoring, academic support programs, or screening, which are designed to improve self-efficacy, cognitive, and social skills, may reduce non-tobacco-related adolescent risks of significant policy concern. Many of the most successful adolescent interventions bring young men and women into sustained contact with knowledgeable adults who provide both support and monitoring to reduce behavioral risk. For example, several studies document the efficacy of home visiting and school-based interventions to prevent child neglect or unintended pregnancies among teen mothers.[20]

Although the focus of this book and of our recommendations is on adolescents, it is important for tobacco control advocates to consider how to change the overall environment that induces adolescents to initiate tobacco use. One problem with targeted prevention strategies is that a single program cannot always or perhaps even often prevent smoking if the environment surrounding the child encourages tobacco use. Cigarette advertising, easy access to tobacco products, and tolerance toward smoking are only some of the issues that may contribute to high rates of youth smoking.

An aggressive approach to changing the social context of smoking would include several dimensions. First, policymakers should emphasize adult cessation programs. To the extent that parental smoking influences or encourages adolescent tobacco use, it is important to involve entire families in smoking cessation programs. For example, managed care programs can emphasize the need for parents to quit, both to protect other family members from exposure to environmental tobacco smoke and to discourage adolescent smoking. Second, the expansion of state and local clean indoor air laws would serve a variety of purposes in discouraging adolescent tobacco use. Such laws send the message that smoking in public places is socially unacceptable, and they may well encourage voluntary clean indoor air restrictions in the private sector, which could help reduce adult smoking. Third, a major challenge is responding to the increased tobacco use rates among young adults. Because tobacco marketing to young adults has a clear spillover effect on underage adolescents, and because young adult culture generates considerable media attention, strategies to discourage this group from smoking are urgently needed.

One key to reducing adolescent tobacco use is a consistent message and strategy that marginalizes tobacco use throughout society, much as has already occurred among the most highly educated members of society. Adult and adolescent antitobacco messages and policies need to be mutually reinforcing. For example, a school-based no-smoking policy will not likely be effective if teachers are permitted to smoke. If schools become no-smoking zones for everyone, the message will at least be consistent, and the public health justification is most easily communicated.

Adolescent tobacco use has been linked with a low level of academic performance, lower self-esteem, lower self-image, and a lack of skills in resisting influences to use tobacco or take other health risks. At this point, we do not know what proportion of the overall adolescent smoking population is affected by these problems. If the policies being implemented are effective in reducing overall adolescent tobacco use, it will leave an important subset more vulnerable than ever. Over the long-term, therefore, policymakers will need to develop a strategy to address this subgroup of adolescent smokers.

Indeed, public policy would be well-served by interventions that effectively assist adolescent smokers who experience multiple needs. For example, some research has demonstrated that better after-school programs for adolescents would lead to positive outcomes that would reduce a range of risky behaviors, including smoking.[21] Programs designed to improve academic performance are also likely to have an ancillary benefit of reducing adolescent smoking and other risky behaviors. Programs designed to teach adolescents better refusal skills may help improve their social competency and reduce the likelihood of their using tobacco.[22]

In this sense, policymakers can take actions that would simultaneously address multiple problem behaviors that emerge in adolescence, though policymakers can do little directly to relieve the stress adolescents feel in their lives. In thinking about school-based interventions, some funds might be allocated for developing programs that enhance adolescent self-esteem and self-image while simultaneously providing a tobacco control message. If successful, this could influence adolescent tobacco consumption and may also affect other risk-taking behaviors.

Establishing a Policy-Oriented Research Agenda

As academics, we may appear self-serving by recommending that states allocate the states' tobacco litigation settlement funds for more research. After all, we have witnessed a significant expansion of tobacco-related research during the past decade, much of it reviewed in part 2. We believe strongly that this research has substantially enhanced our understanding of adolescent tobacco use and has contributed to better policy formulation. Yet much remains to be learned that can be translated into effective public policy. In this section, we outline a research strategy based on our analysis in part 2. We hope to engage other tobacco policy researchers in refining, expanding, and implementing this agenda.

Evaluations of Intervention Effectiveness

The most pressing research need is to determine whether interventions reduce adolescent tobacco use. Until recently, most research studies have investigated whether program or policy interventions work by measuring changes in attitude, reductions in sales to minors, and so on. What has not been measured adequately is whether programs also reduce actual smoking behavior. To assist policymakers in choosing which programs to support, information on the interventions that are more likely to reduce overall tobacco consumption would be invaluable.[23] This is particularly important for identifying the most cost-effective interventions.

Evaluating Multiple-Component Intervention Strategies
Many policies and programs aimed at reducing adolescent smoking are implemented simultaneously. The need for multiple, simultaneous (i.e., comprehensive) interventions, however, poses difficult challenges for evaluation efforts. How does one determine whether or not each specific intervention component had a significant effect and which specific combination of intervention strategies and policies is responsible for any observed improvement in youth smoking behavior?

The only way to ascertain with scientific certainty the unique contributions of different interventions or programs is to a conduct a randomized trial for each specific strategy. Not surprisingly, a vast array of logistical, ethical, and resource concerns preclude this from happening. Thus, evaluators are faced with the need to use quasi-experimental designs in their assessments of intervention worth. Such designs, when supported by data of high validity and reliability, can provide compelling evaluation evidence. These designs include time series analysis (in which researchers observe a trend before an intervention and look for a significant change in the trend line after the intervention implementation) and community-intervention designs (in which communities receiving a set of interventions are compared with communities that did not receive any intervention or that received a different type of intervention). When different intervention components are implemented in different communities at varying times, researchers can take advantage of this timing in what amounts to a "natural experiment." For example, evaluators of the effects of California's tobacco control program were able to disentangle the impact of the increased excise tax from the impact of the resources devoted to the statewide media campaign.[24]

The fact remains that it is often quite difficult to ascertain the exact impact of different intervention strategies that are occurring at the same time. We recommend that each intervention in a multiple-component approach have its own process evaluation. A process evaluation focuses on how an intervention was implemented and whether or not it had the quality, content, and coverage intended. For example, a process evaluation of a media campaign would look at whether youth in the target groups actually were exposed to the messages of the campaign and whether they understood them.

Rather than focusing solely on tobacco use as the evaluation outcome under study, researchers should also look at the "targeted mediators," or the mechanisms by which interventions are expected to have an impact on smoking behavior. If an intervention is intended to reduce youth smoking by improving adolescents' self-efficacy skills, evaluation efforts should attempt to measure changes in self-efficacy. While the goal of all of these interventions is the same—a reduction in youth smoking—the paths or mechanisms by which different intervention components reach this goal are different. Without such a careful and detailed evaluation strategy, the important task of separating worthwhile intervention strategies from those that are benign (or perhaps even detrimental) will not be possible.

Cost-Effectiveness

One question that recurred throughout writing this book is, Which interventions are cost-effective? To a policymaker faced with allocating scarce resources, choosing programs that are likely to be cost-effective is imperative. While not every program must meet a rigorous cost-effectiveness test, the overall expenditures must bear some reasonable relationship to cost-effectiveness to retain public support. The absence of attempts to quantify program effectiveness is troublesome and diminishes the persuasiveness of the case for investing in tobacco control prevention. It also effectively prohibits estimating the return on social investments.

At this point, there is very little research on the cost-effectiveness of the various interventions. The absence of such information makes it difficult to make a persuasive case for particular interventions, let alone to convince policymakers that money should be spent on tobacco control as opposed to competing state-level needs. By definition, cost-effectiveness analysis presupposes the existence of knowledge regarding overall effectiveness. This problem plagues many areas of tobacco control, helping to explain why few cost-effectiveness analyses (CEA) have been completed outside of the area of cessation. There is yet another important reason many central tobacco control interventions have not been subjected to CEA: they represent the type of intervention for which costs are so hard to quantify that CEA may be meaningless or at least controversial. For example, although taxation is documented to be a highly effective intervention, how does one value the cost of violating the economic neutrality of the fiscal system? How does one measure the cost of possible inequities associated with the burdens placed on poor smokers by tax increases?

Another reason for the dearth of CEA in tobacco control programs is that serious methodological issues must be addressed. Given the number of interventions simultaneously occurring, it is very difficult to separate the effects of one program from another. Evaluating the effectiveness of specific interventions is a precursor to CEA. California faced this difficulty in attempting to quantify the effects of its comprehensive tobacco control program and has funded two separate attempts to do so. Still, methodological challenges remain in conducting evaluations of intervention efficacy, and these are compounded by the number of assumptions and data challenges that accompany any cost-effectiveness study. Evaluation designs that attempt to address methodological concerns and also attempt to gather the appropriate amount of information necessary for CEA are expensive. Nonetheless, with the resources available at this point in time, we recommend that investments be made in rigorous evaluation designs that include cost analyses.

Adolescent Cessation

As described earlier, our knowledge regarding the process of nicotine dependence and effective smoking cessation interventions among adolescents is severely limited at this point in time. Thus, more research on adolescent smoking cessation should be a priority. For example, we need to ascertain the tolerance and effectiveness of pharmaceutical products for adolescent use, evaluating, for example, the benefits of nicotine replacement therapies in adolescent smokers (though early results have been disappointing).

We also need to conduct a variety of interventions to determine how to translate adolescent desires to quit into successful cessation programs. How should adult cessation programs be modified to serve adolescents? What pharmaceutical products need to be approved for adolescent use to reinforce other efforts? How can physicians be involved in prescribing available NRTs to adolescents? An important aspect of this research is to examine unexplored social or other barriers to participation. Another important aspect is to determine how various cessation programs might apply at the various stages of adolescent smoking. Smoking cessation programs must also be prepared to address other potential behaviors among adolescent smokers, particularly alcohol and illicit substance use.

Transition Stages

Further research into transition stages regarding adolescent smoking behavior is essential. We know that somewhere between the sixth and ninth grades, adolescent smokers often shift from casual to more regular use. What motivates the transition from sporadic smoking to habitual use? What interventions can be developed to block this transition, especially among middle school students? We know, for example, that elementary school students find smoking unpleasant. By middle school, though, many of them begin to smoke. In this context, our review of the literature suggests the importance of peer group leaders in discouraging other youths from smoking. A case study on how peer group leader programs operate would be timely, as would interventions designed to encourage the formation of nonsmoking peer groups.

Why Children Do Not Smoke
On one level, the question of why a majority of adolescents do not smoke should be easy enough to answer: it is the inverse of why others smoke. In fact, however, there is much to be learned by studying why most children do not move beyond experimenting with tobacco products. Although some researchers have conducted focus groups to address this aspect of the problem, few results have been published. It would be worthwhile to conduct focus groups and other types of research to understand better why adolescent nonsmokers resist the influences that others find so appealing.

As a related research area, research to identify ways to improve adolescent self-image with reference to tobacco use could help address several concerns. How adolescents see themselves and the world around them in the context of smoking is an important indicator of smoking status. For example, a series of focus group interviews showed that reasons for not smoking varied across gender and ethnic subgroups. We share the researchers' suggestion that "we need to understand more about how positive non-smoking identities and attributes could be made part of an adolescent's ideal self-image."[25]

Penalties

A controversial strategy has been to fine underage tobacco users or refer them to tobacco court. A multisite case study or quantitative assessment of these programs would be very important for determining whether such programs lead to reduced adolescent smoking. The research should attempt to determine whether the effectiveness of such policies varies as a function of an adolescent's age or smoking status (i.e., experimenter vs. routine user) or by type of program. Does a smoking court have advantages over other alternatives, such as suspending a driver's license? If so, is it more cost-effective than other options? The effectiveness of penalties could also be evaluated within a single state, with different counties adopting different penalty strategies.

System Dynamics of Smoking

James Koopman argues that epidemiologic models of human interaction are needed to understand the process of smoking progression across populations.[26] In his view, epidemiologic principles from population system dynamics might provide a formal structure for analyzing the different influences that affect transition stages. A formal systems model, he argues, will help make "predictions regarding the micro- and macro-distribution of different stages of smoking under alternative theories and where to gather information to test those theories."[27] For example, Koopman hypothesizes that increasing the social mixing between smoking and nonsmoking cliques will dramatically affect smoking levels and presumably transition stages. These ideas seem well worth pursuing.

Computer-Based Programs

The effectiveness of using computer-based programs to reach adolescents has not been systematically evaluated. An important line of research would be to conduct a series of evaluations to determine the effectiveness of different computer-based approaches to adolescent smoking behavior. For example, the tailored computer interventions described in chapter 4 need to be assessed for their efficacy over time. Another set of research questions would assess the effects of different ways of providing the computer-based information to different population groups.

Specific research questions would include examining the level of exposure (i.e., the number of times the computer program is used), time interval between sessions, and the optimal session length needed for tailored behavior change computer programs to be effective. The increasing availability of the Web as a delivery system for cessation programs highlights this issue. Smokers could access the programs on the Web conveniently at any time, as often and as long as they want to, at minimal cost. In the past, researchers have been forced to study only a limited variety of comparisons between different levels of exposure to the similar programs delivered through traditional, more expensive channels. Consequently, we have very limited empirical data on a minimal or optimal amount of program exposure that is needed to help different types of smokers quit or make progress in their quit effort. Research addressing these issues would be worthwhile.

Biomedical Research

One potential factor for explaining why some children smoke while others exposed to the same factors do not is genetic susceptibility to nicotine. To date, most of the reported research on nicotine addiction deals with adults. Since there is adequate research funding and interest in this issue through traditional biomedical research channels (e.g., the National Institutes of Health process), we do not recommend that states allocate tobacco control funding to this area.

At the federal funding level, three general issues should be explored. First, what is the relationship between genetic predisposition to nicotine dependence and social/environmental factors influencing a decision to smoke? It is important to conduct interdisciplinary research to address this issue.[28] Second, what are the genetic influences on transition stages? One of our interview respondents suggested that there may be genetic explanations for responses to the various transition stages; that is, among experimental smokers, some will be biologically susceptible to nicotine dependence. Researchers need to identify what percentage might be genetically susceptible and what the biological markers are for genetic susceptibility to nicotine.[29] Third, how might genetic predisposition to nicotine dependence affect adolescent prevention and cessation programs? In particular, several researchers have noted the limited understanding of genetic factors influencing adolescent smoking decisions.

Physician Involvement

Additional research on physician involvement in tobacco prevention activities might be worth considering, especially in the context of reducing family smoking patterns. Although many physicians have not been active in counseling patients against smoking, recent research indicating the importance of family smoking may be helpful in developing physician interventions regarding parental tobacco use. What happens to children's smoking patterns when parents quit? Parental modeling could emerge as a key issue in preventing youth smoking. If so, physician intervention with parents might be an effective strategy and more attractive to physicians than the paternalistic interventions now being used.

In the early 1990s, the National Cancer Institute developed an initiative to promote physicians' use of brief counseling interventions. The cornerstone of the intervention is the "Four A's": (1) ask all patients about their smoking behavior, (2) advise smokers on the ill effects of smoking and benefits of cessation, (3) assist in choosing and implementing a cessation method, and (4) arrange to follow up with patients for further support and reinforcement. Meta-analyses of this type of intervention suggest that the most successful results occur when a team of physician and nonphysician providers combine intervention strategies to deliver individualized advice on a number of occasions.[30] Yet evidence suggests that most physicians have not adopted this strategy. What changes need to be made to invigorate physicians' willingness to counsel patients against smoking?

Another important area to pursue is the involvement of pediatricians in direct counseling with adolescents. As a group, pediatricians may be well positioned to address low self-esteem and other threats to adolescent well-being that are also smoking risks.[31]

Relationship to Other Problem Behaviors
Because tobacco use is associated with adolescent problems, physicians should screen adolescent smokers to identify problems that might otherwise go undetected. In traditional health care settings, research indi-

cates that adolescent depression is underdiagnosed and undertreated. Given the strong linkage between depression, substance use, and tobacco use, improved screening for depression may also reduce adolescent tobacco use.

Media Strategies

The American Legacy Foundation and various states (including Massachusetts, California, and Florida) are currently implementing and evaluating countermarketing strategies. Research needs to be conducted on how advertisers and marketers view adolescent smoking and the messages conveyed by tobacco advertising. According to K. Michael Cummings, who has been studying tobacco industry documents, most tobacco advertising strategies were developed by advertisers and marketers rather than by the tobacco industry.[32] If so, understanding better how "Madison Avenue" marketers think about appealing to adolescents may help construct more effective antitobacco marketing strategies.[33]

Adopting a Comprehensive Strategy

The rationale for recommending a comprehensive strategy is straightforward. To begin with, a comprehensive approach benefits from synergies across various interventions. To take just one example, adult smoking cessation has resulted from dissemination of information about the dangers of smoking, from increased excise taxes, from responses to media antismoking campaigns, and from participation in formal smoking cessation programs. No one of these interventions could have successfully prompted all of the adult smoking cessation that has occurred. The diversity of interventions was essential to bring us to the point where half of all Americans who have ever smoked have quit. In the absence of any one of these interventions, a significant number of now former smokers might have remained smokers.

Also, the interventions almost certainly reinforce each other. Information dissemination on the hazards of smoking may move smokers from the precontemplation stage to contemplation of quitting.[34] A media campaign mocking smoking may move the now ambivalent smoker toward action. A cigarette tax increase may push the smoker "over the top," toward successful quitting. The elimination of tobacco billboards in 1999 may aid that former smoker's resolve to continue abstaining. More generally, through specific interventions (e.g., clean indoor air laws) and the norms they help to create (a nonsmoking ethos), the social environment becomes increasingly conducive to quitting.

A balanced program that deals with both adults and adolescents is likely to be more sustainable and more effective than one targeted primarily at either adults or adolescents. As we have shown in chapter 3, the social context in which adolescents contemplate tobacco use is suffused with influences from parents, peers, and popular cultural figures, along with individually predisposing factors. Some of these can be addressed through short-term strategies, while others may be amenable to change, if at all, only through long-term approaches. But focusing on youth or adults alone misses the essential insight that to be effective, policies must address all of the factors influencing adolescents' smoking decisions. As adolescents negotiate the boundaries between adolescence and adulthood, they will inevitably attempt to emulate adult behaviors. For this reason, such policies as clean indoor air laws that affect all tobacco consumers are likely to be more effective than age-specific policies designed to reinforce strong boundaries between adolescent and adult behaviors.

Several recent studies support the comprehensive strategy. First, the National Research Council of the Institute of Medicine released a summary document arguing that state-level tobacco control programs are effective; counteradvertising should be expanded; clean indoor air restrictions reduce smoking, as do increased cigarette taxes; youth access restrictions should be enforced; and tobacco control programs should be evaluated. Second, CDC has issued best practices for tobacco control that are comprehensive in nature and similar to the Institute of Medicine's program.[35] For instance, CDC recommends the expansion of local community prevention programs, school-based programs, and smoking cessation efforts. Third, the initial successes of the comprehensive interventions being implemented in California, Florida, and Massachusetts are more promising than the previously limited interventions being replaced.[36]

Nevertheless, the arguments raised in chapter 1 regarding the rationale for specific adolescent-centered policies are important to keep in mind. As a political matter, such policies command wide public support, so that policymakers will be able to "sell" them more easily to the public and to each other. The advances in adult-oriented antismoking policies, such as worksite smoking restrictions, have not come without

controversy. Further advances, including increased taxes, may be difficult to achieve unless framed as a means of reducing adolescent
tobacco use.

Smoking initiation usually occurs in early adolescence, with heavy
smoking and related problem behaviors arising among the earliest
tobacco-initiating individuals. Devising and implementing strategies
and policies to interfere with this pattern must remain a priority. Even
though tremendous reductions in adolescent tobacco initiation will not
result in dramatically reduced smoking prevalence rates immediately,[37] reduced adolescent tobacco initiation remains a critical strategy
for ensuring a long-term secular decline in tobacco's staggering health
and human costs.

Another reason for a comprehensive approach is the potential for
intergenerational interactions. If smoking declines among parents of
teens, we have reason to believe that adolescent smoking will also
decline. Conversely, if teens can be convinced that smoking is dangerous and stupid, they may influence their parents to quit. In short, one
generation's behavior can influence another's. Something quite similar
has been happening in the environmental movement. With greater
attention to environmental protection in schools, children bring the
message home and influence their parents' outlook toward environmental issues. For instance, more parents are participating in recycling
thanks to their children's interest.

A Thought Experiment

Suppose, for the purposes of a thought experiment, that we are successful beyond expectations in reducing teen smoking. Does this mean
that the problem has been solved or just postponed? There is some reason to believe that the problem would only be postponed. In China,
most people start smoking in their twenties, as was the case in the
United States in the early 1900s. Even now, we have documented some
disturbing trends about the increase in smoking initiation among U.S.
college-age young adults (see chap. 4). Another disturbing trend is the
boomlet in cigar smoking. Previously, cigar smoking was almost exclusively the province of elderly men. Now, young adults, both men and
women, smoke cigars as a status symbol for the glamour and wealth of
high society.

Consider, as well, "Joe's kids," the generation raised on Joe Camel
advertisements. They are now in their 20s and likely to respond to a
more sophisticated marketing approach. That appears to be exactly the

strategy the tobacco industry is pursuing—to make smoking a young adult activity. Tobacco ads have been appearing in publications that focus on the young adult market, knowing that the ads will be widely viewed by an under-18 audience. The new ads emphasize more overtly sexual and sophisticated imagery. Camel also advertises flavored variations in brightly colored packs, presumably to compete with flavored bidis that are gaining sales among adolescents. By appealing to a young adult audience, it is also likely that the industry's campaign will appeal to adolescents.

These potential crossover appeals are exactly why a comprehensive tobacco control strategy is needed. Tobacco control advocates and policymakers need to begin thinking about how to counter the industry's marketing to young adults.

Conclusion

The most obvious conclusion from this book is that while adolescent smoking prevention efforts have had mixed results to date, there are many promising interventions and strategies that may show more positive results in the near future. It is also clear that no one approach is likely to reverse the finding of mixed results, although the few comprehensive programs that have been tried in the states have shown generally positive results in decreasing adolescent tobacco use.

We hope that the reader is convinced by now that there is a wide range of available activities that will discourage adolescent tobacco use. A reader may remain somewhat skeptical and would no doubt be correct to argue that the evidence we have presented does not reveal an absolutely conclusive answer. As one author of this book has written previously: "Ultimately, however, the need for a definitive assessment may prove as unnecessary as it is elusive. Certainty, or the search for it, is the life-blood of the scholar; ambiguity, and probability, are both the dominant realities of life and the currency of politics and the law."[38] Taken in its entirety, the evidence is compelling that tobacco control activities can reduce adolescent tobacco use. At a minimum, it is quite possible that without the measures already taken to discourage adolescent tobacco use, the problem might be much worse than it already is. Even if the specifics of those interventions remain open to dispute, available programs are sufficiently promising to justify continuing investment in tobacco control.

Our view, in short, is that neither doing nothing nor waiting for perfect information on program effectiveness is a viable option. Given the health consequences of routine or habitual tobacco use, we believe that society has an obligation to keep trying different policy strategies to discourage adolescent tobacco use. Tobacco initiation remains largely an adolescent phenomenon that, at least in part, can be disrupted through targeted interventions.

We believe that previous calls for youth-centered tobacco control efforts remain relevant and critically important as we move into the twenty-first century. This book suggests that a number of interventions and strategies deserve further consideration, dissemination, and evaluation. The resources available through the settlement with the tobacco industry provide an unprecedented opportunity to meet the adolescent smoking challenge by investing in youth tobacco control.

We are optimistic about the potential for reducing adolescent tobacco use. The social environment in which tobacco use occurs has changed for the better during the past decade. As recently as the late 1980s, the tobacco industry dominated the policy realm. Since then, the industry has become much more vulnerable to public policy oversight; while it remains a creative and powerful force, its vulnerabilities have been exposed. At least for the foreseeable future, tobacco control advocates will have an enormous opportunity to influence the policy environment. The question for tobacco control advocates is how best to take advantage of this opportunity. From a public health perspective, we are appropriately concerned that the prevalence of youth smoking remains high despite the attention already devoted to this problem and the wide array of interventions that have been tried. Yet it is possible that without these interventions, rates of both experimental and habitual smoking among youth would be even higher.

In this book, we have synthesized what we know about adolescent tobacco use and how we might direct future efforts to discourage and reduce smoking among teens. Without doubt, the social and policy environments for these efforts are more favorable than they have been since the turn of the twentieth century. But history tells us that these favorable trends are not irreversible. By the mid-1920s, the 14 preexisting state laws against smoking had been repealed.[39] Though we do not foresee the same type of reversal in the twenty-first century, it is important to capitalize on the current window of opportunity.

We have also explored what we know about adolescent tobacco use and ways of discouraging teen smoking behavior. We have recommended that states adopt a comprehensive strategy, balancing interventions that directly affect adolescent tobacco use and those that do so indirectly through reducing adult use. In the end, the most important reason for supporting adolescent tobacco control measures is that the impact of tobacco use on the future of children's health is too great simply to abandon the effort.

We close with a final thought about adolescent tobacco control: it is not a short-term fight. When entering the battle against tobacco use, one should be prepared to stay for the long haul. After 35 years, tobacco control has achieved a great deal, enough that it is justifiably ranked among the great public health triumphs of the past 50 years.[40] Yet despite this success, the toll of tobacco remains almost inconceivably high—higher in body count in the United States than the sum total of all other drugs, licit and illicit; all injuries, intentional and otherwise; and all the major infectious diseases, including AIDS. This is hardly the time to declare victory and go home, and few tobacco control advocates have done so.

Battles, often small battles, have been won, and the victories should be savored. But they are never an excuse to lose sight of the bigger picture. Further, the small triumphs should never be considered immutable: just as the smoker who quits faces months and even years of risk of relapse, tobacco control successes are not necessarily ultimate victories. Witness, for example, how the industry converted federally mandated warning labels, which have never been demonstrated to discourage smoking, into successful product liability defenses and protection (preemption) against scores of more draconian and expensive state-based warning systems. Tobacco control—and by extension, other behavioral health intervention issues—demands constant vigilance, evaluation and reevaluation, and creativity in looking forward to the next stages of intervention.

NOTES

1. Warner 1986.

2. Policymakers might consider that one reason why the tobacco industry agreed to remove its advertising from television was the power of antismoking public service announcements

3. The American Legacy Foundation will also sponsor targeted advertising that may not be national in scope.

4. Patten 2000.

5. It is, of course, possible that younger adolescents will smoke more if they know that cessation programs work.

6. The Clinton administration has proposed such a program through Medicaid in its budget request to Congress for fiscal year 2001. Even if enacted, this would leave those not covered by Medicaid without access to cessation therapies involving pharmaceuticals.

7. McCormick and Thompkins 1998; Crossett, Everett, and Brener 1999.

8. Sutton 2000.

9. It is unlikely that the public would support laws restricting smoking in the home. In some cases, family law judges have taken smoking into account in awarding custody and conditioning visitation rights. So far, these are random decisions that do not indicate broad public support for overcoming what most Americans view as the right to conduct their home life with considerable freedom from governmental interference.

10. Gilpin et al. 1999.

11. Ashley et al. 1998.

12. Massing 1998.

13. One analyst predicts that in five years, the Internet will account for as much as 20 percent of all cigarette sales (Armstrong 1999).

14. We thank Mike Pertshuk for this observation.

15. In previous work, two authors of this book indicated opposition to fines and penalties for use and possession (Jacobson and Wasserman 1997). In rethinking this issue, these authors have come to believe that the concerns expressed by tobacco control advocates can be mitigated. Therefore, we now collectively support these programs if they prove to be effective in reducing adolescent tobacco use.

16. Warner, Slade, and Sweanor 1997.

17. Sorensen et al. 1998; Fortmann et al. 1995.

18. Recent CDC efforts, such as the Racial and Ethnic Approaches to Community Health (REACH) initiative to reduce race/ethnic health disparities and HIV prevention community planning, provide useful models of technology transfer to local community groups.

19. Hawkins, Catalano, Miller 1992.

20. Olds et al. 1997; Seitz and Apfel 1994.

21. See, further, Behrman 1999.

22. See, e.g., Epstein, Griffin, and Botvin 2000.

23. One of our interview respondents also suggests focusing on which intervention might have the largest impact: an intervention reaching 90 percent of the population with a small change at the margin or an intervention reaching a smaller population but with greater marginal benefits.

24. Hu, Sung, and Keeler 1995.

25. Mermelstein and the Tobacco Control Network Writing Group 1999. In a personal interview with Peter Jacobson (June 1998), Robin Mermelstein added that various ethnic subgroups respond to different messages. Based on her research, whites are more influenced by traditional advertising than are African Americans.

26. James Koopman, personal communication, September 1999.

27. James Koopman, E-mail message, September 15, 1999.

28. Swan 1999.

29. We thank Michael McGinnis for these suggestions.
30. Epps and Manley 1993.
31. See, e.g., Zellman, Jacobson, and Bell 1997.
32. K. Michael Cummings, personal conversation, June 1999.
33. The American Legacy Foundation's advertising agencies are doing so.
34. Prochaska et al. 1993; Velicer et al. 1993.
35. IOM 2000.
36. As discussed in chapter 4, these programs represent varying levels of comprehensiveness, with Florida's program being considerably less comprehensive than those in California and Massachusetts. See Wakefield and Chaloupka (2000) for further discussion.
37. Mendez and Warner 1998.
38. Warner 1986.
39. Jacobson, Wasserman, and Anderson 1997.
40. USDHHS 1989; CDC 1999a.

Bibliography

Abernathy, T. 1997. Differences in the reported prevalence of adolescents who have never smoked. *American Journal of Public Health* 87:298–99.

Abernathy, T. J., L. Massad, and L. Romano-Dwyer. 1995. The relationship between smoking and self-esteem. *Adolescence* 30:899–907.

Aguirre-Molina, M., and D. M. Gorman. 1996. Community-based approaches for the prevention of alcohol, tobacco, and other drug use. *Annual Review of Public Health* 17:337–58.

AHRQ [Agency for Healthcare Research and Quality]. 2000. AHRQ cessation guidelines. <http://www.ahcpr.gov/clinic/> (June 12, 2000).

Aitken, P. P., and D. R. Eadie. 1990. Reinforcing effects of cigarette advertising on underage smoking. *British Journal of Addiction* 85:399–412.

Aitken, P. P., et al. 1991. Predisposing effects of cigarette ads on children's intent to smoke when older. *British Journal of Addiction* 86:383–90.

Akerlof, G., and W. Dickens. 1982. Economic consequences of cognitive dissonance. *American Economic Review* 72:307–19.

Allen, K., A. Moss, G. A. Giovino, D. Shopland, and J. P. Pierce. 1993. Teenage smoking data. Estimates from the teenage attitudes and practices survey— United States, 1989. *Advance Data from Vital and Health Statistics* 224. Hyattsville, Md.: National Center for Health Statistics.

Aloise-Young, P. A., and K. M. Hennigan. 1996. Self-image, the smoker stereotype, and cigarette smoking: Development patterns from fifth through eighth grade. *Journal of Adolescence* 19:163–77.

Aloise-Young, P. A., K. M. Hennigan, and J. W. Graham. 1996. Role of the self-image and smoker stereotype in smoking onset during early adolescence: A longitudinal study. *Health Psychology* 15:494–97.

Altman, D. G., D. W. Levine, R. Coeytaux, J. Slade, and R. Jaffe. 1996. Tobacco promotion and susceptibility to tobacco use among adolescents aged 12 through 17 years in a nationally representative sample. *American Journal of Public Health* 86:1590–93.

Altman, D. G., A. Y. Wheelis, M. McFarlane, H. Lee, and S. P. Fortmann. 1999. The relationship between tobacco access and use among adolescents: A four-community study. *Social Science and Medicine* 48:759–75.

American Legacy Foundation. The Public Education Campaign. <http://www.americanlegacy.org/grants/marketing.html>.

261

Anda, R., et al. 1990. Depression and the dynamics of smoking. *Journal of the American Medical Association* 264:1541–45.

Anda, R. F., J. B. Croft, V. J. Felitti, D. Nordenberg, W. H. Giles, D. F. Williamson, and G. A. Giovino. 1999. Adverse childhood experiences and smoking during adolescence and adulthood. *Journal of the American Medical Association* 282:1652–58.

Annas, G. J. 1997. Tobacco litigation as cancer prevention: Dealing with the devil. *New England Journal of Medicine* 336 (4): 304–8.

Anonymous. 1999. Tobacco Wars Still. *Washington Post,* December 29, p. A26.

Armstrong, L. 1999. All the tar and none of the taxes. *Business Week,* December 13, p. 8.

Arnett, J. J., and G. Terhanian. 1998. Adolescents' responses to cigarette advertisements: Links between exposure, liking, and the appeal of smoking. *Tobacco Control* 7:129–33.

Ashley, M. J., J. Cohen, R. Ferrence et al. 1998. Smoking in the home: changing attitudes and current practices. *American Journal of Public Health* 1998, 88:797–800.

Aveyard, P., K. K. Cheng, J. Almond, E. Sherratt, R. Lancashire, T. Lawrence, C. Griffin, and O. Evans. 1999. Cluster randomised controlled trial of expert system based on the transtheoretical ("stages of change") model for smoking prevention and cessation in schools. *British Medical Journal* 319:948–53.

Bachman, J. G., L. D. Johnston, and P. M. O'Malley. 1990. Explaining the recent decline in cocaine use among young adults: Further evidence that perceived risks and disapproval lead to reduced drug use. *Journal of Health and Social Behavior* 31:173–84.

Bachman, J. G., L. D. Johnston, P. M. O'Malley, and R. H. Humphrey. 1988. Explaining the recent decline in marijuana use: Differentiating the effects of perceived risks, disapproval, and general lifestyle factors. *Journal of Health and Social Behavior* 29:92–112.

Bachman, J. G., K. N. Wadsworth, P. M. O'Malley, L. D. Johnston, and J. Schulenberg. 1997. *Smoking, Drinking, and Drug Use in Young Adulthood: The Impacts of New Freedoms and Responsibilities.* Mahway, N.J.: Lawrence Erlbaum Associates.

Bailey, S. I., S. T. Ennett, and C. L. Ringwalt. 1993. Potential mediators, moderators, or independent effects in the relationship between parents' former and current cigarette use and their children's cigarette use. *Addictive Behaviors* 18:601–21.

Baker, L. S., G. E. Morley, and D. C. Barker. 1995. Health-care provider advice on tobacco use to persons aged 10–12–22 years—United States, 1993. *Morbidity & Mortality Weekley Report* 44 (44): 826–30.

Balbach, E. D., and S. A. Glantz. 1998. Tobacco control advocates must demand high-quality media campaigns: The California experience. *Tobacco Control* 7:397–408.

Baltagi, B. H., and D. Levin. 1977. Estimating dynamic demand for cigarettes using panel data: The effects of bootlegging, taxation, and advertising reconsidered. In *Review of social learning theory.* Englewood Cliffs: Prentice-Hall.

————. 1986. Estimating dynamic demand for cigarettes using panel data: The effects of bootlegging, taxation and advertising reconsidered. *Review of Economics and Statistics* 68:148–55.

Bandura, A. 1977. *Social Learning Theory.* Englewood Cliffs: Prentice-Hall.

Barnett, P. G., T. E. Keeler, and T. W. Hu. 1995. Oligopoly structure and the incidence of cigarette excise taxes. *Journal of Public Economics* 57:457–70.

Barzel, Y. 1976. An alternative approach to the analysis of taxation. *Journal of Political Economy* 84:1177–97.

Bauman, K. E., G. J. Botvin, E. M. Botvin, and E. Baker. 1992. Normative expectations and the behavior of significant others: An integration of traditions in research on adolescents' cigarette smoking. *Psychological Reports* 71:568–70.

Bauman, K. E., V. A. Foshee, M. A. Linzer, and G. G. Koch. 1990. Effect of parental smoking classification on the association between parental and adolescent smoking. *Addictive Behaviors* 15:413–22.

Bearman, N. S., A. O. Goldstein, and D. C. Bryan. 1995. Legislating clean air: Politics, preemption, and the health of the public. *North Carolina Medical Journal* 56:14–19.

Becker, G. S., M. Grossman, and K. M. Murphy. 1994. An Empirical Analysis of Cigarette Addiction. *American Economic Review* 84:396–418.

Becker, G. S., and K. M. Murphy. 1988. A theory of rational addiction. *Journal of Political Economy* 96 (4): 675–700.

Behrman, R. E., ed. 1999. When school is out. *Future of Children* 9 (2): 1–160 .

Benowitz, N. L. 1992. The genetics of drug dependence: Tobacco addiction. *New England Journal of Medicine* 327:881–83.

Benowitz, N. L., and J. E. Henningfield. 1994. Establishing a nicotine threshold for addiction. *New England Journal of Medicine* 331:123–25.

Bental, D. S., A. Cawsey, and R. Jones. 1999. Patient information systems that tailor to the individual. *Patient Education and Counseling* 36:171–80.

Bhonsle, R. B., R. P. Murti, and P. C. Gupta. 1992. Tobacco habits in India. In *Control of tobacco-related cancers and other diseases,* ed. P. C. Gupta, J. E. Hamner III, and P. R. Muri. Bombay: Oxford University Press.

Biener, L., and G. Fitzgerald. 1999. Smoky bars and restaurants: Who avoids them and why? *Journal of Public Health Management Practice* 5:74–78.

Biener, L. W. 1999. *Progress toward reducing smoking in the Commonwealth of Massachusetts from 1993 through FY 1999.* Boston: Center for Survey Research, University of Massachusetts at Boston.

Biglan, A., D. Ary, V. Koehn, et al. 1996. Mobilizing positive reinforcement in communities to reduce youth access to tobacco. *American Journal of Community Psychology* 24:625–38.

Biglan, A., D. V. Ary, K. Smolkowski, T. Duncan, and C. Black. 1999. A randomized controlled trial of a community intervention to prevent adolescent tobacco use. *Tobacco Control* 9:24–32.

Biglan, A., D. Ary, H. Yudelson, et al. 1996. Experimental evaluation of a modular approach to mobilizing antitobacco influences of peers and parents. *American Journal of Community Psychology* 24:311–39.

Biglan A., et al. 1995. Peer and parental influences on adolescent tobacco use. *Journal of Behavioral Medicine* 18:315–30.

Biglan, A., and C. W. Metzler. 1998. A public health perspective for research on family-focused interventions. In *National Institute of Drug Addiction Monographs*, no. 177. Bethesda, MD: U.S. Department of Health and Human Services.

Black, D. R., N. S. Tobler, and J. P. Sciacca. 1998. Peer helping/involvement: An efficacious way to meet the challenge of reducing alcohol, tobacco, and other drug use among youth? *Journal of School Health* 68 (3): 87–93.

Bloom, P. N., and W. D. Novelli. 1981. Problems and challenges in social marketing. *Journal of Marketing* 45:79–88.

Borden, N. 1942. *The Economic Effects of Advertising*. Chicago: Richard D. Irwin.

Borrelli, B., et al. 1996. The impact of depression on smoking cessation in women. *American Journal of Preventive Medicine* 12:378–87.

Botvin, G. J., E. Baker, L. Dusenbury, E. M. Botvin, and T. Diaz. 1995. Long-term follow-up results of a randomized drug abuse prevention trial in a white middle-class population. *Journal of the American Medical Association* 273:1106–12.

Botvin, G. J., E. M. Botvin, E. Baker, L. Dusenbury, and C. J. Goldberg. 1992. The false consensus effect: Predicting adolescents' tobacco use from normative expectations. *Psychological Reports* 70:171–78.

Botvin, G. J., C. J. Goldberg, E. M. Botvin, and L. Dusenbury. 1993. Smoking behavior of adolescents exposed to cigarette advertising. *Public Health Reports* 108:217–24.

Bowen, D. J., S. Kinne, and M. Orlandi. 1995. School policy in COMMIT: A promising strategy to reduce smoking by youth. *Journal of School Health* 65:140–44.

Boyum, D., and M. Kleiman. 1995. Alcohol and other drugs. In *Crime*, ed. J. Q. Wilson and J. Petersilia. San Francisco: Institute for Contemporary Studies.

Breslau, N., and E. L. Peterson. 1996. Smoking cessation in young adults: Age at initiation of cigarette smoking and other suspected influences. *American Journal of Public Health* 86:214–20.

Brown and Williamson. 2000. <http://www.brownandwilliamson.com> (9/26/2000).

Brown and Williamson Collection CD-ROM, The University of California, San Francisco, Library and Center for Knowledge Management.

Brownson, R. C., J. R. Davis, J. Jackson-Thompson, and J. C. Wilkerson. 1995. Environmental tobacco smoke awareness and exposure: Impact of a statewide clean indoor air law and the report of the U.S. Environmental Protection Agency. *Tobacco Control* 4:132–44.

Brownson, R. C., M. P. Eriksen, R. M. Davis, and K. E. Warner. 1997. Environmental tobacco smoke: Health effects and policies to reduce exposure. *Annual Review of Public Health* 18:163–85.

Bruvold, W. H. 1993. A meta-analysis of adolescent smoking prevention programs. *American Journal of Public Health* 83 (6): 872–80.

Burt, R. D., and A. V. Peterson. 1998. Smoking cessation among high school seniors. *Preventive Medicine* 27:319–27.

Business Wire. 2000. Ten-year report hails the California anti-tobacco program for saving lives and millions in taxpayers' dollars. <http// biz .yahoo.com/bw/000217/ca_cali_de_l.html> (March 2000).

California documents from the State of Minnesota depository. 1999. <http://www.library.ucsf.edu/tobacco/calminnesota> (9/26/2000).

California EPA [Environmental Protection Agency]. 1997. Health effects of exposure to environmental tobacco smoke. *Tobacco Control* 6:346–53.

Camp, D. E., R. C. Klesges, and G. Relyea. 1993. The relationship between body weight concerns and adolescent smoking. *Health Psychology* 12:24–32.

Carmelli, D., G. E. Swan, D. Robinette, and R. Fabsitz. 1992. Genetic influence on smoking—a study of male twins. *New England Journal of Medicine* 327:829–33.

Caulkins, J. P., and P. Reuter. 1998. What price data tell us about drug markets. *Journal of Drug Issues* 28:593–612.

CDC [Centers for Disease Control and Prevention]. 1999j. Life Skills Training. <http://www.cdc.gov/nccdphp/dash/rtc/curric6.html> (March 2000).

———. 1991. Cigarette smoking among youth—United States, 1989. *MMWR* 40:712–15.

———. 1994. Guidelines for school health programs to prevent tobacco use and addiction. *MMWR* 43 (RR-2): 1–18. Available at <http://aepo-xdv -www.epo.cdc.gov/wonder/prevguid/m0026213/mo0026213.html> (March 2000).

———. 1995. Minors' access to smokeless tobacco—Florida, 1994. *MMWR* 44:839–41.

———. 1996a. Accessibility to minors of smokeless tobacco products— Broward County, Florida. *MMWR* 45:1079–82.

———. 1996b. Estimates of retailers willing to sell tobacco to minors—California, August–September 1995 and June–July 1996. *MMWR* 45:1095–99.

———. 1996c. Youth risk behavior surveillance—United States, 1995. *MMWR* 45 (SS04): 181–84.

———. 1996d. Accessibility of tobacco products to youths ages 12–17 years— United States, 1989 and 1993. *MMWR* 45:125–30.

———. 1996e. Tobacco use and usual source of cigarettes among high school students—United States, 1995. *MMWR* 45:413–18.

———. 1997a. Cigar smoking among teenagers—United States, Massachusetts, and New York, 1996. *MMWR* 46:433–40.

———. 1997b. Smoking-attributable mortality and years of potential life lost— United States, 1984. *MMWR* 46:444–51.

———. 1998a. Youth risk behavior surveillance—United States, 1997. *MMWR* 47 (SS03): 1–89.

———. 1998b. Incidence of initiation of cigarette smoking—United States, 1965–1996. *MMWR* 47:837–40.

———. 1998c. State-specific prevalence among adults of current cigarette smoking and smokeless tobacco use and per capita tax-paid sales of cigarettes—United States, 1997. *MMWR* 47:922–26.

———. 1999a. Tobacco use among middle and high school students—Florida, 1998 and 1999. *MMWR* 48:248–53.

————. 1999b. Bidi use among urban youth—Massachusetts. *MMWR* 48: 796–99.

————. 1999c. Cigarette smoking among high school students—11 states, 1991–1997. *MMWR* 48:686–92.

————. 1999d. State tobacco activities tracking and evaluation. <http://www2.cdc.gov/nccdphp/osh/state> (9/26/2000).

————. 1999e. Youth risk behavior surveillance—national alternative high school youth risk behavior survey, United States, 1998. *MMWR* 48 (SS07): 1–44.

————. 1999f. Cigarette smoking among adults—United States, 1997. *MMWR* 48:993–96.

————. 1999g. Preemptive state tobacco-control laws—United States, 1982–1998. *MMWR* 47:1112–14.

————. 1999h. Achievements in public health, 1900–1999: Tobacco use—United States, 1900–1999. *MMWR* 48:986–93.

————. 1999i. State laws on tobacco control—United States, 1998. *MMWR.* 48 (SS03): 21–62.

————. 1999j. *Best practices for comprehensive tobacco control programs.* Atlanta, GA: U.S. Department of Health and Human Services, Centers for Disease Control and Prevention, National Center for Chronic Disease Prevention and Health Promotion, Office on Smoking and Health.

————. 1999k. Tobacco use prevention curriculum and evaluation fact sheets. <http://www.cdc.gov/nccdphp/dash/rtc/tob-curric.html> (March 2000).

————. 2000a. Tobacco use among middle and high school students—United States, 1999. *MMWR* 49 (3): 49–53.

————. 2000b. Youth risk behavior surveillance—United States, 1999. *MMWR* 49 (SS05): 1–96.

————. 1999j. Project Towards No Tobacco Use <http://www.cdc.gov/nccdphp/dash/rtc/curric7.html> (6/12/2000).

————. 2000d. CDC cessation guidelines. <http://www.cdc.gov/tobacco/how2quit.htm> (June 12, 2000).

Chaloupka, F. J. 1988. An economic analysis of addictive behavior: The case of cigarette smoking. Ph.D. diss., City University of New York.

————. 1990. Rational addictive behavior and cigarette smoking. Working paper no. 3268, National Bureau of Economic Research, Cambridge, MA.

————. 1991. Rational addictive behavior and cigarette smoking. *Journal of Political Economy* 99:722–42.

————. 1998. *The impact of proposed cigarette price increases.* Health Science Analysis Project, Policy Analysis 9. Washington, DC: Advocacy Institute.

————. 1999. Macro-social influences: The effects of prices and tobacco-control policies on the demand for tobacco products. *Nicotine and Tobacco Research* 1 (supp. 1): 105–9.

Chaloupka, F. J. 1990. Rational addictive behavior and cigarette smoking. National Bureau of Economic Research. Working paper 3268.

Chaloupka, F. J., and M. Grossman. 1996. Price, tobacco control policies, and youth smoking. Working paper no. 5740, National Bureau of Economic Research, Cambridge, MA.

Chaloupka, F. J., and A. Laixuthai. 1997. Do youths substitute alcohol and marijuana? Some econometric evidence. *Eastern Economic Journal* 23:253–76.

Chaloupka, F. J., and R. L. Pacula. 1999. Sex and race differences in young people's responsiveness to price and tobacco control policies. *Tobacco Control* 8:373–77.

Chaloupka, F., H. Saffer, and M. Grossman. 1993. Alcohol-control policies and motor-vehicle fatalities. *Journal of Legal Studies* 22:161–86.

Chaloupka, F. J., and K. E. Warner. 2000. The economics of smoking. In *Handbook of health economics,* ed. J. P. Newhouse and A. Cuyler. New York: Elsevier.

Chaloupka, F. J., and H. Wechsler. 1997. Price, tobacco control policies, and smoking among young adults. *Journal of Health Economics* 16:359–73.

Chapman Walsh, D., R. E. Rudd, B. A. Moeykens, and T. W. Moloney. 1993. Social marketing for public health. *Health Affairs,* summer, 104–19.

Charlton, A., K. E. Minagawa, and D. While. 1999. Saying "no" to cigarettes: A reappraisal of adolescent refusal skills. *Journal of Adolescence* 22:695–707.

Chassin, L. 1996. The natural history of cigarette smoking from adolescence to adulthood: Demographic predictors of continuity and change. *Health Psychology* 15:478–84.

Chen, K., and D. B. Kandel. 1995. The natural history of drug use from adolescence to the mid-thirties in a general population sample. *American Journal of Public Health* 85:41–47.

Choi, W. S., J. P. Pierce, E. A. Gilpin, A. J. Farkas, and C. C. Berry. 1997. Which adolescent experimenters progress to established smoking in the United States. *American Journal of Preventive Medicine* 13:385–91.

Cigarette makers lift wholesale prices 8%. 1999. *New York Times,* August 31, p. C-5.

Cimons, M. 2000. State programs credited for dip in lung cancer. *Los Angeles Times,* December 1, 2000, P. A-1.

COMMIT Research Group. 1995a. Community Intervention Trial for Smoking Cessation (COMMIT). Part 1, Cohort results from a four-year community intervention. *American Journal of Public Health* 85:183–92.

———. 1995b. Community Intervention Trial for Smoking Cessation (COMMIT). Part 2, Changes in adult cigarette smoking prevalence. *American Journal of Public Health* 85:193–200.

Connolly, G., and H. Robbins. 1998. Designing an effective statewide tobacco control program—Massachusetts. *Cancer* 83 (supp.): 2722–27.

Conrad, K. M., B. R. Flay, and D. Hill. 1992. Why children start smoking cigarettes: Predictors of onset. *British Journal of Addiction* 87:1711–24.

Cook, P. J., and M. Moore. 1994. This tax's for you: The case for higher beer taxes. *National Tax Journal* 47:559–73.

———. 1999. Alcohol. Working paper no. W6905, National Bureau of Economic Research, Cambridge, MA.

Crisp, A., P. Sedgwick, C. Halek, N. Joughin, and H. Humphrey. 1999. Why may teenage girls persist in smoking? *Journal of Adolescence* 22:657–72.

Cromwell, J., W. J. Bartosch, M. C. Fiore, V. Hasselblad, and T. Baker. 1997. Cost-effectiveness of the clinical practice recommendations in the AHCPR guideline for smoking cessation. *Journal of the American Medical Association* 278:1759–66.

Crossett, L., S. A. Everett, and N. D. Brener. 1999. Adherence to the CDC guidelines for school health programs to prevent tobacco use and addiction. *Journal of Health Education* Sept/Oct supp. 1999, vol. 30, no. 5, S4–S11.

Cummings, K. M., A. Hyland, T. F. Pechacek, M. Orlandi, and W. R. Lynn. 1997. Comparison of recent trends in adolescent and adult cigarette smoking behaviour and brand preferences. *Tobacco Control* 6 (supp. 2): S31–S37.

Cummings, K. M., A. Hyland, T. Saunders-Martin, J. Perla, P. R. Coppola, and T. F. Pechacek. 1998. Evaluation of an enforcement program to reduce tobacco sales to minors. *American Journal of Public Health* 88:932–36.

Currie, J. 1995. *Welfare and the well-being of children.* Chur, Switzerland: Harwood Academic.

DeCicca, P., D. Kenkel, and A. Mathios. 1998. Putting out the fires: Will higher cigarette taxes reduce youth smoking? Working paper, Department of Policy Analysis and Management, Cornell University.

Dee, T., and W. Evans. 1997. Teen drinking and education attainment: Evidence from two-sample instrumental variables (TSIV) estimates. Working paper no. 6082, National Bureau of Economic Research, Cambridge, MA.

———. 1998. A comment on DeCicca, Kenkel, and Mathios. Working paper, School of Economics, Georgia Institute of Technology.

Derzon, J. H., and M. W. Lipsey. 1999. Predicting tobacco use to age 18: A synthesis of longitudinal research. *Addiction* 94:995–1006.

Des Jarlais, D. C. 1995. Harm reduction—a framework for incorporating science into drug policy. *American Journal of Public Health* 85:10–12.

DiFranza, J. R. 1999. Are the federal and state governments complying with the Synar Amendment? *Archives of Pediatrics and Adolescent Medicine* 153:1089–97.

DiFranza, J. R., and L. J. Brown. 1992. The tobacco institute's "It's the Law" campaign: Has it halted illegal sales of tobacco to children? *American Journal of Public Health* 82:1271–73.

DiFranza, J. R., et al. 1991. RJR Nabisco's cartoon camel promotes Camel cigarettes to children. *Journal of the American Medical Association* 266:3149–53.

DiFranza, J. R., and N. A. Rigotti. 1999. Impediments to the enforcement of youth access laws. *Tobacco Control* 8:152–55.

DiFranza, J. R., J. A. Savageau, and B. F. Aisquit. 1996. Youth access to tobacco: The effects of age, gender, vending matching locks and "It's the Law" programs. *American Journal of Public Health* 86:221–24.

Dijkstra, M., I. Mesters, H. De Vries, G. Van Breukelen, and G. S. Parcel. 1999. Effectiveness of a social influence approach and boosters to smoking prevention. *Health Education Research* 14:791–802.

Dinh, K. T., I. G. Sarason, and A. V. Peterson. 1995. Children's perceptions of smokers and nonsmokers: A longitudinal study. *Health Psychology* 14:32–40.

Distefan, J. M., E. A. Gilpin, W. S. Choi, and J. P. Pierce. 1998. Parental influences predict adolescent smoking in the United States—1989–1993. *Journal of Adolescent Health* 22:466–74.

Distefan, J. M., E. A. Gilpin, J. D. Sargent, and J. P. Pierce. 1999. Do movie stars encourage adolescents to start smoking? Evidence from California. *Preventive Medicine* 28:1–11.

Dolcini, M. M., and N. E. Adler. 1994. Perceived competencies, peer group affiliations, and risk behavior among early adolescents. *Health Psychology* 13:496–506.

Donovan, J. E., R. Jessor, and F. M. Costa. 1991. Adolescent health behavior and conventionality-unconventionality: An extension of problem-behavior theory. *Health Psychology* 10:52–61.

Douglas, S. 1998. The duration of the smoking habit. *Economic Inquiry* 36:49–64.

Douglas, S., and G. Hariharan. 1994. The hazard of starting smoking: Estimates from a split population duration model. *Journal of Health Economics* 13:213–30.

Drew, C. 1998. RJR Nabisco unit admits smuggling: Cigarette seller evaded taxes, using Mohawk reservation. *New York Times*, 12/23/98, p. A1.

Elder, J. P., J. F. Sallis, S. I. Woodruff, and M. B. Wildey. 1993. Tobacco-refusal skills and tobacco use among high-risk adolescents. *Journal of Behavioral Medicine* 16:629–42.

Elders, M. J., C. L. Perry, M. P. Eriksen, and G. A. Giovino. 1994. The report of the surgeon general: Preventing tobacco use among young people. *American Journal of Public Health* 84:542–47.

Ellickson, P. L., and R. D. Hays. 1992. On becoming involved with drugs: Modeling adolescent drug use over time. *Health Psychiatry* 11:377–85.

Enforcement policy guidelines for North Carolina. 2000. <http://www.communityhealth.dhhs.state.nc.us/tobacco/grguide/enforce.html> (March 2000).

Engels, R. C., R. A. Knibbe, H. de Vries, and M. J. Drop. 1998. Antecedents of smoking cessation among adolescents: Who is motivated to change? *Preventive Medicine* 27:348–57.

Engels, R. C., R. A. Knibbe, M. J. Drop, and Y. T. de Haan. 1997. Homogeneity of cigarette smoking within groups: Influence or selection? *Health Education and Behavior* 24:801–11.

Ennett, S. T., and K. E. Bauman. 1994. The contribution of influence and selection to adolescent peer group homogeneity: The case of adolescent cigarette smoking. *Journal of Personality and Social Psychology* 67:653–63.

Ennett, S. T., K. E. Bauman, and G. G. Koch. 1994. Variability in cigarette smoking within and between adolescent friendship cliques. *Addictive Behaviors* 19:295–305.

Ennett, S. T., N. S. Tobler, C. L. Ringwalt, and R. L. Flewelling. 1994. How effective is drug abuse resistance education? A meta-analysis of Project DARE outcome evaluations. *American Journal of Public Health* 84:1394–401.

Ennett, S. T., D. P. Rosenbaum, R. L. Flewelling, G. S. Bieler, C. L. Ringwalt, and S. L. Bailey. 1994. Long-term evaluation of drug abuse resistance education. *Addictive Behaviors* 19:113–25.

EPA [Environmental Protection Agency]. 1993. *EPA fact sheet—respiratory health effects of passive smoking.* EPA-43-F-93–003. Washington, DC.

Epps, R. P., and M. W. Manley. 1992. The clinician's role in preventing smoking initiation. *Medical Clinics of North America* 76:439–50.

———. 1993. Prevention of tobacco use during childhood and adolescence: Five steps to prevent the onset of smoking. *Cancer* 72:1002–4.

Epps, R. P., M. W. Manley, and T. J. Glynn. 1995. Tobacco use among adolescents: Strategies for prevention. *Pediatric Clinics of North America* 42:389–402.

Epstein, J. A., G. J. Botvin, and T. Diaz. 1998a. Ethnic and gender differences in smoking prevalence among a longitudinal sample of inner-city adolescents. *Journal of Adolescent Health* 23:160–66.

———. 1998b. Linguistic acculturation and gender effects on smoking among Hispanic youth. *Preventive Medicine* 27:583–89.

Epstein, J. A., K. W. Griffin, and G. J. Botvin. 2000. Competence skills help deter smoking among inner city adolescents. *Tobacco Control* 9:33–39.

Epstein, J. A., C. Williams, G. J. Botvin, T. Diaz, and M. Ifill-Williams. 1999. Psychosocial predictors of cigarette smoking among adolescents living in public housing developments. *Tobacco Control* 8:45–52.

Escobedo, L. G., S. E. Marcus, D. Holtzman, and G. A. Giovino. 1993. Sports participation, age at smoking initiation, and the risk of smoking among US high school students. *Journal of the American Medical Association* 269:1391–95.

Evans, N., A. Farkas, E. Gilpin, C. Berry, and J. Pierce. 1995. Influence of tobacco marketing and exposure to smokers on adolescent susceptibility to smoking. *Journal of the National Cancer Institute* 87:1538–45.

Evans, W. N., and M. C. Farrelly. 1998. The Compensating Behavior of Smokers: Taxes, Tar, and Nicotine. *RAND Journal of Economics* 29:578–95.

Evans, W. N., and L. X. Huang. 1998. Cigarette taxes and teen smoking: New evidence from panels of repeated cross-sections. Working paper, Department of Economics, University of Maryland.

Everett, S. A., G. A. Giovino, C. W. Warren, L. Crossett, and L. Kann. 1998. Other substance use among high school students who use tobacco. *Journal of Adolescent Health* 23:289–96.

Everett, S. A., C. W. Warren, D. Sharp, L. Kann, C. G. Husten, and L. S. Crossett. 1999. Initiation of cigarette smoking behavior among U.S. high school students. *Preventive Medicine* 29:327–33.

Farkas, A. J., E. A. Gilpin, J. M. Distefan, and J. P. Pierce. 1999. The effects of household and workplace smoking restrictions on quitting behaviors. *Tobacco Control* 8:261–65.

Farkas, A. J., E. A. Gilpin, M. M. White, J. P. Pierce. 2000. Association between household and workplace smoking restrictions and adolescent smoking. *Journal of the American Medical Association* 284:717–22.

Farrell, A. D., S. J. Danish, and C. W. Howard. 1992. Risk factors for drug use in urban adolescents: Identification and cross-validation. *American Journal of Community Psychology* 20:263–86.

Farrelly, M. C., and J. W. Bray. 1998. Response to increases in cigarette prices by race/ethnicity, income, and age groups—United States, 1976–1993. *MMWR* 47:605–9.

Farrelly, M. C., W. N. Evans, and A. E. S. Sfekas. 1999. The impact of workplace smoking bans: Results from a national survey. *Tobacco Control* 8:272–77.

FDA [Food and Drug Administration]. 1996. Regulations restricting the sale and distribution of cigarettes and smokeless tobacco to protect children and adolescents; final rule. *Federal Register* 61:44396–5318.

Feigelman, W., and J. Lee. 1995. Probing the paradoxical pattern of cigarette smoking among African-Americans: Low teenage consumption and high adult use. *Journal of Drug Education* 25:307–20.

Feighery, E., D. G. Altman, and G. Shaffer. 1991. The effects of combining education and enforcements to reduce tobacco sales to minors. *Journal of the American Medical Association* 266:3168–71.

Feighery, E., D. L. Borzekowski, C. Schooler, and J. Flora. 1998. Seeing, wanting, owning: The relationship between receptivity to tobacco marketing and smoking susceptibility in young people. *Tobacco Control* 7:123–28.

Felitti, V. J., R. F. Anda, D. Nordenberg, D. F. Williamson, A. M. Spitz, V. Edwards, M. P. Koss, and J. S. Marks. 1998. Relationship of childhood abuse and household dysfunction to many of the leading causes of death in adults, The Adverse Childhood Experiences (ACE) Study. *American Journal of Preventive Medicine* 14:245–58.

Fennell, T. 1994. Risky business: Tax-weary Canadians help support a boom in smuggled alcohol. *MacLean's,* July 11, pp. 14–16.

Fergusson, D. M., and L. J. Horwood. 1995. Transitions to cigarette smoking during adolescence. *Addictive Behaviors* 20:627–42.

Fergusson, D. M., M. T. Lynskey, and L. J. Horwood. 1995. The role of peer affiliations, social, family and individual factors in continuities in cigarette smoking between childhood and adolescence. *Addiction* 90:647–59.

Ferrence, R., J. Slade, R. Room, and M. Pope, eds. 2000. *Nicotine and public health.* Washington, DC: American Public Health Association.

Fichtenberg, C. M., and S. A. Glantz. 2000. Association of the California tobacco control program with declines in cigarette consumption and mortality from heart disease. *New England Journal of Medicine* 343:1772–77.

Fighting Back. 2000. <http://www.rwjf.org/nation/jnation.htm> (June 12, 2000).

Flay, B. R., F. B. Hu, and J. Richardson. 1998. Psychosocial predictors of different stages of cigarette smoking among high school students. *Preventive Medicine* 27:A9–A18.

Flay, B. R., F. B. Hu, O. Siddiqui, L. E. Day, D. Hedeker, J. Petraitis, J. Richardson, and S. Sussman. 1994. Differential influence of parental smoking and friends' smoking on adolescent initiation and escalation of smoking. *Journal of Health and Social Behavior* 35:248–65.

Flay, B. R., J. Petraitis, and F. B. Hu. 1999. Psychosocial risk and protective factors for adolescent tobacco use. *Nicotine and Tobacco Research* 1 (supp. 1): 59–65.

Florida Department of Health, Office of Tobacco Control. 2000. Report regarding the progress of the Tobacco Pilot Program, March 17.

Floyd, R., et al. 1993. Review of smoking in pregnancy: Effects on pregnancy outcomes and cessation efforts. *Annual Review of Public Health* 14:379–411.

Flynn, B. S., J. K. Worden, and R. H. Secker-Walker. 1994. Mass media and school interventions for cigarette smoking prevention: Effects two years after completion. *American Journal of Public Health* 84 (7): 1148–50.

Flynn, B. S., J. K. Worden, R. H. Secker-Walker, G. J. Badger, B. M. Geller, and M. C. Costanza. 1992. Prevention of cigarette smoking through mass media intervention and school programs. *American Journal of Public Health* 82 (6): 827–34.

Forster, J. L., D. M. Murray, M. Wolfson, T. M. Blaine, A. C. Wagenaar, and D. J. Hennrikus. 1998. The effects of community policies to reduce youth access to tobacco. *American Journal of Public Health* 88:1193–98.

Forster, J. L., and M. Wolfson. 1998. Youth access to tobacco: Policies and politics. *Annual Review of Public Health* 19:203–35.

Forster, J. L., M. Wolfson, D. M. Murray, A. C. Wagenaar, and A. J. Claxton. 1997. Perceived and measured availability of tobacco to youth in 14 Minnesota communities: The TPOP Study. *American Journal of Preventive Medicine* 13:167–74.

Fortmann, S. P., J. A. Flora, M. A.Winkleby, C. Schooler, C. B. Taylor, and J. W. Farquar. 1995. Community-intervention trials: Reflections on the Stanford Five-City Project experience. *American Journal of Epidemiology* 142:576–86.

Frank, E., M. A. Winkleby, D. G. Altman, B. Rockhill, and S. P. Fortmann. 1991. Predictors of physicians' smoking cessation advice. *Journal of the American Medical Association* 266:3139–44.

Frankowski, B. L., and R. H. Secker-Walker. 1989. Advising parents to stop smoking: Opportunities and barriers in pediatric practice. *American Journal of Diseases in Children* 143 (9): 1091–94.

Frankowski, B. L., S. O. Weaver, and R. H. Secker-Walker. 1993. Advising parents to stop smoking: Pediatricians' and parents' attitudes. *Pediatrics* 91:296–300.

French, S. A., C. L. Perry, G. R. Leon, and J. A. Fulkerson. 1994. Weight concerns, dieting behavior, and smoking initiation among adolescents: A prospective study. *American Journal of Public Health* 84:1818–20.

Fujii, E. T. 1980. The demand for cigarettes: Further empirical evidence and its implications for public policy. *Applied Economics* 12:479–89.

Galbraith, J. W., and M. Kaiserman. 1997. Taxation, smuggling, and demand for cigarettes in Canada: Evidence from time-series data. *Journal of Health Economics* 16:287–301.

Gemson, D. H., H. L. Moats, B. X. Watkins, M. L. Ganz, S. Robinson, and E. Healton. 1998. Laying down the law: Reducing illegal tobacco sales to minors in Central Harlem. *American Journal of Public Health* 88:936–39.

Gilpin, E. A., and J. P. Pierce. 1997. Trends in adolescent smoking initiation in the United States: Is tobacco marketing an influence? *Tobacco Control* 6:122–27.

Gilpin, E. A., J. P. Pierce, and B. Rosbrook. 1997. Are adolescents receptive to current sales promotion practices of the tobacco industry? *Preventive Medicine* 26:14–21.

Gilpin, E. A., M. M. White, A. J. Farkas, and J. P. Pierce. 1999. Home smoking restrictions: which smokers have them and how are they associated with smoking behavior. *Nicotine & Tobacco Research* 1:153–62.

Giovino, G. A. 1999. Epidemiology of tobacco use among US adolescents. *Nicotine and Tobacco Research* 1 (supp 1): 31–40.

Giovino, G. A., J. E. Henningfield, S. L. Tomar, L. G. Escobedo, and J. Slade. 1995. Epidemiology of tobacco use and dependence. *Epidemiologic Reviews* 17:48–65.

Glantz, S. A. 1996. Preventing tobacco use—the youth access trap. *American Journal of Public Health* 86 (2): 1156–58.

Glasgow, R. E., T. M. Vogt, and S. M. Boles. 1999. Evaluating the public health impact of health promotion interventions: The RE-AIM framework. *American Journal of Public Health* 89:1322–27.

Gleckman, H. 1998. Firing up a black market: Illegal cigs may follow tax hikes *Business Week,* 5/25/98, p. 26.

Goldman, L. K., and S. A. Glantz. 1998. Evaluation of antismoking advertising campaigns. *Journal of the American Medical Association* 279:772–77.

Goodman, J. 1994. *Tobacco in history: The cultures of dependence.* New York: Routledge.

Gostin, L. O. Forthcoming. *American public health law.* Berkeley: University of California Press.

Greene, J. M., S. T. Ennett, and C. L. Ringwalt. 1997. Substance use among runaway and homeless youth in three national samples. *American Journal of Public Health* 87:229–35.

Greening, L., and S. J. Dollinger. 1991. Adolescent smoking and perceived vulnerability to smoking-related causes of death. *Journal of Pediatric Psychology* 16:687–99.

Greenlund, K. J., C. C. Johnson, L. S. Webber, and G. S. Berenson. 1997. Cigarette smoking attitudes and first use among third- through sixth-grade students: the Bogalusa Heart Study. *American Journal of Public Health* 87:1345–48.

Greenlund, K. J., K. Liu, C. I. Kiefe, C. Yunis, A. R. Dyer, and G. L. Burke. 1995. Impact of father's education and parental smoking status on smoking behavior in young adults. *American Journal of Epidemiology* 142:1029–33.

Gritz, E. R. 1994. Reaching toward and beyond the year 2000 goals for cigarette smoking: Research and public health priorities. *Cancer* 74 (supp. 4): 1423–32.

Grossman, M., and F. J. Chaloupka. 1997. Cigarette taxes: The straw to break the camel's back. *Public Health Reports* 112:290–97.

Gruber, J., and J. Zinman. 2000. Youth smoking in the U.S.: Evidence and implications. In *Risky behavior among youth: An economic analysis,* ed. J. Gruber. Chicago: University of Chicago Press.

Hamilton, W. L., and G. S. Norton. 1999. Independent evaluation of the Massachusetts Tobacco Control Program. Fifth annual report summary. Abt Associates, Boston.

Han, C., M. K. McGue, and W. G. Iacono. 1999. Lifetime tobacco, alcohol, and other substance use in adolescent Minnesota twins: Univariate and multi-variate behavioral genetic analyses. *Addiction* 94:981–93.

Hansen, W. B., and R. B. McNeal. 1997. How DARE works: An examination of program effects on mediating variables. *Health Education and Behavior* 24:165–76.

Harrell, J. S., S. I. Bangdiwala, S. Deng, J. S. Webb, and C. Bradley. 1998. Smoking initiation in youth: The roles of gender, race, socioeconomics, and developmental status. *Journal of Adolescent Health* 23:271–79.

Harris, J. E. 1980. Taxing tar and nicotine. *American Economic Review* 70:300–311.

———. 1983. Cigarette smoking among successive birth cohorts of men and women in the United States during 1900–80. *Journal of the National Cancer Institute (JNCI)* 71:473–79.

———. 1994. A working model for predicting the consumption and revenue impacts of large increases in the U.S. federal cigarette excise tax. Working paper no. 4803, National Bureau of Economic Research, Cambridge, MA.

Hawkins, J. D., R. F. Catalano, and J. Y. Miller. 1992. Risk and protective factors for alcohol and other drug problems in adolescence and early adulthood. *Psychological Bulletin* 112:64–105.

Hebert, R. 1999. Article summaries. *Nicotine and Tobacco Research* 1 (supp. 1): 25–28.

Heiser, P. F., and M. E. Begay. 1997. The campaign to raise the tobacco tax in Massachusetts. *American Journal of Public Health* 87:968–73.

Henningfield, J. E., C. Cohen, and W. B. Pickworth. 1993. Psychopharmacology of nicotine. In *Nicotine addiction: Principles and management,* ed. C. T. Orleans and J. Slade. New York: Oxford University Press.

Henningfield, J. E., et al. 1998. Reducing the addictiveness of cigarettes. *Tobacco Control* 7:281–93.

Hettema, J. M., L. A. Corey, and K. S. Kendler. 1999. A multivariate genetic analysis of the use of tobacco, alcohol, and caffeine in a population based sample of male and female twins. *Drug and Alcohol Dependence* 57:69–78.

Hill, D. 1999. Why we should tackle adult smoking first. *Tobacco Control* 8:333–35.

Hinds, M. W. 1992. Impact of local ordinance banning tobacco sales to minors. *Public Health Reports* 107:355–58.

Hine, D. W., C. Summers, K. Tilleczek, and J. Lewko. 1997. Expectancies and mental models as determinants of adolescents' smoking decisions. *Journal of Social Issues* 53:35–52.

Hirschman, R. S., H. Leventhal, and K. Glynn. 1984. The development of smoking behavior: Conceptualization and supportive cross-sectional survey data. *Journal of Applied Social Psychology* 14:184–206.

Holmen, T. L., E. Barrett-Connor, J. Holmen, and L. Bjermer. 2000. Health problems in teenage daily smokers versus nonsmokers, Norway, 1995–1997: The Nord-Trondelag Health Study. *American Journal of Epidemiology* 151:148–55.

Houston, T., L. J. Kolbe, and M. P. Eriksen. 1998. Tobacco-use cessation in the '90s—not "adults only" anymore. *Preventive Medicine* 27 (5, pt. 3): A1–2.

Hu, F. B., D. Hedecker, B. R. Flay, S. Sussman, L. E. Day, and O. Siddiqui. 1996.

The patterns and predictors of smokeless tobacco onset among urban public school teenagers. *American Journal of Preventive Medicine* 12:22–28.

Hu, T. W., Z. Lin, and T. E. Keeler. 1998. Teenage smoking, attempts to quit, and school performance. *American Journal of Public Health* 88:940–43.

Hu, T. W., H. Y. Sung, and T. E. Keeler. 1995. Reducing cigarette consumption in California: Tobacco taxes vs. an anti-smoking media campaign. *American Journal of Public Health* 85:1218–22.

Hurt, R. D., G. A. Croghan, S. D. Beede, T. D. Wolter, I. T. Croghan, and C. A. Patten. 2000. Nicotine patch therapy in 101 adolescent smokers. *Archives of Pediatrics & Adolescent Medicine* 154:31–37.

Iannotti, R. J., P. J. Bush, and K. P. Weinfurt. 1996. Perception of friends' use of alcohol, cigarettes, and marijuana among urban schoolchildren: A longitudinal analysis. *Addictive Behaviors* 21:615–32.

Independent Evaluation Consortium. 1998. *Final report of the independent evaluation of the California Tobacco Control Prevention and Education Program: Wave I data, 1996–1997.* Rockville, MD: Gallup Organization.

IOM [Institute of Medicine]. 1994. *Growing up tobacco free: Preventing nicotine addiction in children and youth .* Washington, DC: National Academy Press.

———. 2000. *State programs can reduce tobacco use.* Washington, DC: National Academy Press.

Israel, B. A., A. J. Schulz, E. A. Parker, and A. B. Becker. 1998. Review of community-based research: Assessing partnership approaches to improve public health. *Annual Review of Public Health* 19:173–202.

Jackson, C. 1997. Initial and experimental stages of tobacco and alcohol use during late childhood: Relation to peer, parent, and personal risk factors. *Addictive Behaviors* 22:685–98.

———. 1998. Cognitive susceptibility to smoking and initiation of smoking during childhood: A longitudinal study. *Preventive Medicine* 27:129–34.

Jackson, C., D. J. Bee-Gates, and L. Henriksen. 1994. Authoritative parenting, child competencies, and initiation of cigarette smoking. *Health Education Quarterly* 21:103–16.

Jackson, C., L. Henriksen, D. Dickinson, and D. W. Levine. 1997. The early use of alcohol and tobacco: Its relation to children's competence and parents' behavior. *American Journal of Public Health* 87:359–64.

Jackson, C., L. Henriksen, D. Dickinson, L. Messer, and S. B. Robertson. 1998. A longitudinal study predicting patterns of cigarette smoking in late childhood. *Health Education and Behavior* 25:436–47.

Jacobson, P. D., and K. E. Warner. 1999. Litigation and public health policy making: The case of tobacco control. *Journal of Health Politics, Policy, and Law* 24:769–804.

Jacobson, P. D., and J. Wasserman. 1997. *Tobacco control laws: Implementation and enforcement.* Santa Monica, CA: Rand.

———. 1999. Tobacco control laws: Implementation and enforcement. *Journal of Health Politics, Policy, and Law* 24:567–98.

Jacobson, P. D., J. Wasserman, and J. R. Anderson. 1997. Historical overview of tobacco legislation and regulation. *Journal of Social Issues* 53:75–95.

Jacobson, P. D., J. Wasserman, and K. Raube. 1993. The politics of antismoking legislation: Lessons from six states. *Journal of Health Politics, Policy, and Law* 18:787–819.

Jacobson, P. D., and L. Wu. 2000. The enactment of clean indoor air laws: Trends and policy implications. In *Regulating tobacco: Premises and policy options,* ed. R. L. Rabin and S. S. Sugarman. New York: Oxford University Press.

Jason, L.A. 1998. Tobacco, drug, and HIV preventive media interventions. *American Journal of Community Psychology* 26:151–87.

Jason, L. A., M. Berk, D. L. Schnopp-Wyatt, and B. Talbot. 1999. Effects of enforcement of youth access laws on smoking prevalence. *American Journal of Community Psychology* 27:143–60.

Jason, L. A., W. D. Billows, D. L. Schnopp-Wyatt, and C. King. 1996a. Reducing the illegal sales of cigarettes to minors: Analysis of alternative enforcement schedules. *Journal of Applied Behavioral Analysis* 29:333–44.

———. 1996b. Long-term findings from Woodridge in reducing illegal cigarette sales to older minors. *Evaluation and the Health Professions* 19:3–13.

Jason, L. A., P. Y. Ji, M. D. Anes, and S. C. Birkhead. 1991. Active enforcement of cigarette control laws in the prevention of cigarette sales to minors. *Journal of the American Medical Association* 266:3159–61.

Jellinek, P. S., and R. P. Hearn. 1991. Fighting drug abuse at the local level. *Issues in Science and Technology* 7:78–84.

Jernigan, D. H., and P. A. Wright. 1996. Media advocacy: Lessons from community experiences. *Journal of Public Health Policy* 17:306–30.

Joe Camel Campaign: Mangini v. R. J. Reynolds Tobacco Company Collection. <http://www.library.ucsf.edu/tobacco/mangini> (9/26/2000).

Johnson, T. R. 1978. Additional evidence on the effects of alternative taxes on cigarette prices. *Journal of Political Economy* 86:325–28.

Johnston, L. D., P. M. O'Malley, and J. G. Bachman. 1999. Cigarette smoking among American teens continues gradual decline. *MTF Web site,* <http://www.monitoringthefuture.org> (9/26/2000).

———. 1996. *National survey results on drug use from the Monitoring the Future study, 1975–1995.* Vol. 1. Rockville, MD: NIDA, National Institutes of Health, National Institute on Drug Abuse.

———. 1998a. Drug use by American young people begins to turn downward. *University of Michigan News and Information Services,* December, on-line. Available at <http://www.isr.umich.edu/src/mtf> (9/26/2000).

———. 1998b. Nineteen ninety-eight data tables/figures. *MTF Web site,* <http://www.isr.umich.edu/src/mtf> (9/26/2000).

———. 1999. Nineteen ninety-nine data tables/figures. *MTF Web site,* <http://www.isr.umich.edu/src/mtf> (9/26/2000).

———. Cigarette use and smokeless tobacco use decline substantially among teens. *MTF Web site* (2/14/2000).

Johnston, L. D., P. M. O'Malley, and J. G. Bachman. 1999. *National survey results of drug use from the Monitoring the Future study, 1975–1988.* Vol. 1: Secondary school students (NIH Publication No. 99-4660). Rockville, Md.: National Institute on Drug Abuse.

———. 2000. *The Monitoring the Future National Survey Results on Adolescent*

Drug Use: Overview of Key Findings, 1999. (NIH Publication No. 00-4690). Rockville, Md.: National Institute on Drug Abuse.

Johnston, L. D., P. M. O'Malley, J. G. Bachman, and J. E. Schulenberg. 1999. *Cigarette brand preferences among adolescents.* Monitoring the Future Occasional Paper 45. Institute for Social Research, University of Michigan. <http://www.isr.umich.edu/src/mtf/occpaper45/paper.html> (9/26/2000).

Kadushin, C., E. Reber, L. Saxe, and D. Livert. 1998. The substance use system: Social and neighborhood environments associated with substance use and misuse. *Substance Use and Misuse* 33:1681–710.

Kagan, R. A., and D. Vogel. 1993. The politics of smoking regulation: Canada, France, the United States. In *Smoking policy: Law, politics, and culture,* ed. R. L. Rabin and S. D. Sugarman. New York: Oxford University Press.

Kaufman, J. S., L. A. Jason, L. M. Sawlski, and J. A. Halpert. 1994. A comprehensive multi-media program to prevent smoking among black students. *Journal of Drug Education* 24 (2): 95–108.

Keeler, T. E., T. W. Hu, P. G. Barnett, and W. G. Manning. 1993. Taxation, regulation, addiction: A demand function for cigarettes based on time series evidence. *Journal of Health Economics* 12:1–18.

Keeler, T. E., T. W. Hu, P. G. Barnett, W. G. Manning, and H. Y. Sung. 1996. Do cigarette producers price-discriminate by state? An empirical analysis of local cigarette pricing and taxation. *Journal of Health Economics* 15:499–512.

Kegler, M. Crozier, et al. 1998. Factors that contribute to effective community health promotion coalitions: A study of 10 Project ASSIST coalitions in North Carolina. *Health Education and Behavior* 25 (3): 338–53.

Kelder, G. E., Jr., and R. A. Daynard. 1997. Judicial approaches to tobacco control: The third wave of tobacco litigation as a tobacco control mechanism. *Journal of Social Issues* 53:169–86.

Kellam, S. G., and J. C. Anthony. 1998. Targeting early antecedents to prevent tobacco smoking: Findings from an epidemiologically based randomized field trial. *American Journal of Public Health* 88:1490–95.

Kenkel, D. S. 1993. Prohibition versus taxation: Reconsidering the legal drinking age. *Contemporary Policy Issues* 11:48–57.

Kim, S., C. Crutchfield, C. Williams, and N. Helper. 1998. Toward a new paradigm in substance abuse and other problem behavior prevention for youth: Youth development and empowerment approach. *Journal of Drug Education* 29 (1): 1–17.

King, C., M. Siegel, C. Celebucki, and G. N. Connolly. 1998. Adolescent exposure to cigarette advertising in magazines: An evaluation of brand-specific advertising in relation to youth readership. *Journal of the American Medical Association* 279:516–20.

Kleiman, M. 1993. *Against excess: Drug policy for results.* New York: Basic.

Klesges, R. C., V. E. Elliott, and L. A. Robinson. 1997. Chronic dieting and the belief that smoking controls body weight in a biracial, population-based adolescent sample. *Tobacco Control* 6:89–94.

Kluger, R. 1996. *Ashes to ashes: America's hundred-year cigarette war and the unabashed triumph of Philip Morris.* New York: Alfred A. Knopf.

Koval, J. J., and L. L. Pederson. 1999. Stress-coping and other psychosocial risk factors: A model for smoking in grade 6 students. *Addictive Behaviors* 24:207–18.

Lamkin, L., B. Davis, and A. Kamen. 1998. Rationale for tobacco cessation interventions in youth. *Preventive Medicine* 27:A3–A8.

Landrine, H., J. L. Richardson, E. A. Klonoff, and B. Flay. 1994. Cultural diversity in the predictors of adolescent cigarette smoking: The relative influence of peers. *Journal of Behavioral Medicine* 17:331–45.

Lefebvre, R. C., and J. A. Flora. 1988. Social marketing and public health intervention. *Health Education Quarterly* 15:299–315.

Lerman, C., N. E. Caporaso, J. Audrain, D. Main, E. D. Bowman, B. Lockshin, N. R. Boyd, and P. G. Shields. 1999. Evidence suggesting the role of specific genetic factors in cigarette smoking. *Health Psychology* 18:14–20.

Levy, D. T., and K. Friend. 1999. Strategies for reducing youth access to tobacco: A review of the literature and framework for future research. Pacific Institute for the Research and Evaluation.

Levy, D. T. and K. Friend. 2000. A simulation model of tobacco youth access policies. *Journal of Health Politics, Policy and Law* 25:1023–50.

Lewit, E. M., and D. Coate. 1982. The potential for using excise taxes to reduce smoking. *Journal of Health Economics* 1:121–45.

Lewit, E. M., D. Coate, and M. Grossman. 1981. The effects of government regulation on teenage smoking. *Journal of Law and Economics* 24:545–70.

Lewit, E. M., A. Hyland, N. Kerrebrock, and K. M. Cummings. 1997. Price, public policy, and smoking in young people. *Tobacco Control* 6 (supp. 2): 17–24.

Lifrak, P. D., J. R. McKay, A. Rostain, A. I. Alterman, and C. P. O'Brien. 1997. Relationship of perceived competencies, perceived social support, and gender to substance use in young adolescents. *Journal of the American Academy of Child and Adolescent Psychiatry* 36:933–40.

Ling, J. C., B. A. K. Franklin, J. F. Lindsteadt, and S. A. N. Gearon. 1992. Social marketing: Its place in public health. *Annual Review of Public Health* 13:341–62.

Logan, R. A., and D. R. Longo. 1999. Rethinking anti-smoking media campaigns: Two generations of research and issues for the next. *Journal of Health Care Finance* 25:77–90.

Lucas, K., and B. Lloyd. 1999. Starting smoking: Girls' explanations of the influence of peers. *Journal of Adolescence* 22:647–55.

Luke, D. A., K. A. Stamakis, and R. C. Brownson. 2000. State youth-access tobacco control policies and youth smoking behavior in the United States. *American Journal of Preventive Medicine* 19:180–87.

Lynan, D. R., et al. 1999. Project DARE: No effects at 10-year follow-up. *Journal of Consulting and Clinical Psychology* 67:490–593.

Macaskill, P., J. P. Pierce, J. M. Simpson, and D. M. Lyle. 1992. Mass media–led antismoking campaign can remove the education gap in quitting behavior. *American Journal of Public Health* 82:96–98.

Maibach, E., and D. R. Holtgrave. 1995. Advances in public health communication. *Annual Review of Public Health* 16:219–38.

Majeski, T. 2000. MN: Teen-age smokers need special help to quit/kid smokers need extra help to quit. *Pioneer Press,* January 31.

Males, M. 1995. The influence of parental smoking on youth smoking: Is the recent downplaying justified? *Journal of School Health* 65:228–31.

Manley, M. W., R. P. Epps, and T. J. Glynn. 1992. The clinician's role in promoting smoking cessation among clinic patients. *Medical Clinics of North America* 76:477–94.

Manley, M. W., et al. 1997. Impact of the American Stop Smoking Intervention Study on cigarette consumption. *Tobacco Control* 6 (supp. 2): 12–16.

Manning, W. G., E. B. Keeler, J. P. Newhouse, E. M. Sloss, and J. Wasserman. 1989. The taxes of sin: Do smokers and drinkers pay their way? *Journal of the American Medical Association* 261:1604–9.

Mannino, D. M., M. Siegel, C. Husten, D. Rose, and R. Etzel. 1996. Environmental tobacco smoke exposure and health effects in children: Results from the 1991 National Health Interview Survey. *Tobacco Control* 5:13–18.

Manske, S. R., K. S. Brown, and A. J. Cameron. 1997. School-based smoking control: A research agenda. *Cancer Prevention and Control* 1 (3): 190–91.

Marcus, S., G. A. Giovino, J. P. Pierce, and Y. Harel. 1993. Measuring tobacco use among adolescents. *Public Health Reports* 108 (supp. 1): 20–24.

Marsden, W. 1999. Tobacco insider talks/major firms deeply involved in cross-border smuggling, former executive says. *Montreal Gazette,* December 18. Available at <http://www.montrealgazette.com/news/pages/991218/3316186.html> (12/99).

Massing, M. 1998. *The Fix.* New York: Simon and Schuster.

McBride, C. M., S. J. Curry, A. Cheadle, C. Anderman, E. H. Wagner, P. Diehr, and B. Psaty. 1995. School-level application of a social bonding model to adolescent risk-taking behavior. *Journal of School Health* 65:63–68.

McCormick, L., and N. O. Thompkins. 1998. Diffusion of CDC's guidelines to prevent tobacco use and addiction. *Journal of School Health* 68:43–45.

McGee, R., and W. R. Stanton. 1993. A longitudinal study of reasons for smoking in adolescence. *Addiction* 88:265–71.

McGee, R., S. Williams, and W. Stanton. 1998. Is mental health in childhood a major predictor of smoking in adolescence? *Addiction* 93:1869–74.

McGinnis, J. M., and W. H. Foege. 1993. Actual causes of death in the United States. *Journal of the American Medical Association* 270:2207–12.

McKenna, J. W., and K. N. Williams. 1993. Crafting effective tobacco counter advertisements: Lessons from a failed campaign directed at teenagers. *Public Health Reports* 108 (supp. 1): 85–89.

Mendez, D., and K. E. Warner. 1998. Has smoking cessation ceased? Expected trends in the prevalence of smoking in the United States. *American Journal of Epidemiology* 148:249 58.

Mermelstein, R., and the Tobacco Control Network Writing Group. 1999. Explanations of ethnic and gender differences in youth smoking: A multi-site, qualitative investigation. *Nicotine and Tobacco Research* 1 (supp. 1): 91–98.

Moore, M. C., and C. J. Mikhail. 1996. A new attack on smoking using an old-time remedy. *Public Health Reports* 111:192–203.

MTF [Monitoring the Future]. 1999. <http://www.isr.umich.edu/ src/mtf /t2_1b4.html>.

Mulhall, P. F., D. Stone, and B. Stone. 1996. Home alone: Is it a risk factor for middle school youth and drug use? *Journal of Drug Education* 26:39–48.

Mullahy, J. 1985. Cigarette smoking: Habits, health concerns, and heterogeneous unobservables in a microeconomic analysis of consumer demand. Ph.D. diss., University of Virginia.

Murray, C. J., and A. D. Lopez 1996. Evidence-based health policy—lessons from the Global Burden of Disease study. *Science* 274:740–43.

Murray, D. M., et al. 1992. Results from a statewide approach to adolescent tobacco use prevention. *Preventive Medicine* 21:449–72.

Murray, D. M., P. Pirie, R. V. Leupker, and U. Pallonen. 1989. Five- and six-year follow-up results from four seventh-grade smoking prevention strategies. *Journal of Behavioral Medicine* 12:207–18.

Myers, M. L. 1999. Adults versus teenagers: A false dilemma and a dangerous choice. *Tobacco Control* 8:336–38.

Napier, K. 1996. *Cigarettes—what the warning label doesn't tell you: The first comprehensive guide to the health consequences of smoking.* New York: American Council on Science and Health.

Naquin, M. R., and G. G. Gilbert. 1996. College students' smoking behavior, perceived stress, and coping style. *Journal of Drug Education* 26 (4): 367–76.

National Association of Attorneys General. "Multistate Settlement with the Tobacco Industry." 11/23/98. Found in <http://www.naag.org /tob2 .htm> (3/2000).

National Cancer Institute. 1993. *The impact of cigarette excise taxes on smoking among children and adults.* Atlanta, GA: National Cancer Institute.

National Cancer Policy Board. 2000. *State tobacco programs can reduce tobacco use.* Washington, DC: National Academy Press.

Navarro, M. 1998. Florida gives teen-age smokers a day in court. *New York Times,* July 20, p. A-1.

Nelson, D. E., G. A. Giovino, D. R. Shopland, P. D. Mowery, S. L. Mills, and M. P. Eriksen. 1995. Trends in cigarette smoking among US adolescents, 1974 through 1991. *American Journal of Public Health* 85:34–40.

NHIS [National Health Interview Survey]. 1999. <http://www.cdc.gov/nchs /nhis.htm> (9/26/2000).

Noble, H. B. 1999. He's "gone commercial" to spread gospel of health. *New York Times,* February 2, p. C1.

Norton, E. C., R. C. Lindrooth, and S. T. Ennett. 1998. Controlling for the endogeneity of peer substance use on adolescent alcohol and tobacco use. *Health Economics* 7:439–53.

Ockene, J. K., E. A. Lindsay, N. Hymowitz, C. Giffen, T. Purcell, P. Pomrehn, and T. Pechacek. 1997. Tobacco control activities of primary-care physicians in the Community Intervention Trial for Smoking Cessation. *Tobacco Control* 6 (supp. 2): S49–S56.

Ockene, J. K., and J. G. Zapka. 1997a. Physician-based smoking intervention: A rededication to a five-step strategy to smoking research. *Addictive Behaviors* 22:835–48.

————. 1997b. Changing provider behaviour: Provider education and training. *Tobacco Control* 6 (supp. 1): S63–S67.

Olds, D. L., J. Eckenrode, C. R. Henderson Jr., H. Kitzman, J. Powers, R. Cole, K. Sidora, P. Morris, L. M. Pettitt, and D. Luckey. 1997. Long-term effects of home visitation on maternal life course and child abuse and neglect. Fifteen-year follow-up of a randomized trial. *Journal of the American Medical Association* 278:637–43.

Pacula, R. L. 1998. Does increasing the beer tax reduce marijuana consumption? *Journal of Health Economics* 17:557–85.

Pallonen, U. E. 1998. Transtheoretical measures for adolescent and adult smokers. *Preventive Medicine* 27:A29–A38.

Pallonen, U. E., J. O. Prochaska, et al. 1998. Stages of acquisition and cessation for adolescent smoking: An empirical integration. *Addictive Behaviors* 23:303–24.

Pallonen, U. E., W. F. Velicer, et al. 1998. Computer-based smoking cessation interventions in adolescents: Description, feasibility, and six-month follow-up findings. *Substance Use and Misuse* 33:935–65.

Parent, R. 1999. Newton psychologists eye CD-ROM's as effective health educators. *Boston Globe*, January 24, p. 8.

Patton, G. C., J. B. Carlin, C. Coffrey, R. Wolfe, M. Hibbert, and G. Bowes. 1998a. Depression, anxiety, and smoking initiation: A prospective study over three years. *American Journal of Public Health* 88:1518–22.

————. 1998b. The course of early smoking: A population-based cohort study over three years. *Addiction* 93:1251–60.

Pechmann, C., and E. T. Reibling. 2000. Anti-smoking advertising campaigns targeting youth: case studies from USA and Canada. *Tobacco Control* 9 Suppl. 2:18–31.

Pederson, L. L., J. J. Koval, G. A. McGrady, and S. L. Tyas. 1998. The degree and type of relationship between psychosocial variables and smoking status for students in grade 8: Is there a dose-response relationship? *Preventive Medicine* 27:337–47.

Pederson, L. L., J. J. Koval, and K. O'Connor. 1997. Are psychosocial factors related to smoking in grade-6 students? *Addictive Behaviors* 22:169–81.

Penn Advertising of Baltimore v. Mayor and City Council of Baltimore, 63 F3d 1318 (4th Cir 1995).

Pentz, M. A., B. R. Brannon, et al. 1989. The power of policy: The relationship of smoking policy to adolescent smoking. *American Journal of Public Health* 79:857–62.

Pentz, M. A., J. H. Dwyer, et al. 1989. A multicommunity trial for primary prevention of adolescent drug abuse: Effects on drug use prevalence. *Journal of the American Medical Association* 261 (22): 3259–66.

Pentz, M. A., D. P. MacKinnon, J. H. Dwyer, et al. 1989. Longitudinal effects of the Midwestern Prevention Project on regular and experimental smoking in adolescents. *Preventive Medicine* 18:304–21.

Pentz, M. A., S. P. MacKinnon, B. R. Flay, et al. 1989. Primary prevention of chronic diseases in adolescence: Effects of the Midwestern Prevention Project on tobacco use. *American Journal of Epidemiology* 130:713–24.

Perez-Stable, E. J., M. Juarez-Reyes, C. P. Klaplan, et al. 2001. Counseling smoking parents of young children. *Archives of Pediatric Adolescent Medicine* 155:25–31.

Perry, C. L. 1999. The tobacco industry and underage youth smoking: Tobacco industry documents from the Minnesota litigation. *Archives of Pediatrics and Adolescent Medicine* 153:935–41.

Perry C. L., et al. 1992. Community-wide smoking prevention: Long-term outcomes of the Minnesota Heart Health Program and the Class of 1989 Study. *American Journal of Public Health* 82 (9): 1210–16.

Peterson, A. V., K. A. Kealey, S. L. Mann, P. M. Marek, and I. G. Sarason. 2000. Hutchinson Smoking Prevention Project: Long-term randomized trial in school-based tobacco use prevention—results on smoking. *Journal of the National Cancer Institute* 92:1979–91.

Petoskey, E. L., K. R. Van Stelle, and J. A. DeJong. 1998. Prevention through empowerment in a Native American community. *Drugs and Society* 12:147–62.

Philip Morris. 2000. Youth smoking prevention. <http://www.philipmorris .com/tobacco_bus/tobacco_issues/youth_smoking_prevention.html> (9/26/2000).

Pianezza, M. L., E. M. Sellers, and R. F. Tyndale. 1998. Nicotine metabolism defect reduces smoking. *Nature* 393:750.

Pierce, J. P., W. S. Choi, E. A. Gilpin, A. J. Farkas, and C. C. Berry. 1998. Tobacco industry promotion of cigarettes and adolescent smoking. *Journal of the American Medical Association* 279:511–15.

Pierce, J. P., et al. 1991. Does tobacco advertising target young people to start smoking? Evidence from California. *Journal of the American Medical Association* 266:3154–58.

Pierce, J. P., and E. A. Gilpin. 1994. Smoking initiation by adolescent girls, 1944 through 1988: An association with targeted advertising. *Journal of the American Medical Association* 271:608–11.

———. 1996. How long will today's new adolescent smoker be addicted to cigarettes? *American Journal of Public Health* 86:253–56.

Pierce, J. P., E. A. Gilpin, and W. S. Choi. 1999. Sharing the blame: Smoking experimentation and future smoking-attributable mortality due to Joe Camel and Marlboro advertising and promotions. *Tobacco Control* 8:37–44.

Pierce, J. P., E. A. Gilpin, S. L. Emery, A. J. Farkas, S. H. Zhu, W. S. Choi, C. C. Berry, J. M. Distefan, M. M. White, S. Soroko, and A. Navarro. 1998. *Tobacco control in California: Who's winning the war? An evaluation of the Tobacco Control Program, 1989–1996.* La Jolla, CA: University of California, San Diego.

Pierce, J. P., E. A. Gilpin, S. L. Emery, M. W. White, B. Rosbrook, C. C. Berry. 1998. Has the California Tobacco Control Program reduced smoking? *Journal of the American Medical Association* 280:893–99.

Pierce, J. P., L. Lee, and F. A. Gilpin. 1994. Smoking initiation by adolescent girls, 1944 through 1988: An association with targeted advertising. *Journal of the American Medical Association* 271:608–11.

Pomerleau, O. F. 1995. Individual differences in sensitivity to nicotine: Implications for genetic research on nicotine dependence. *Behavior Genetics* 25:161–77.

Popham, W. J., et al. 1994. Effectiveness of the California 1990–1991 tobacco education media campaign. *American Journal of Preventive Medicine* 10:319–26.

Prochaska, J. O., C. C. DiClemente, W. F. Velicer, J. S. Rossi. 1993. Standardized, individualized, interactive, and personalized self-help programs for smoking cessation. *Health Psychology* 12:399–405.

Proescholdbell, R. J., L. Chassin, and D. P. MacKinnon. 2000. Home smoking restrictions and adolescent smoking. *Nicotine & Tobacco Research* 2:159–67.

Pucci, L. G., and M. Siegel. 1999. Exposure to brand-specific cigarette advertising in magazines and its impact on youth smoking. *Preventive Medicine* 29:313–20.

R. J. Reynolds. 1988. *Chemical and biological studies of new cigarette prototypes that heat instead of burn tobacco.* Winston-Salem, NC.

———. 2000. <http://www.rjrt.com/TI/Pages/Ticover.asp> (9/26/2000).

Rabin, R. L. 1991. Some thoughts on smoking regulation. *Stanford Law Review* 43:475–96.

Ramirez, A. G., and K. J. Gallion. 1993. Nicotine dependence among Blacks and Hispanics. In *Nicotine addiction: Principles and management,* ed. C. T. Orleans and J. Slade. New York: Oxford University Press.

Reuter, P. 1985. *The organization of illegal markets: An economic analysis.* Washington, DC: National Institute of Justice.

Richards, J. W., J. B. Tye, and P. M. Fischer. 1996. The tobacco industry's code of advertising in the United States: Myth and reality. *Tobacco Control* 5:295–311.

Richardson, J. L., K. Dwyer, K. McGuigan, W. Hansen, C. Dent, C. A. Johnson, S. Y. Sussman, B. Brannon, and B. Flay. 1989. Substance use among eighth-grade students who take care of themselves after school. *Pediatrics* 84:556–66.

Richardson, J. L., B. Radziszewska, C. W. Dent, and B. R. Flay. 1993. Relationship between after-school care of adolescents and substance use, risk taking, depressed mood, and academic achievement. *Pediatrics* 92:32–38.

Rigotti, N. A., J. R. DiFranza, Y. C. Chang, T. Tisdale, B. Kemp, and D. E. Singer. 1997. The effect of enforcing tobacco-sales laws on adolescents' access to tobacco and smoking behavior. *New England Journal of Medicine* 337:1044–51.

Rigotti, N. A., and C. L. Pashos. 1991. No-smoking laws in the United States: An analysis of state and city actions to limit smoking in public places and workplaces. *Journal of the American Medical Association* 266:3162–67.

Rooney, B. L., and D. M. Murray. 1996. A meta-analysis of smoking prevention programs after adjustment for errors in the unit of analysis. *Health Education Quarterly* 23:48–64.

Rose-Ackerman, S. 1978. *Corruption : A study in political economy.* New York: Academic Press.

Ross, N. A., and S. M. Taylor. 1998. Geographical variation in attitudes towards smoking: Findings from the COMMIT communities. *Social Science and Medicine* 46:3–17.

Rossi, P., et al. 1999. *Evaluation: A systematic approach.* Thousand Oaks, CA: Sage.

Rowe, D. C., L. Chassin, C. Presson, and S. J. Sherman. 1996. Parental smoking and the "epidemic" spread of cigarette smoking. *Journal of Applied Social Psychology* 26:437–54.

Rust, L. 1999. Tobacco prevention advertising: Lessons from the commercial world. *Nicotine and Tobacco Marketing* 1 (supp.): 81–89.

Saba, R. P., et al. 1995. The demand for cigarette smuggling. *Economic Inquiry* 33:189–202.

Sabol, S. Z., M. L. Nelson, C. Fisher, L. Gunzerath, C. L. Brody, S. Hu, L. A. Sirota, S. E. Marcus, B. D. Greenberg, F. R. Lucas, J. Benjamin, D. L. Murphy, and D. H. Hamer. 1999. Genetic association for cigarette smoking behavior. *Health Psychology* 18:7–13.

Saffer, H., and F. Chaloupka. 1999. Tobacco advertising: Economic theory and international evidence. Working paper no. 6958, National Bureau of Economic Research, Cambridge, MA.

SAMHSA [Substance Abuse and Mental Health Services Administration]. 1998. Preliminary results from the 1997 National Household Survey on Drug Abuse.<http:// www.samhsa.gov/ oas/ nhsda/ nhsda97/ httoc .html> (10/99).

———. 1999. Summary of findings from the 1998 National Household Survey on Drug Abuse. <http://www.samhsa.gov/OAS/NHSDA /98SummHtml/NHSDA98Summ08.htm#P539_42390> (10/99).

Samuels, B. E., and S. A. Glantz. 1991. The politics of local tobacco control. *Journal of the American Medical Association* 266:2110–17.

Sanchez, L., S. Sanchez, and A. Goldberg. 2000. Tobacco and alcohol advertisements in magazines: Are young readers being targeted? *Journal of the American Medical Association* 283 (16):2106–7.

Sarason, I. G., E. S. Mankowski, A. V. Peterson, Jr., and K. T. Dinh. 1992. Adolescents' reasons for smoking. *Journal of School Health* 62:185–90.

Sargent, J. D., M. Dalton, and M. Beach. 2000. Exposure to cigarette promotions and smoking uptake in adolescents: Evidence of a dose-response relation. *Tobacco Control* 9:163–68.

Sargent, J. D., L. A. Mott, and M. Stevens. 1998. Predictors of smoking cessation in adolescents. *Archives of Pediatrics and Adolescent Medicine* 152:388–93.

Schooler, C., E. Feighery, and J. A. Flora. 1996. Seventh graders' self-reported exposure to cigarette marketing and its relationship to their smoking behavior. *American Journal of Public Health* 86:1216–21.

Schorling, J. B., M. Gutgesell, P. Klas, D. Smith, and A. Keller. 1994. Tobacco, alcohol, and other drug use among college students. *Journal of Substance Abuse* 6:105–15.

Schubiner, H., A. Herrold, and R. Hurt. 1998. Tobacco cessation and youth: The feasibility of brief office interventions for adolescents. *Preventive Medicine* 27:47–54.

Schwartz, G. T. 1993. Tobacco liability in the courts. In *Smoking policy: Law, pol-*

itics, and culture, ed. R. L. Rabin and S. D. Sugarman. New York: Oxford University Press.

Secker-Walker, R. H., J. K. Worden, B. R. Holland, B. S. Flynn, and A. S. Detsky. 1997. A mass media program to prevent smoking among adolescents: Costs and cost-effectiveness. *Tobacco Control* 6:207–12.

Seidel-Marks, A. 1998. Behavioral management of tobacco addiction: What does social marketing have to offer? In *The economics of tobacco control: Towards an optimal policy mix,* ed. Abedian, I., R. van der Merwe, N. Wilkins, and P. Jha. Rondesbosch, South Africa: Applied Fiscal Research Center, University of Cape Town.

Seitz, V., and N. H. Apfel. 1994. Parent-focused intervention: Diffusion effects on siblings. *Child Development* 65:677–83.

Siegel, M. 1998. Mass media antismoking campaigns: A powerful tool for health promotion. *Annals of Internal Medicine* 129:128–32.

Siegel, M., and L. Biener. 2000. The impact of anti-smoking media campaigns on progression to established smoking: Results of a longitudinal youth study in Massachusetts. *American Journal of Public Health* 90:380–86.

Siegel, M., L. Biener, and N. A. Rigotti. 1999. The effect of local tobacco sales laws on adolescent smoking initiation. *Preventive Medicine* 29:334–42.

Siegel, M., and L. Doner. 1998. *Marketing public health: Strategies to promote social change.* Gaithersburg, MD: Aspen.

Siegel, M., et al. 1997. Preemption in tobacco control: Review of an emerging public health problem. *Journal of the American Medical Association* 28:858–63.

Slovic, P. 2000. What does it mean to know a cumulative risk? Adolescents' perceptions of short-term and long-term consequences of smoking. *Journal of Behavioral Decision Making* 13:259–66.

Smith, T. A., et al. 1996. Nicotine patch therapy in adolescent smokers. *Pediatrics* 98:659–67.

Sorensen, G., E. Emmons, M. K. Hunt, and D. Johnston. 1998. Implications of the results of community intervention trials. *Annual Review of Public Health* 19:379–416.

Sowden, A., and L. Arblaster. 2000. Community interventions for preventing smoking in young people. *Cochrane Database of Systematic Reviews* (computer file).

Stanton, W. R., J. B. Lowe, and P. A. Silva. 1995. Antecedents of vulnerability and resilience to smoking among adolescents. *Journal of Adolescent Health* 16:71–77.

Stanton, W. R., and R. McGee. 1996. Adolescents' promotion of nonsmoking and smoking. *Addictive Behaviors* 21:47–56.

Stanton, W. R., and P. A. Silva. 1992. A longitudinal study of the influence of parents and friends on children's initiation of smoking. *Journal of Applied Developmental Psychology* 13:423–34.

Stead, L. F., and T. Lancaster. 2000. A systematic review of interventions for preventing tobacco sales to minors. *Tobacco Control* 9:169–76.

Stein, J. A., M. D. Newcomb, and P. M. Bentler. 1996. Initiation and maintenance of tobacco smoking: Changing personality correlates in adolescence and young adulthood. *Journal of Applied Social Psychology* 26:160–87.

Stone, S. L., and J. L. Kristeller. 1992. Attitudes of adolescents toward smoking cessation. *American Journal of Preventive Medicine* 14:405–7.

Strecher, V. J. 1999. Computer-tailored smoking cessation materials: A review and discussion. *Patient Education and Counseling* 36:107–17.

Study finds alarming smoking rates at University of Minnesota. 1999. *USA Today,* November 18. Available at <http://www.usatoday.com/news/states/mnmain.htm> (11/99).

Sullum, J. 1998. *For your own good: The anti-smoking crusade and the tyranny of public health.* New York: Free Press.

Sumner, D. A., and J. M. Alston. 1984. The impact of removal of price supports and supply controls for tobacco in the United States. *Research in Domestic and Agribusiness Management* 5:107–64.

Sussman, S., et al. 1993. Project Towards No Tobacco Use: 1-year behavior outcomes. *American Journal of Public Health* 83:1245–50.

Sussman, S., K. Lichtman, A. Ritt, and U. E. Pallonen. 1999. Effects of thirty-four adolescent tobacco use cessation and prevention trials on regular users of tobacco products. *Substance Use and Misuse* 34:1469–503.

Sutton, C. D. 2000. A hard road: Finding ways to reduce teen tobacco use. *Tobacco Control* 9:1–2.

Swan, G. E. 1999. Implications of genetic epidemiology for the prevention of tobacco use. *Nicotine and Tobacco Research* 1 (supp. 1): 49–56.

Swartz, S. 1999. Removing the cool from cigarettes. *Fort Worth Star Telegram,* November 26.

Syme, S. L., and R. Alcalay. 1982. Control of cigarette smoking from a social perspective. *Annual Review of Public Health* 3:179–99.

Tansey, B. 1999. In pursuit of smoke-free living space—apartment dwellers fear health risks from neighbors' cigarettes. *San Francisco Chronicle,* June 28, p. A1.

Tauras, J. A., and F. J. Chaloupka. 1998. Price, clean indoor air laws, and cigarette smoking: Evidence from longitudinal data for young adults. Working paper, University of Michigan, Department of Health Management and Policy.

———. 1999. Determinants of smoking cessation: An analysis of young adult men and women. Working paper no. 7262, National Bureau of Economic Research, Cambridge, MA.

Teen courts connect. 2000. *Oregonian,* January 30. Available at <http://www.oregonlive.com/news/00/01/st013115.h5ml> (2/2000).

Teinowitz, I. 1998. After the tobacco settlement. *Washington Post,* December 6, p. C1.

———. 2000. Philip Morris USA slams "Truth" ads from foundation. *Advertising Age,* February 14, p. 3.

Thorlindsson, T., R. Vilhjalmsson, and G. Valgeirsson. 1990. Sport participation and perceived health status: A study of adolescents. *Social Science and Medicine* 30:551–56.

Thorndike, A. N., T. G. Ferris, R. S. Stafford, and N. A. Rigotti. 1999. Rates of U.S. physicians counseling adolescents about smoking. *Journal of the National Cancer Institute* 91:1857–62.

Thorndike, A. N., N. A. Rigotti, and R. S. Stafford. 1998. National patterns in the treatment of smokers by physicians. *Journal of the American Medical Association* 279:604–8.

Thrush, D., C. Fife-Schaw, and G. M. Breakwell. 1997. Young people's representations of others' views of smoking: Is there a link with smoking behaviour? *Journal of Adolescence* 20:57–70.

Thursby, J. G., and M. C. Thursby. 1994. *Interstate cigarette bootlegging: Extent, revenue losses, and effects of federal intervention.* Cambridge, MA: National Bureau of Economic Research.

Tilley, N. M. 1985. *The R. J. Reynolds Tobacco Company.* Chapel Hill, NC: University of North Carolina Press.

Tobacco dependence: Innovative regulatory approaches to reduce death and disease. 1998. *Food and Drug Law Journal* 53 (supp.): special issue.

Tobacco Institute. 1998. *The tax burden on tobacco,* historical compilation 1995. Vol. 30. Washington, DC: Tobacco Institute.

Tobler, N. S. 1986. Meta-analysis of 143 adolescent drug prevention programs: Quantitative outcomes results of program participants compared to a control or comparison group. *Journal of Drug Issues* 16:537–67.

———. 1992. Drug prevention programs can work: Research findings. *Journal of Addictive Diseases* 11 (3): 1–28.

———. 1997. Meta-analysis of adolescent drug prevention programs: Results of the 1993 meta-analysis. *NIDA Research Monograph* 170:5–68.

Tomar, S. L., and G. A. Giovino. 1998. Incidence and predictors of smokeless tobacco use among US youth. *American Journal of Public Health* 88:20–26.

Tomeo, C. A., A. E. Field, C. S. Berkey, G. A. Colditz, and A. L. Frazier. 1999. Weight concerns, weight control behaviors, and smoking initiation. *Pediatrics* 104:918–24.

Townsend, J. L. 1987. Cigarette tax, economic welfare, and social class patterns of smoking. *Applied Economics* 19:355–65.

Townsend, J. L., P. Roderick, and J. Cooper. 1994. Cigarette smoking by socio-economic group, sex, and age: Effects of price, income, and health publicity. *British Medical Journal* 309:923–26.

Traynor, M. P., and S. A. Glantz. 1996. California's tobacco tax initiative: The development and passage of Proposition 99. *Journal of Health Politics, Policy, and Law* 21:543–85.

Tschann, J. M., N. E. Adler, C. E. Irwin Jr., S. G. Millstein, R. A. Turner, and S. M. Kegeles. 1994. Initiation of substance use in early adolescence: The roles of pubertal timing and emotional distress. *Health Psychology* 13:326–33.

Tuakli, N., M. A. Smith, and C. Heaton. 1990. Smoking in adolescence: Methods for health education and smoking cessation. *Journal of Family Practice* 31:369–74.

Turco, R. M. 1997. Effects of exposure to cigarette advertisements on adolescents' attitudes toward smoking. *Journal of Applied Social Psychology* 27:1115–30.

Turner, R. A., C. E. Irwin Jr., and S. G. Millstein. 1991. Family structure, family processes, and experimenting with substances during adolescence. *Journal of Research on Adolescence* 1:93–106.

Turner-Bowker, D., and W. Hamilton. 2000. Ad money moves from billboards to print: Cigarette advertising expenditures before and after the master settlement agreement—preliminary findings. <http://www.tobacco.org/News/000515ma.html> (9/26/2000).

Tyas, S. L., and L. L. Pederson. 1998. Psychosocial factors related to adolescent smoking: A critical review of the literature. *Tobacco Control* 7:409–20.

Tye, J. B., K. E. Warner, and S. A. Glantz. 1987. Tobacco advertising and consumption: Evidence of a causal relationship. *Journal of Public Health Policy* 8:492–508.

Unger, J. B., C. A. Johnson, and L. A. Rohrbach. 1995. Recognition and liking of tobacco and alcohol advertisements among adolescents: Relationships with susceptibility to substance use. *Preventive Medicine* 24:461–66.

Urberg, K. A. 1992. Locus of peer influence: Social crowd or best friend. *Journal of Youth and Adolescence* 21:439–50.

Urberg, K. A., S. M. Degirmencioglu, and C. Pilgrim. 1997. Close friend and group influence on adolescent cigarette smoking and alcohol use. *Developmental Psychiatry* 33:834–44.

Urberg, K. A., S. J. Shyu, and J. Liang. 1990. Peer influence in adolescent cigarette smoking. *Addictive Behaviors* 15:247–55.

U.S. Bureau of the Census. 1994. *County and city data book, 1994.* Washington, DC: U.S. Government Printing Office.

USDHEW [U.S. Department of Health, Education, and Welfare]. 1964. *Smoking and health.* Report of the advisory committee to the surgeon general of the Public Health Service. PHS Publication 1103 U.S. Government Printing Office, Washington, D.C.

USDHHS [U.S. Department of Health and Human Services]. 1988. *The health consequences of smoking: Nicotine addiction.* Report of the surgeon general. DHHS Publication (CDC) 88-8406. U.S. Government Printing Office, Washington, D.C.

———. 1989. *Reducing the health consequences of smoking: Twenty-five years of progress.* Report of the surgeon general. DHHS Publication (CDC) 89-8411. Atlanta, GA: U.S. Public Health Services, Department of Health and Human Services.

———. 1992. *Smoking and health in the Americas.* Report of the surgeon general in collaboration with the Pan American Health Organization. DHHS Publication (CDC) 92-8419. Atlanta, GA: U.S. Public Health Services, Dept. of Health and Human Services.

———. 1994. *Preventing tobacco use among young people.* Report of the surgeon general. Washington, DC: U.S. Government Printing Office.

———. 1996a. Tobacco regulation for substance abuse prevention and treatment block grants: Final rule. *Federal Register* 61:1491–1509.

———. 1996b. Regulations restricting the sale and distribution of cigarettes and smokeless tobacco to protect children and adolescents. *Federal Register* 61:44395–445.

————. 1999. Healthy people 2010 objectives: Draft for public comment. <http://web.health.gov/healthypeople> (9/2000).

Vega, W. A., A. G. Gil, and R. S. Zimmerman. 1993. Patterns of drug use among Cuban-American, African-American, and White non-Hispanic boys. *American Journal of Public Health* 83:257–59.

Vega, W. A., R. S. Zimmerman, G. J. Warheit, E. Apospori, and A. G. Gil. 1993. Risk factors for early adolescent drug use in four ethnic and racial groups. *American Journal of Public Health* 83:185–89.

Velicer, W. F., J. O. Prochaska, J. M. Bellis, C. C. DiClemente, J. S. Rossi, J. L. Fava, J. H. Steiger. 1993. An expert system intervention for smoking cessation. *Addictive Behaviors* 18:269–90.

Velicer, W. F., J. O. Prochaska, J. L. Fava, R. G. Laforge, and J. S. Rossi. 1999. Interactive versus noninteractive interventions and dose-response relationship for stage-matched smoking cessation programs in a managed care setting. *Health Psychology* 18:21–28.

Viscusi, W. 2000. Comment: The perils of qualitative smoking risk measures. *Journal of Behavioral Decision Making* 13:267–71.

Wagner, S. 1971. *Cigarette country: Tobacco in American history and politics.* New York: Praeger.

Wakefield, M., and Chaloupka, F. 2000. Effectiveness of comprehensive tobacco control programmes in reducing teenage smoking in the USA. *Tobacco Control* 9:177–86.

Wakefield, M. A., F. J. Chaloupka, N. J. Kaufman, et al. 2000. Effect of restrictions on smoking at home, at school, and in public places on teenage smoking: Cross-Sectional Study. *British Medical Journal* 321:333–37.

Walack, L., L. Dorfman, D. Jernigan, and M. Themba. 1993. *Media advocacy and public health: Power for prevention.* Newbury Hills, CA: Sage.

Walsh, M. M., J. F. Hilton, C. M. Masouredis, L. Gee, M. A. Chesney, and V. L. Ernster. 1999. Smokeless tobacco cessation intervention for college athletes: Results after one year. *American Journal of Public Health* 89:228–34.

Wang, M. Q., E. C. Fitzhugh, J. E. Cowdery, and J. Trucks. 1995. Developmental influences of attitudes and beliefs on adolescents' smoking. *Psychological Reports* 76:399–402.

Wang, M. Q., E. C. Fitzhugh, J. M. Eddy, R. C. Westerfield, and Q. Fu. 1998. Tobacco use among school adolescents: National sociodemographic risk profiles. *Journal of Health Education* 29:174–78.

Wang, M. Q., E. C. Fitzhugh, J. Trucks, J. Cowdery, and M. Perko. 1995. Physiological sensations of initial smoking in the development of regular smoking behavior. *Perceptual and Motor Skills* 80:1131–34.

Wang, M. Q., E. C. Fitzhugh, L. Turner, and Q. Fu. 1997. Social influence on southern adolescents' smoking transition: A retrospective study. *Southern Medical Journal* 90:218–22.

Wang, M. Q., E. C. Fitzhugh, L. Turner, Q. Fu, and R. C. Westerfield. 1996. Association of depressive symptoms and school adolescents' smoking: A cross-legged analysis. *Psychological Reports* 79:127–30.

Wang, M. Q., E. C. Fitzhugh, C. Westerfield, and J. M. Eddy. 1995. Family and peer influences on smoking behavior among American adolescents: An age trend. *Journal of Adolescent Health* 16:200–203.

Warner, K. 1978. Possible increases in the underreporting of cigarette consumption. *Journal of the American Statistical Association* 73:314–17.

———. 1981. Cigarette smoking in the 1970's: The impact of the antismoking campaign on consumption. *Science* 211:729–31.

———. 1986. *Selling smoke: Cigarette advertising and public health.* Washington, DC: American Public Health Association.

———. 1989. Effects of the antismoking campaign: An update. *American Journal of Public Health* 79:144–51.

———. 1997. Cost-effectiveness of smoking cessation therapies: Interpretation of the evidence and implications for coverage. *PharmacoEconomics* 11:538–49.

———. 2000a. The economics of tobacco: Myths and realities. *Tobacco Control* 9:78–89.

———. 2000b. Example of a multilevel approach to intervention: Tobacco control. Paper prepared for the symposium "Capitalizing on Social Science and Behavioral Research to Improve the Public's Health" sponsored by the Institute of Medicine and the National Research Council's Commission on Behavioral and Social Sciences and Education, Atlanta, GA, February 2–3.

———. In press. Reducing harms to smokers: Methods, their effectiveness, and the role of policy. In *Regulating tobacco: Premises and policy options,* ed. R. L Rabin and S. D. Sugarman. New York: Oxford University Press.

Warner, K. E., F. J. Chaloupka, P. J. Cook, W. G. Manning, J. P. Newhouse, T. E. Novotny, T. C. Schelling, and J. Townsend. 1995. Criteria for determining an optimal cigarette tax: The economist's perspective. *Tobacco Control* 4: 380–86.

Warner, K. E., et al. 1986. Promotion of tobacco products: Issues and policy options. *Journal of Health Policy, Politics and Law* 11:367–92.

Warner, K. E., and H. A. Murt. 1982. Impact of the antismoking campaign on smoking prevalence: A cohort analysis. *Journal of Public Health Policy* 3:374–89.

———. 1984. Economic incentives for health. *Annual Review of Public Health* 5:107–33.

Warner, K. E., J. Slade, and D. T. Sweanor. 1997. The emerging market for long-term nicotine maintenance. *Journal of the American Medical Association* 278:1087–92.

Wasserman, J. 1988. Excise taxes, regulation, and the demand for cigarettes. Ph.D. diss., RAND Graduate School, Santa Monica, CA.

Wasserman, J., W. G. Manning, P. D. Jacobson, and M. Oshiro. 1998. The impact of cigarette prices, regulations, and parental smoking on teenage smoking behavior. Working Paper. School of Public Health, University of Michigan.

Wasserman, J., W. G. Manning, J. P. Newhouse, and J. D. Winkler. 1991. The effects of excise taxes and regulations on adult and teenage cigarette smoking. *Journal of Health Economics* 10:43–64.

Wechsler, H., N. A. Rigotti, J. Gledhill-Hoyt, and H. Lee. 1998. Increased levels of cigarette use among college students: A cause for national concern. *Journal of the American Medical Association* 280:1673–78.

Werch, E. E., D. M. Pappas, and E. A. Castellon-Vogel. 1996. Drug use prevention efforts at colleges and universities in the United States. *Substance Use and Misuse.* 31 (1): 65–80.

Wills, T. A., and S. D. Cleary. 1996. How are social support effects mediated? A test with parental support and adolescent substance use. *Journal of Personality and Social Psychiatry* 71:937–52.

Wines, M. 1996. White House is given plan to ban cigarettes sales to the young. *New York Times,* Aug 15, p. D20.

Winick, C., and M. J. Larson. 1997. Community action program. In *Substance Abuse: A Comprehensive Textbook,* 3d ed., ed. J. H. Lowinson, P. Ruiz, R. B. Millman, and J. G. Langrod. Baltimore, Md.: Williams and Wilkins.

Worden, J. K. 1999. Research in using mass media to prevent smoking. *Nicotine and Tobacco Research* 1 (supp. 1): 117–21.

Worden, J. K., B. S. Flynn, L. J. Solomon, R. H. Secker-Walker, G. J. Badger, and J. H. Carpenter. 1996. Using mass media to prevent cigarette smoking among adolescent girls. *Health Education Quarterly* 23:453–68.

World Bank. 1999. *Curbing the epidemic: Governments and the economics of tobacco control.* Washington, DC: World Bank.

Wu, L., and J. C. Anthony. 1999. Tobacco smoking and depressed mood in late childhood and early adolescence. *American Journal of Public Health* 89 (12): 1837–40.

Zapka, J. G., K. Fletcher, L. Pbert, et al. 1999. The perceptions and practices of pediatricians: Tobacco intervention. *Pediatrics* 103:1022–23.

Zellman, G. L., P. D. Jacobson, and R. M. Bell. 1997. Influencing physician response to prenatal substance exposure through state legislation and workplace policies. *Addiction* 92:1123–31.

Zhang, P., and C. Husten. 1998. The impact of the tobacco price support program on tobacco control in the United States. *Tobacco Control* 7:176–82.

Index